Treating Dementia

Treating Dementia

Do We Have a Pill for It?

Edited by

Jesse F. Ballenger, Ph.D.

Peter J. Whitehouse, M.D., Ph.D.

Constantine G. Lyketsos, M.D., M.H.S.

Peter V. Rabins, M.D., M.P.H.

Jason H. T. Karlawish, M.D.

The Johns Hopkins University Press

Baltimore

© 2009 The Johns Hopkins University Press
All rights reserved. Published 2009
Printed in the United States of America on acid-free paper
9 8 7 6 5 4 3 2 1

Copyright in this volume excludes the content of chapter 6,
which is copyright Judith Levine.

The Johns Hopkins University Press
2715 North Charles Street
Baltimore, Maryland 21218-4363
www.press.jhu.edu

Library of Congress Cataloging-in-Publication Data

Treating dementia : do we have a pill for it? / edited by Jesse F. Ballenger . . . [et al.].
    p. ; cm.
  Includes bibliographical references and index.
  ISBN-13: 978-0-8018-9365-0 (hardcover : alk. paper)
  ISBN-10: 0-8018-9365-8 (hardcover : alk. paper)
1. Dementia—Chemotherapy. I. Ballenger, Jesse F.
[DNLM: 1. Alzheimer Disease—drug therapy. 2. Alzheimer Vaccines—economics.
3. Alzheimer Vaccines—therapeutic use. 4. Drug Discovery—ethics.
5. Marketing—ethics. WT 155 D7945 2009]
  RC521.D78 2009
  616.8′306—dc22   2008054587

A catalog record for this book is available from the British Library.

*Special discounts are available for bulk purchases of this book. For more information,
please contact Special Sales at 410-516-6936 or specialsales@press.jhu.edu.*

The Johns Hopkins University Press uses environmentally friendly book materials,
including recycled text paper that is composed of at least 30 percent post-consumer
waste, whenever possible. All of our book papers are acid-free, and our jackets and
covers are printed on paper with recycled content.

Contents

Preface

The development and use of drugs has become a focal point of hope and controversy in medicine. That drugs excite hope is not surprising. The hope that medicine will deliver meaningful treatment to the afflicted is ancient. With the development of so-called magic bullets such as penicillin and of preventative therapeutics such as the polio vaccine in the twentieth century, as well as the steady growth in biomedicine's knowledge and technical sophistication, that hope increasingly seems like a reasonable expectation. Scientists, clinicians, policy makers, and the general public have come to believe firmly and often fervently in an orderly pathway from basic science research that identifies disease mechanisms and appropriate targets for intervention to applied science that must eventually produce an effective treatment for every human affliction. This belief is embodied in the steady growth of the National Institutes of Health (NIH) budget since the 1970s, an era in which most other federal agencies have experienced budgetary constraints.

That drugs would provoke controversy may, at first glance, seem puzzling. Shouldn't the increasing power and sophistication of biomedicine lead to greater certainty? Likewise, shouldn't the parallel rise in prestige of biomedical science, clinical practice, and health care policy have also led to increasing scientific certainty? To formulate this question slightly differently, shouldn't it be a straightforward matter, in the era of evidence-based clinical medicine, to determine whether a drug works well enough to be worth the expense and risk its use entails?

The problem that has emerged is that the many parties with an interest in the development of a given drug come to the process with different hopes. People with the disease may take the pill hoping for relief from their symptoms, but their hopes may also include a validation of their suffering that biomedicine can bestow. Clinicians prescribing the pills hope that they will provide relief if not cure for their patients but may also hope that doing so will support their professional legitimacy and authority. Researchers who develop and test the pills hope they will improve human lives but also hope to further their career. The drug companies that manufacture the pills hope their product will be a powerful addition to the therapeutic armamentarium but also hope that it will provide a profitable return investment. All these hopes and many more are understandable and legitimate, but they greatly complicate the process of detecting and evaluating the effects of drugs. Given the powerful and conflicting hopes that are invested in drugs, controversy seems inevitable.

Perhaps nowhere is the dynamic of hope and controversy more clearly operative than in the field of aging and dementia. The development of pharmaceutical treatments for age-related dementias such as Alzheimer's brings together a number of complex and powerful issues—the complexity of the disease itself, with its heterogeneous symptoms and causes, which has led many researchers to question whether it should even be considered a unified disease entity; biomedicine's subsequent difficulty defining suitable targets for drugs and ongoing difficulty with clearly defining the boundaries between aging and disease; the economic, social, and political pressures of an aging population in the United States; deeply rooted cultural attitudes toward aging, decline, cognition, memory, and selfhood; the continued stigmatization of dementia; and, bound up with all of these, the often-conflicting interests and hopes of patients, their caregivers, clinicians, researchers, policy makers, and the pharmaceutical industry.

This book aims to elucidate this dense matrix of hope and controversy. It brings together the perspectives of researchers, clinicians, and scholars from a broad range of disciplines who have studied or been directly involved in different aspects of the development, evaluation, and use of drugs for dementia. But we do not claim that these perspectives constitute a collective consensus, nor do we necessarily endorse the ideas of each author. Rather, as the reader will soon discover, the perspectives in this book are diverse and often conflicting.

We have tried to include the broadest possible spectrum of opinion on the development and use of drugs in dementia. There are multiple perspectives on how, why, and even whether drugs for dementia should be developed, evaluated, and used. Some of the chapters articulate mainstream positions, widely accepted throughout the dementia field. Allan Anderson (chapter 5) describes what he sees as the benefits that currently available drugs bring to patients in his clinical practice, and Donald Price and colleagues (chapter 3) describe the approach of mainstream research that aims to understand the biological mechanisms of dementia and develop pharmacological therapies that act on these mechanisms rather than merely on symptoms. At the other end of the spectrum, Judith Levine (chapter 6) describes the limits of the pharmacologically oriented treatment her father received for his dementia and longs for treatment approaches that would be more respectful of the subjectivity of the person with dementia. Danny George and Peter Whitehouse (chapter 1) critique the medicalization of dementia and the pharmacological strategies that follow logically from it, arguing that there are other equally valid ways to understand dementia and extol the value of nonpharmacological approaches to prevention and treatment. Still other chapters attempt to negotiate some kind of pragmatic middle ground between wholesale acceptance and complete rejection of mainstream approaches.

The book presents an equally diverse array of explanations of how and why the development and use of drugs for dementia have taken the shape they have. Some chapters advance arguments about the power of drug companies to shape the direction of the field, while others explain drug development and clinical practice by situating them in broader historical and cultural contexts. We believe that all of these perspectives are important and capture different aspects of the problem.

Most of the contributors to this book participated in a conference on historical and clinical perspectives on drug development presented at the Johns Hopkins University School of Medicine in 2004, though each of the chapters is significantly altered from what the authors presented. The changes reflect both the challenging interdisciplinary exchange that occurred at the conference and subsequent developments in the field. The two-day conference was highly unusual in that the first day focused on social, cultural, and political analyses of the development of dementia drugs, while the second day presented a primer and continuing medical education update on the state of the art in dementia treatment. Thus, conference participants were challenged to balance theoretical, analytical, and practical issues. In addition to conference participants, we asked a number of authors (Anderson, George, Leibing, Levine, and Moreira) to write chapters that would supply particular perspectives that were missing or that would address issues that emerged at the conference as deserving additional attention. On the whole, the chapters in this book address the essential questions about the past, present, and future of drug treatment for dementia.

We recognize, however, that these perspectives do not add up to a tidy whole. Nor will it be possible to create from this diversity some Archimedean point from which to forge a resolution of the controversies that surround them. The clearest message this book offers is that simplicity should be distrusted.

But acknowledging complexity need not produce paralysis. Greater awareness and appreciation of the different perspectives on the goals and processes of developing, evaluating, and using drugs for dementia will not make disagreements go away. But it may make the controversies that will continue to surround them less bitter and divisive. Our hope is thus not that this book will end disagreement among the various parties whose perspectives it presents; indeed, working on it has made our own differences too clear for us to entertain such a hope. Rather, we hope this book will encourage the kinds of conversation that we have enjoyed in putting it together, exchanges in which disagreement not only divides but also enlightens and generates respectful consideration rather than arrogant dismissal of alternative views. Ultimately, we would like this book to be a resource that helps the different parties with a stake in the development, evaluation, and use of drugs for dementia move toward the fulfillment of their diverse hopes with a heightened sense of humility, respect, and wisdom.

This book is organized in four thematic sections: concepts of dementia and their implications for the development of drug treatments; perspectives on the use and evaluation of drug treatments for dementia; issues surrounding language, values, and objectivity; and ethical and policy issues revolving around our conflicting hopes for these drugs. A detailed introduction to the individual chapters precedes each section.

Acknowledgments

This project began as an interdisciplinary conference held at the Johns Hopkins University School of Medicine in March 2004, entitled Drug Development for Alzheimer's Disease: Historical and Clinical Perspectives, part of the 10th Anniversary Update on the Treatment of Alzheimer's Disease and Other Dementias. The conference was presented by the Department of the History of Medicine, the Division of Geriatric Psychiatry and Neuropsychiatry of the Department of Psychiatry and Behavioral Sciences, and the Alzheimer's Disease Research Center at the Johns Hopkins University, co-sponsored by the Copper Ridge Institute, the greater Maryland chapter of the Alzheimer's Association, the University Memory and Aging Center of the University Hospitals of Cleveland / Case Western Reserve University, the University of Pennsylvania's Alzheimer's Disease Center, and the American Geriatrics Society. Financial support for the conference was provided by Forest Laboratories, Inc.; Novartis; Pfizer, Inc.; EISAI; Janssen Pharmaceutica; and Eli Lilly and Company. Additional support for this book was provided by Forest Laboratories, Inc., and Novartis.

We thank Konrad and Ulrike Maurer for granting us permission to use their play, *The Augusta File*, at the conference, and Anne Basting, director of the Center on Age and Community at the University of Wisconsin–Milwaukee, for her excellent job of editing, producing, and directing the staged reading of the play. We also thank Wendy Harris, the book's editor at the Johns Hopkins University Press, for her patience and encouragement when it seemed this project would never be completed.

Jesse Ballenger thanks a number of people at the Johns Hopkins University. At every stage of this project, Constantine Lyketsos and Peter Rabins have shown the kind of willingness to engage in broad interdisciplinary conversation that is all too rare in any quarter of the modern university; Randall Packard, chair of the Department of the History of Medicine and William Welch Professor of the History of Medicine at Johns Hopkins, provided crucial support and encouragement in the formative stages of this project; and Christine Ruggere, associate director and curator of the Institute of the History of Medicine, gave invaluable advice and support in planning the conference. He also thanks his colleagues in the Science, Technology, and Society Program at Penn State University for their encouragement of his work on this book.

Peter Whitehouse thanks all who keep an open mind and heart about brain aging conditions. Such openness may well prevent the lack of cognitive flexibility and moral imagination that can accompany aging.

Constantine (Kostas) Lyketsos thanks the other editors and contributors to this volume for being excellent collaborators; his colleagues in the dementia field, who are such a stimulating group to work with; and Paul McHugh and Marshall Folstein, whose work and ideas continue to shape his own work.

Peter Rabins thanks his many colleagues with whom discussions over the years have shaped and challenged his ideas about these issues.

Contributors

Allan A. Anderson, M.D., Medical Director and Director of Geriatric Psychiatry, Shore Behavioral Health Services, Cambridge, Maryland; Assistant Professor of Psychiatry, the Johns Hopkins University, Baltimore, Maryland

Jesse F. Ballenger, Ph.D., Assistant Professor, Science, Technology, and Society Program, Penn State University, University Park, Pennsylvania

Mohamed H. Farah, Ph.D., Research Associate, Department of Pathology, the Johns Hopkins University, Baltimore, Maryland

Thomas E. Finucane, M.D., Professor of Medicine, the Johns Hopkins University and Johns Hopkins Berman Institute of Bioethics, Baltimore, Maryland

Danny George, M.Sc., Ph.D. candidate, medical anthropology, Oxford University, Oxford, United Kingdom

John R. Gilstad, M.D., Commander, Medical Corps, U.S. Navy; Chairman, Executive Committee of the Medical Staff, U.S. Naval Hospital, Yokosuka, Japan

David Healy, M.D., FRCPsych, Director, North Wales Department of Psychological Medicine, Cardiff University, Cardiff, Wales

Adam Hedgecoe, Ph.D., Associate Director, ESRC Centre for Economic and Social Aspects of Genomics, Cardiff University, Cardiff, Wales

Jason H. T. Karlawish, M.D., Associate Professor of Medicine and Medical Ethics at the University of Pennsylvania; Associate Director of the PENN Memory Center, University Park, Pennsylvania

Vassilis E. Koliatsos, M.D., Associate Professor of Pathology, the Johns Hopkins University, Baltimore, Maryland

Fiona M. Laird, Ph.D., Research Associate, Department of Pathology, the Johns Hopkins University, Baltimore, Maryland

Annette Leibing, Ph.D., Professor of Medical Anthropology, Faculty of Nursing, Université de Montréal, Montreal, Quebec, Canada

Judith Levine, freelance writer, Brooklyn, New York; winner of the *Los Angeles Times* Book Prize in 2002 for *Harmful to Minors: The Perils of Protecting Children from Sex* (University of Minnesota Press). Author of *Do You Remember Me? A Father, A Daughter, and a Search for the Self* (Free Press, 2004)

Tong Li, Ph.D., Assistant Professor of Pathology, the Johns Hopkins University, Baltimore, Maryland

Margaret Lock, Ph.D., Marjorie Bronfman Professor Emerita in Social Studies in Medicine in the Department of Social Studies of Medicine and the Department of Anthropology at McGill University, Montreal, Quebec, Canada

Constantine G. Lyketsos, M.D., M.H.S., Professor of Psychiatry and Behavioral Sciences, Codirector, Division of Geriatric Psychiatry and Neuropsychiatry, the Johns Hopkins University, Baltimore, Maryland

Tiago Moreira, M.Sc., Ph.D., Lecturer in Sociology, School of Applied Social Sciences, Durham University, United Kingdom

Donald L. Price, M.D., Professor of Pathology, Neuropathology, and Neuroscience, the Johns Hopkins University, Baltimore, Maryland

Peter V. Rabins, M.D., M.P.H., Professor, Department of Psychiatry and Behavioral Sciences, the Johns Hopkins University, Baltimore, Maryland; Senior Faculty, Copper Ridge Institute

Alena V. Savonenko, M.D., Ph.D., Assistant Professor of Pathology, the Johns Hopkins University, Baltimore, Maryland

Juan C. Troncoso, M.D., Professor of Pathology, the Johns Hopkins University, Baltimore, Maryland

Rein Vos, M.D., Ph.D., Professor of Health, Ethics and Philosophy and Chair, Department of Health, Ethics and Society, Faculty of Health, Medicine and Life Sciences, Maastricht University, The Netherlands

Peter J. Whitehouse, M.D., Ph.D., Professor of Neurology, Psychiatry, Neuroscience, Psychology, Nursing, Organizational Behavior, Cognitive Science, and History at Case Western Reserve University; Director, Integrative Studies, Case Western Reserve University, Cleveland Ohio

Philip C. Wong, Ph.D., Professor of Pathology and Neuroscience, the Johns Hopkins University, Baltimore, Maryland

PART I

CONCEPTS OF DEMENTIA AND TREATMENT

In some ways disease does not exist until we have agreed that
it does, by perceiving, naming and responding to it.
                                        —*Charles Rosenberg, 1992*

Medicine begins with disease. Illness is a universal human experience, and medicine has developed as a special body of knowledge and practice in response to it. In the ideal medical encounter, the patient presents an
account of how a mysterious illness disrupts his or her life, and the physician—perhaps with the aid of technologically sophisticated diagnostic procedures—explains that illness in terms of a disease concept with an understandable and predictable course. And, if patient and physician are lucky,
identifying the disease will suggest a course of treatment that can restore
the patient to health.

But disease concepts are complex. They are not simply the product of the
scientific investigation of the pathological processes involved in the patient's
experience of illness, though that is clearly an essential part of their creation. They are also the product of complex negotiations among a wide
number of interested parties—including patients, caregivers, physicians,
researchers, corporations, and policy makers—who all have a stake in how
we perceive, name, and respond to illness.

Given the sea change that has occurred in thinking about dementia since
the 1970s, perhaps nowhere in medicine are disease concepts more compli-

cated and important than in the case of dementia. Reconceptualizing age-associated progressive dementia as the product of disease processes rather than aging has been the core idea driving the creation and development of the Alzheimer's disease (AD) field over the past three decades (Fox 1989; Katzman and Bick 2000). A significant body of historical, cultural, and sociological work has shown how the AD concept itself is intertwined with powerful social and cultural processes such as the aging of society, anxieties about autonomy and selfhood, and the concrete interests of medical institutions and pharmaceutical corporations (Holstein 1997; Whitehouse, Maurer, and Ballenger 2000; Ballenger 2006).

This opening section of our book aims to extend this inquiry by focusing on how concepts of dementia and concepts of treatment have been interrelated and on the implications of some of the more recent conceptual shifts in the dementia field for the future of therapeutics in dementia. If the old adage is true, that give a person a hammer and every problem looks like a nail, it may also be true that when a person believes the problem is a nail, he or she will focus efforts on making and using a hammer. Disease concepts are not merely descriptive; they have prescriptive implications, too.

The first two chapters trace the historical evolution of some of the core concepts related to drug treatment for dementia. The chapter by Danny George and Peter Whitehouse reflects the broader critique of the concept of Alzheimer's disease they have developed (Whitehouse and George 2008), pointing out that the conceptual shift from senility to Alzheimer's disease has not been without cost. They pay particular attention to the ramifications of the emergence of the concept of mild cognitive impairment (MCI). MCI describes a state, measurable by psychometric tests but with little if any functional disability, between normal cognition and dementia. Ostensibly, MCI is a distinct entity that may or may not progress to full-blown dementia, though George and Whitehouse point out that interest in it has been driven by its status as a putative prodromal state, which would allow clinicians to identify patients who may be amenable to treatment and prevention and researchers to better study the pathological mechanisms of the disease. George and Whitehouse argue, however, that the concept of MCI is inherently arbitrary and unstable, obscuring the tremendous variability in the cognitive changes people experience as they age. Thus, like the concept of AD itself, MCI is ultimately no more than a label arbitrarily applied to a position on a continuum of cognitive brain aging. They urge us to see the debate over the concept of MCI as an invitation to ask fundamental questions about the concept of AD and the way it has explicitly privileged a biomedical approach to treating dementia, concluding with a call to reimagine Alzheimer's in a way that would make room for more socially oriented approaches that are currently marginalized.

David Healy suggests that the major conceptual approaches that have defined the history of pharmacological treatment of dementia fall into three periods. In the early period, extending back well into the nineteenth century, a wide range of compounds were claimed to be effective treatments for age-associated cognitive failure on the general notion that cerebral stimulation would enhance whatever brain function remained. Because these compounds found their way into medical practice without the sort of clinical trial evidence that would be required today, they were removed from the market when the 1962 amendment to the Food, Drug, and Cosmetics Act charged the FDA with reviewing the efficacy of all drugs then on the market. Because these drugs were long off patent, pharmaceutical industries did not find it worthwhile to undertake the clinical trials needed to gain approval, and Healy provocatively suggests that a number of promising therapeutic leads may have been abandoned. In the middle period, ranging from the 1960s through the development of the currently available acetylcholinesterase inhibitors, approaches to the development of antidementia drugs followed the pattern established by the development of antidepressants, conceiving of AD as a cholinergic deficit disorder. In the third period, which Healy argues is under way, research on neurodegenerative disorders may lead to more effective drugs that act on the glutamatergic or other neural systems enhancing cognitive function and directly alter the pathological processes underpinning dementia.

The chapter by Donald L. Price, one of the leading neuropathologists in AD research, and coauthors also emphasizes how contemporary research developments are transforming concepts of dementia and approaches to drug treatment. Price and colleagues describe the more narrow transformation of Alzheimer's into a molecular disease. They provide an extensive review of the identification of AD-related genes and make the case that the more precise definitions of MCI and early AD and the increased understanding of the pathological role and molecular composition of amyloid beta (Aβ), the main constituent of the plaques that accumulate in the brains of people with Alzheimer's disease, have created new therapeutic pathways that aim at disease mechanisms rather than relief of symptoms. Price and colleagues' story is of the success researchers have had in focusing narrowly on basic mechanisms of the disease to identify new potential therapeutic targets that they hope will benefit patients.

In contrast, the final chapter in this section describes the expansion of the boundaries of the dementia concept to include a broader range of symptoms. Medical anthropologist Annette Leibing argues that behavioral and psychological symptoms have moved from being regarded as peripheral to dementia, which from the 1970s at least has been defined primarily as a cognitive disorder, to being regarded by many clinicians and researchers as some of its central features. The impetus for this change comes from a number of directions: patients and caregivers striving to bring attention to some of the most distressing aspects of their experience, clinicians working to provide treatment that will improve the quality of life of patients and caregivers even if unable to arrest cognitive decline, and pharmaceutical companies looking to expand uses and markets for their products.

Taken as a whole, the chapters in this section demonstrate that the construct of dementia and the development of treatments for it have followed a circuitous route that is still evolving. They suggest that any evaluation of strategies of drug development and treatment must begin by attending to the complex prescriptive implications of concepts of dementia.

REFERENCES

Ballenger, J. F. 2006. *Self, senility, and Alzheimer's disease in modern America.* Baltimore: Johns Hopkins University Press.

Fox, P. 1989. From senility to Alzheimer's disease: The rise of the Alzheimer's disease movement. *Milbank Quarterly* 67 (1): 58–102.

Holstein, M. 1997. Alzheimer's disease and senile dementia, 1885–1920: An interpretive history of disease negotiation. *Journal of Aging Studies* 11 (1): 1–13.

Katzman, R., and K. L. Bick. 2000. *Alzheimer disease: The changing view.* San Diego, Calif.: Academic.

Rosenberg, C. E. 1992. Framing disease: Illness, society and history. In *Framing disease: Studies in cultural history,* ed. C. E. Rosenberg and J. L. Golden. New Brunswick, N.J.: Rutgers University Press.

Whitehouse, P. J., and D. George. 2008. *The myth of Alzheimer's disease: What you aren't being told about today's most dreaded diagnosis.* New York: St. Martin's Press.

Whitehouse, P. J., K. Maurer, and J. F. Ballenger. 2000. *Concepts of Alzheimer disease: Biological, clinical, and cultural perspectives.* Baltimore: Johns Hopkins University Press.

CHAPTER 1

The Classification of Alzheimer's Disease and Mild Cognitive Impairment

Enriching Therapeutic Models through Moral Imagination

DANNY GEORGE, M.SC.

PETER J. WHITEHOUSE, M.D., PH.D.

Even the briefest reflection on the history of any disease will reveal that knowledge about a particular physiological condition does not divulge itself over time in a slow, ordered process and that our classificatory categories often evolve through a series of corrections and elisions rather than a progressive unfolding of "the truth." In the annals of medical knowledge, disease classifications—be they for malaria, HIV/AIDS, hysteria, homosexuality, or "Alzheimer's disease" (AD)—are far from immutable, and the statements, theories, diagnoses, and norms that seem firm and canonical to one generation are worn away by the passage of time and replaced by more persuasive explanatory classifications. Disease, as it were, enters and leaves mankind as through a door (Canguilhem 1989, p. 39).

A careful and sustained engagement with the history of dementia of the Alzheimer's type reveals that the condition that has come to be known as "the disease of the twentieth century" is a shaky, vulnerable, and vacillating construct and suggests that humanity's understanding of the brain aging process is likely to keep changing over time. This chapter will tell the story of Alzheimer's disease over the past 100 years and will ultimately suggest that society is in need of a new strategy for diagnosing and treating persons whose brains are aging—a strategy that will save us from our faith in pharmacological cures for Alzheimer's and open up new therapeutic options for individuals and families who are coping with the challenges of cognitive loss.

The Birth of the AD Classification

Alzheimer's disease is named after Dr. Alois Alzheimer, a Bavarian-born neurologist who worked in late-nineteenth- and early-twentieth-century Germany. In 1906, Dr. Alzheimer presented a lecture entitled "On a Peculiar, Severe Disease Process of the Cerebral Cortex" to the 37th Assembly of Southwest German Alienists (psychologists) in Tübingen, Germany. In his talk, Dr. Alzheimer detailed his observations of a 51-year-old woman named Auguste D., who presented a multitude of symptoms relating to progressive cognitive impairment and was found to have high concentrations of protein plaques and neurofibrillary tangles on her brain in postmortem investigation. Alzheimer raised the question of whether Auguste D.'s case represented a condition that could be distinguished from senile dementia. Those on hand were not persuaded by Alzheimer's evidence, and in fact, the minutes of the proceedings reported that the lecture had been "inappropriate for a brief report" (Maurer 2003, p. 169).

Nevertheless, Alzheimer continued to be intrigued by Auguste D.'s case. The response to his presentation *had* illuminated an intractable classificatory dilemma: did his patient's symptoms simply represent an atypical, early onset form of "senile dementia," or could they possibly represent a separate disease entity altogether? (Maurer et al. 2000, p. 24). Because Auguste D.'s range of behavioral and pathological symptoms were also observed in a great number of older persons with senile dementia, Alzheimer—despite his fascination with the patient—was apprehensive about formally classifying her condition as a specific disease process. His boss, Emil Kraepelin—a man nicknamed by his peers the "Linnaeus of psychiatry"—was not so hesitant. In 1910, Kraepelin officially coined the term "Alzheimer's krankheit" (Alzheimer's disease), including it on page 627 of the eighth edition of his authoritative *Textbook of Psychiatry*. Ironically, the illustrious history of what has become the "disease of the century" commences with this not-so-illustrious sentence: "The clinical interpretation of Alzheimer's disease is still unclear at the moment . . . whereas the anatomic findings suggest that we are dealing with a severe form of senile dementia, the fact that the disease from time to time begins at the end of the patient's forties speaks against it. In such cases at least one would therefore have to assume a presenile dementia, if we are not in fact dealing with a peculiar disease process that is largely independent of age" (translation by Bick et al. 1987).

Although the description was small and obscurely placed in the nether regions of Kraepelin's massive textbook, Alzheimer's reaction to the promulgation of the eponym was ambivalence. In an article he submitted to the *Zeitschrift fur die Gesamte Neurologie and Psychiatrie* in 1911, he wrote: "Thus the question arises whether these cases of disease, which I have considered as peculiar, still show characteristic features in clinical and histological aspects that distinguish them from senile dementia or whether they must be assigned instead to senile dementia itself" (Maurer and Maurer 2003, p. 218). Toward the beginning of the report, Alzheimer alludes to the ambivalence of his boss, writing that "Kraepelin still considers that the position of these cases is unclear." And later he answers the question that he initially posed by concluding that "there is, then, *no tenable reason to consider these cases as caused by a specific disease process.* They are senile psychoses, atypical forms of senile dementia. Nevertheless, they do assume a certain separate position so that one has to know of their existence" (Möller and Graeber 2000, p. 41, emphasis added).

The Evolution of the "Alzheimer's" Classification

For the next several decades after the publication of Kraepelin's textbook, the diagnosis of "Alzheimer's disease" remained obscure and was rarely applied by those in the medical profession. Its symptoms were mainly attributed to the common effects of old age rather than to an adverse pathology, and the medical community largely refused to diagnose patients as having "AD." In 1925, Dr. Ernst Grunthal, who worked at the Clinic for Psychiatric Illnesses in Wurzburg, published an extensive work on AD. In it, he came to a profound conclusion: "At the moment, at least without methods, a differential diagnosis between senile dementia and Alzheimer's disease cannot be made on the basis of histopathological images" (Maurer and Maurer 2003, p. 221). And so the tenuous line between Kraepelin's disease classification and the normal symptoms of aging observed in senile dementia continued to blur.

It shouldn't have been surprising that the clinicopathological boundaries described in Kraepelin's textbook were being called into question. After all, in many cases, the senile plaques and neurofibrillary tangles held to be the distinctive pathological features of patients with alleged Alzheimer's disease were also found in the brains of older patients who had shown no behavioral signs of dementia in life. In fact, in 1912, just two years after the publication of Kraepelin's textbook, more than 45 articles representing examinations of material from at least 500 brains appeared in psychiatric literature reporting senile plaques and neurofibrillary tangles in all forms of dementing disease, and similar reports continued well into the twentieth century (Torack 1978, p. 1). Other conditions in which plaques and tangles were found included post-traumatic stress dementia, cerebral arteriosclerosis, cerebrocerebellar arteriolar amyloidosis, amyotrophic lateral sclerosis, Down syndrome, toxic conditions, dementia pugilistica, postencephalitic parkinsonism, and phenacetin abuse (Fox 1989, p. 64). Muddying the classificatory waters further was the fact that sometimes those who died severely demented were found at autopsy to have few if any of the pathological hallmarks of AD.

Though on the wane in the 1920s, the "AD" classification never vanished completely from medical discourse. From 1926 to 1935, the *American Journal of Psychiatry* and the *Archives of Neurology and Psychiatry*, the two leading professional journals of American psychiatry and neurology, ran nine articles concerning Alzheimer's disease (Ballenger 2000, p. 83). The biomedical model of Alzheimer's disease was ostensibly giving way to a more psychodynamic model of care that predominated in the mid-twentieth century, opening up a greater range of treatment options for elder persons with aging brains. Psychiatrists such as David Rothschild argued that society should stop dwelling on the problems of old age and focus instead on its opportunities; perhaps biomedicine could not solve the problems of old age for elderly people, but society could allow elderly people to create meaningful roles for themselves.

Rothschild made it clear that the social pathology of aging could be damaging to modern society: "In our present social set-up, with its loosening of family ties, unsettled living conditions and fast economic pace, there are many hazards for individuals who are growing old," he wrote. "Many of these persons have not had adequate psychological preparation for their inevitable loss of flexibility, restriction of outlets, and loss of friends or relatives; they are individuals who are facing the prospect of retirement from their life-long activities with few mental assets and perhaps meager material resources" (Rothschild 1947, p. 125). The perils of aging were hard enough without society making it more difficult to deal with, Rothschild seemed to be saying.

In the middle of the twentieth century, then, little mention was made of AD, and only a small number of clinicians used the term, reserving it for younger patients in their fifth decade who presented the clinical and neuropathological signs of senile dementia. It wasn't until the 1960s that the eponym began resurfacing in common literature. In 1964, Elfriede Albert of Düsseldorf published a lecture she had given two years previous entitled "Senile Dementia and Alzheimer's Disease as Expressions of the Same Disease Event." In it, she acknowledged no distinction, either anatomically or clinically, between AD and senile dementia: "Alzheimer himself had already decided against a distinction in principle between presenile stupor and senile dementia," she wrote, seeming to allude to Kraepelin's role in the classification of a specific disease entity (Maurer 2003, pp. 227, 228).

Renascent interest in the term can be traced to the 1950s, when the genetics of "Alzheimer's disease" had begun to emerge and foreshadow modern issues of genetic medicine. Even so, in the first version of *Diagnostic and Statistical Manual of Mental Disorders* (DSM), published in 1952, the term "chronic brain syndrome" was used in place of "dementia," relegating "Alzheimer's disease" to the periphery of classificatory discourse (American Psychiatric Association 1952, p. 128). The diagnosis of AD might have remained rare and insignificant if it weren't for two unprecedented developments in human history that began affecting human populations in the mid- to late twentieth century: the gradual increase of mean life expectancy in industrialized countries and the advent of modern technology. By the late 1960s, thanks to improvements in hygienic and social conditions and the astounding successes of public health efforts in controlling epidemics and improving nutrition in the Western world, an increasing number of individuals were living to be 85 or older and made up the most rapidly growing part of the population.

As society was becoming more and more populated by men and women whose brains were moving deeper into senescence along with their aging bodies, technical developments in various aspects of neuropathological and biochemical research—including electron microscope studies of plaques and tangles and the ability to measure neurotransmitter levels in aging brains— had advanced our ability to study the biology of dementia and paved the way for a return to dominance of a biomedical classificatory approach to AD. The combination of an aging society and the proliferation of technological tools that held the promise of ameliorating the travails of old age created the impetus for a reinvestment in geriatric research and a rethinking of classificatory categories. And the application of technology occurred in the context of academic medicine, which, as any researcher will tell you, rewards productive research and publication through various means such as personal prestige, economic incentives, and economic security (Fox 1989, p. 64). Consequently, many neuroscientists working in academic medicine became some of the most avid supporters of the Alzheimer's disease movement and advocated distilling the broad concept of senile dementia into discreet categories on the basis of putative biological causes. This, of course, harkened back to Kraepelin's earlier attempts at establishing a nosology, which had seemed to be in vain for the greater part of the early to mid-twentieth century.

AD as a Political Entity: A "Politics of Anguish"

In 1974, the National Institute on Aging (NIA) was born in the United States. Initially, President Richard Nixon vetoed the NIA-establishment bill in an effort to reduce the size of the federal government, but two months before leaving office after the Watergate scandals, he withdrew his opposition, presumably to avoid alienating a Congress that was deliberating on his impeachment. And so on May 31, 1974, the NIA became an official subsidiary of the National Institutes of Health, which had the responsibility of developing a plan for a program designed to promote research into the biological, medical, psychological, social, educational, and economic aspects of aging (Butler and Engel 1978).

Immediately, the NIA, under the leadership of Dr. Robert Butler, a practicing clinical psychiatrist and gerontologist, began promoting AD as its primary research area, enabling federal funding for the "disease" to be channeled from federal coffers to individual researchers. Said Butler: "I decided that we had to make it [Alzheimer's disease] a household word. And the reason I felt that, is that's how the pieces get identified as a national priority. And I call it the health politics of anguish" (Fox 1989, p. 82). The organization's ability to aggregate money and labor that could be mobilized to support further investigation of the illness provided much-needed infrastructure for the Alzheimer's movement and multiplied research efforts nationally.

Butler and the NIA staff were acutely aware of the importance of involving the media in their quest for funding and made continued efforts to keep the press apprised of NIA-sponsored research results. Zaven Khachaturian, hired by Butler to establish the Neurobiology of Aging program, realized how vital the media would be in spreading and normalizing the disease label and put together a systematic strategy for disseminating information to journalists: "Around here [in Washington] Congress tends to pay more attention to popular media than scientific journals . . . part of the strategy was to inform the public, using the media, about major scientific accomplishments in Alzheimer's disease research and the implications of the scientific findings in terms that lay people could understand" (Fox 1989, p. 89).

Advocates for the "disease" soon surfaced in the media, attempting to educate Americans about the new "epidemic." Robert Katzman, one of the most notable advocates for AD research, wrote in an April 1976 editorial that Alzheimer's disease ranked as the fourth or fifth most common cause of death in the United States and called for the country to mobilize resources to address a growing social and health problem. Katzman questioned the overlaps between normal aging and Alzheimer's disease, challenging the long-held assumption that cognitive decline was an inevitable effect of old age (Katzman and Bick 2000, p. 272). As Arthur Kleinman observed, Alzheimer's disease quickly became "an unacceptable index of the final assault of aging on the autonomy [of aging individuals]" (Kleinman 1988, pp. 25, 26).

In 1978, Katzman (who has been dubbed by some as an "issue entrepreneur" (McCarthy and Zald 1987, p. 48) and others created the first AD lay organization: the Alzheimer's Disease Society, which was granted tax exempt status by the government. And in 1979, the Alzheimer's Disease and Related Disorders Association (ADRDA) was created in Washington, D.C. Suddenly, the American public, which had long accepted cognitive impairment as an ineluctable accessory of old age, was coming to learn and fear the *real* scourge of elderly people: Alzheimer's disease. Still, the eminent classificatory texts were hesitant to demarcate AD as a discreet disease. The DSM-III, published in 1980, urged that Alzheimer's disease be referred to as a "presenile dementia." The manual says that because "nearly all cases of these Dementias are associated with Alzheimer's and the identification of Alzheimer's and Pick's diseases is largely or entirely dependent on histopathological data, it seems more useful to have in a clinical classification of mental disorders a single category that encompasses the syndrome of Primary Degenerative Dementia" (American Psychiatric Association 1980, p. 125).

In 1982, in an effort to increase visibility in Washington, the ADRDA hired a consulting firm to organize its lobbying efforts and so increased its access to representatives and senators. It wasn't long before Alzheimer's became a fashionable talking point in Congress. On September 15, 1983, the U.S. House of Representatives proposed a resolution declaring November of that year to be "National Alzheimer's Disease Month." Congress passed the resolution in the hope that "an increase in the national awareness of the problem of Alzheimer's disease may stimulate the interests and concern of the American people, which may lead, in turn, to increased research and eventually to the discovery of a cure" (Ballenger 2006, p. 113). Within a week, President Ronald Reagan, who would later become the world's most famous patient with Alzheimer's, issued a proclamation declaring the resolution official. When November rolled around, he held a formal signing ceremony and photo opportunity in the Oval Office for leaders of the campaign, with the intent of raising awareness of the disease.

And so the war on a disease classified as Alzheimer's was launched. Classificatory texts seem to reflect this large-scale political shift. The 1987 DSM-III (revised) distinguished AD as an "organic mental disorder," and it was given the subcategorization 290.xx: "primary degenerative dementia of the Alzheimer type" (American Psychiatric Association 1987, p. 119). One can only imagine what Alois Alzheimer—who himself concluded that there was "no tenable reason to consider [his] cases as caused by a specific disease process"—would have said had he been alive to see this classificatory *redux* in the late twentieth century.

The reconceptualization of senility as Alzheimer's disease and the large-scale financial commitments bestowed by the government generated excitement among researchers and trickled down to family members and caregivers of "Alzheimer's victims," who spoke passionately of its ravages in the mass media and helped shape the contemporary story of AD. Not only did Alzheimer's disease begin to replace senility as a societal marker for cognitive impairments associated with age, but also a cultural "vernacular of anguish" began to emerge around the concept of AD, which quickly became known as the "never-ending funeral," the "mind-robber," the "slow death of the mind," and "a loss of selfhood" and was described as a "ravaging," "tragic," "degenerative," "devastating" disease. Wildly successful books with titles such as *Loss of Self* (Cohen and Eisdorfer 1986) and *The 36-Hour Day* (Mace and Rabins 1981) began to proliferate on bookshelves in the United States and abroad and became "must-reads" for patients and caregivers alike. Dozens of community-based organizations were created to help Americans cope with the care and treatment of diseased relatives; by 1985, the NIA had established ten Alzheimer's Disease Research Centers across the country, and the government passed a law authorizing the director of the institute to make grants specifically for AD-related research—the first such disease-specific mandate in public health law.

The mainstream acceptance of the Alzheimer's disease classification was supported by celebrity involvement with the emerging "cause." Princess Yasmin Aga Kahn—the daughter of film star Rita Hayworth, who had been diagnosed with AD in 1981—was a highly visible advocate for the disease. When her mother, the world-famous "love goddess," died on May 14, 1987, Yasmin Kahn released the doctors from their confidentiality obligations, ensuring that her famous mother would make the term "Alzheimer's disease" known throughout the world. This surging public awareness was only reinforced by the stunning revelation in 1994 that Ronald Reagan had developed AD. In his letter to the public, he wrote:

> My fellow Americans, I have recently been told that I am one of the millions of Americans who will be afflicted with Alzheimer's disease. Upon learning this news, Nancy and I had to decide whether as private citizens we would keep this a private matter or whether we would make this news known in a public way . . . now we feel it is important to share it with you. In opening our hearts, we hope this might promote greater awareness of this condition. Perhaps it will encourage a clear understanding of the individuals and families who are affected by it. (Reagan 1994)

Reagan's continued advocacy of AD research throughout the 1990s helped aim an even more acute spotlight on Alzheimer's disease and contributed to the '90s being declared "the decade of the brain." Over the years, the public uptake of AD as a disease-cause has correlated with drastically increased federal funding. In 1976, federal funding for AD was less than $1 million (Ballenger 2006); by 2005, the Alzheimer's Association estimated that federal expenditures for AD research were $647 million (Alzheimer's Association 2006).

The AD Classification Today

The DSM-IV, the Alzheimer's Association, and indeed nearly all other current classification authorities refer to Alzheimer's disease as the most common cause of dementia (American Psychiatric Association 1994, p. 139). Interestingly, AD is called a "diagnosis of exclusion" because no direct pathological evidence of its presence can be obtained, and other etiologies for cognitive deficits (hypothyroidism, stroke, vitamin B_{12} deficiency, folic acid deficiency, niacin deficiency, hypercalcemia, neurosyphillis depression, head trauma, cerebrovascular disease, Parkinson's disease, Huntington's disease, subdural hematoma, normal-pressure hydrocephalus, brain tumor, malingering and factitious disorder, schizophrenia, HIV infection, or the persisting effects of a substance (such as alcohol) must first be ruled out (American Psychiatric Association 1994, pp. 138–40; Alzheimer's Association 2004, p. 2).

Because the disease diagnosis is the result of an attempt to eliminate all other causes of the presenting symptoms, many times patients with dementia for which no specific cause can be identified are labeled with the presumptive diagnosis of Alzheimer's disease. Based on commonly used research criteria, a diagnosis of AD can formally be made only after death, when autopsy tissue is available (although this classification is still suspect because the key pathological features of AD are also the features of normal brain aging) (American Psychiatric Association 1994, p. 141).

A Diagnosis under Construction: Mild Cognitive Impairment

The relatively newly identified condition mild cognitive impairment (MCI) dramatically illustrates the difficulties in differentiating normal aging from so-called AD. MCI is, as the name suggests, a condition (although best considered plural, as many types of MCI are now claimed to exist) in which cognitive (usually memory but also other) abilities are not severely enough affected to impair significantly activities of living. MCI is being actively socially constructed at the interfaces of science, clinical, work, and business (Whitehouse 2004a, 2004b; Whitehouse and Juengst 2005; Gaines and Whitehouse 2006). Individuals and groups of people are exploring the use of the term to serve their own purposes and, it is hoped, those of society at large. A language game is in full play, with academics claiming that MCI is a great discovery. Innumerable consensus conferences are debating the merit of the concept, while social scientists study how professionals and laypersons are using the term "mild cognitive impairment" (Corner and Bond 2006). Government and lay organizations are mounting public-information campaigns to change the story of these age-related conditions. Industry is hoping to expand the markets for their currently approved treatments for Alzheimer's disease. Perhaps patients and families want a gentler label than mild Alzheimer's or dementia.

MCI of the proprietary technical type is different than our academic confusion, however, which may be considered more than mild. Here, three ordinary words in our language—"mild," "cognitive," and "impairment"—have been appropriated by physician experts to try to create a specific condition from the highly variable phenomenology of age-related cognitive change. MCI is said to be a state in between normality and dementia in which a subjective concern is validated by some psychometric evidence of impairment but no, or relatively little, functional disability exists (Petersen et al., 2001). Logically speaking, all those who progress from a state of normal intellect to a disabling state of dementia must pass through a time when their cognitive impairments are intermediate—present but not of sufficient magnitude to warrant the label "dementia." Such an appropriation of language comes with advantages and disadvantages for the profession and society, not to mention for the people at risk of having the label applied.

When used as a general expression of speech, "mild cognitive impairment" is a condition that any human being might experience. A night of partying; jet lag from traveling to a foreign country; or taking on a challenging academic task could create a sense of mild confusion or cognitive limitation. MCI emerged from a long history of recognizing the obvious: that most, if not all, older persons develop some changes in cognition as they age. "Benign senile forgetfulness" was the first term popularized in the medical literature to describe this unfortunate metamorphosis, although the broadly used concept of senility preceded any usage of medical terms (Kral 1962). "Senility" deftly captured the ambiguity of the cognitive aging phenomenology: is memory loss a disease or the normal accompaniment of aging? It is a term that human beings have used for centuries to describe and honor changes in cognitive vitality without imposing a pathological condition.

Following "benign senile forgetfulness," "aging-associated memory impairment" (AAMI) emerged, and it remains of interest today (Crook et al. 1986). Older people were said to have AAMI if they complained of memory problems and performed on psychological tests below one standard deviation of younger individuals (creating a large number of elders with AAMI). This category created some of the same dilemmas faced by those who invented the label "MCI"; namely, are cognitive changes reducible to memory alone, or are they manifest in other areas of cognition beyond memory? Do you need a subjective complaint from someone (the "patient" or their family) in order to label them with AAMI or MCI? Are activities of daily living affected? How impaired psychometrically (how many standard deviations lower than a referent population norms, and which population?) must an individual be before a label is applied?

Yet another classificatory push led to the creation of the label "aging associated cognitive decline," which emphasized cognitive rather than memory impairment (Levy 1994). Each of the given examples represents an arbitrary decision and involve "experts" setting thresholds on the continuum of aging that demarcate "the normal and the pathological." The unifying goal is to identify people as early as possible who are likely to progress to frank dementia. However, the cutoff points for concern will always be fuzzy. Different groups propose different thresholds, and no number of quasi-consensus conferences can eliminate the essentially fragile and fluid nature of these predementia categories. The wide variability in the phenomenology of cognitive aging is simply an intractable conundrum for the diagnostic community.

The strongest motivation for the clinical usage of MCI is that the phenomenology exists (in other words, some older people have symptoms of cognitive decline that meet criteria for MCI, and some practicing physicians appear to like using the term). In our opinion, clinicians favor the term because they can avoid using the "A" word (Alzheimer's). But even though the phenomenology of cognitive impairment exists, it is not necessary to label it with a particular biomedical term. Some clinicians, for instance, John Morris at Washington University of St. Louis, believe that MCI is a euphemism for early dementia, most likely AD, if memory impairment is predominant (Morris 2006). Others, such as Ron Petersen, try to identify MCI as a discrete category with its own diagnostic threshold on the continuum of aging. Some in Petersen's group have further reified the concept of MCI by defining a precondition called pre-MCI. Defining a "pre" form of MCI perhaps reinforces the idea that MCI itself is real, just as the existence of MCI substantiates AD. Perhaps in the future we will have pre-pre-MCI, which would in turn represent, for some, pre-pre-pre-AD, and so on down the slippery slope of arbitrary labeling.

Clinicians are often left with a diagnostic dilemma as to whether a person has normal age-related cognitive changes, depression, MCI, or AD. Even the Alzheimer's Association concedes on their website that "there is no single test to detect Alzheimer's"[1] or distinguish it from other causes. There is hope in the field that multiple tests—cerebrospinal fluid (CSF) taps and high-tech neuroimaging, which could potentially measure levels of tau and amyloid proteins—might be combined to increase diagnostic certainty. But all tests have inherent variability, and multiple tests might actually increase diagnostic uncertainty. Furthermore, both classes of test are expensive and invasive (involving needles with risk of bleeding and infection), and deploying multiple tests on patients can be cumbersome both to individuals who are tested and to society, which must bear the burden of costs without clear proof of scientific value.

AD has also been linked to a susceptibility gene called APOE4 (which helps carry cholesterol through the blood) on chromosomes 21, 14, and 19, but the link between the gene and the disease is not causal, and problematic ethical implications surround disclosing such sensitive (and uncertain) information to patients who may not be prepared to reconcile it. Now, just as in the days of

Dr. Alzheimer, the only variable that seems to correlate with increased cases of AD is age, and classifying a "disease process" along the continuum of brain aging has proven a virtual impossibility. Thus, AD and now MCI continue to exist as a terrifying and stigmatizing signifier in our language without there being any agreed-upon disease etiology or any common method for diagnosing the condition in individuals. There always has been and will be a need to establish arbitrary thresholds to apply labels. We doubt that there will ever be a biological marker for AD. It will always remain a sociomarker. People "get" MCI or AD not when a biological test proves it but when a doctor makes the diagnosis.

It is instructive to consider the parallel with prostate cancer. When does a patient get prostate cancer? The "abnormal" cells that can be labeled cancerous are found in most men who die in late age—most of whom will have neither been diagnosed in life nor suffered any consequences from the cells. On the basis of fairly nonspecific blood tests, some men will have had surgery that impairs their quality of life without clear evidence that the cancer would have been life threatening. Yet others may well have had both the quality and the length of their lives enhanced by early treatment. These boundary issues concerning health and disease are evident in many areas of geriatric medicine. The critical challenges appear to be whether one can predict progression, whether the treatments are effective, and at what stage of illness they are effective. MCI seems to fail on all counts.

Reimagining "Alzheimer's Disease": A New Story of Quality of Life at the End of Life

As the twentieth century clearly revealed, Alzheimer's is a chameleonic concept. Lacking in diagnostic clarity, the classification and its myriad subclassifications have been captive to the vicissitudes of larger political, technological, and cultural forces. As we approach the 100th anniversary of the first publication of AD in 1910, we should remind ourselves that just as MCI is a social construct, so too is AD. AD is also a diagnosis based on arbitrary and culturally variable thresholds on clinical assessments. Human beings have had varying degrees of cognitive impairment as they age for probably the life of the species (certainly since the start of recorded history). What is the evidence that having labeled this as a disease since 1910 helps? Is the cost of currently available therapies worth it? Are the hopes created by research true or false? We at least need to ask these questions, particularly as our populations age and health care costs increase. Labeling something a disease makes care expensive and puts the power in the hands of doctors (and to a lesser extent other health care professionals). The opportunity costs of focusing on fixing brains also diminishes the values of and resources for more home- and commuting-based efforts to improve quality of life through psychosocial interventions.

In fact, we should be able to agree that every illness manifests in both the body and the mind. Everything humans declare a disease is marked by some kind of suffering and must have a biological substrate, perhaps relatively simple or perhaps complex. However, we must also recognize that every disease process, whether we call it by one name (a diagnostic label) or several, represents an agreed-upon category and hence is socially constructed. A biological foundation does not imply that a simple biological approach (for example, a pill) is necessarily the best (the most cost-effective and safe) solution.

Although the AD label has matured into one of the most formidable biomedical markers in the Western world, it should not be forgotten that in the mid-twentieth century, practitioners such as Rothschild succeeded in deemphasizing the biomedical approach to brain aging and advocating a psychosocial model of care that offered more dynamic therapeutic options to elderly individuals. In turn, a fundamental alteration in medicine's classificatory "story" led to an enrichment in therapeutic strategy. As we contemplate the increasing diagnostic confusion of "Alzheimer's" today, it would seem that such a paradigmatic shift is once again possible—if not altogether necessary.

It may be helpful to reflect on the therapies that currently exist for the millions of elderly persons who are labeled as having Alzheimer's disease. Once allocated the label, individuals are traditionally put on one of five pills currently on the market. Cholinesterase-inhibiting pills (brand names Aricept, Exelon, Razadyne, and Cognex) and a glutamate receptor antagonist (Namenda) are all approved by the FDA but have drawn criticism for their limited efficacy, and in the case of the cholinergic drugs, side effects that include gastrointestinal upset such as nausea, vomiting, diarrhea, and muscle cramps as well as sleep disturbances such as insomnia and nightmares. Namenda's side effects include constipation, dizziness, and confusion.[2] Biomedicine promises a bright future with disease-modifying drugs to treat Alzheimer's pathology, but until these therapies are proven safe and efficacious, they are merely science fiction and offer more hype than hope. So for most patients labeled with an Alzheimer's diagnosis, the predicament is thus: they are given a socially stigmatized "disease" for which there is no cure, put on dosages of modestly effective pills with known side effects, and told that science is working hard to find a "magic-bullet" cure for their condition but that this cure is nowhere near fruition. Surely, as a human community we can devise a better therapeutic strategy to help individuals and their families cope with brain aging.

Indeed, when we approach memory loss as an adverse pathological condition called Alzheimer's, we end up aiming our treatments at the disease rather than at the persons who are experiencing it. Because we have come to understand Alzheimer's disease in purely mechanical and molecular terms (in other words, as a biological fact), our public resources are disproportionately expended on the biological war against disease rather than on long-term care strategies for those living with a disease for which there is no current or foreseeable cure. We are so enamored with how we may treat people in the future that we have lost sight of those who require treatment at present. Cure has usurped care.

By changing the biomedical story we tell about Alzheimer's disease—primarily by eliminating the specious classificatory boundary between AD and brain aging and ceasing to extend the pathology of Alzheimer's onto millions of patients each year—we can make the range of therapeutic options available to aging individuals far more dynamic and indeed more effective at promoting quality of life. By ceasing to label people with a stigmatizing disease that not only implies ineptitude and incompetence but also narrows the therapeutic options to a range of moderately effective and potentially deleterious pharmacological interventions, we can begin to offer aging persons a comprehensive strategy of biopsychosocial care that will allow them to maintain independent functioning and feel a personal sense of normality, connectedness, and physical, social, and familial usefulness despite their cognitive challenges. Our efforts to reimagine the brain aging process must first challenge the heavily entrenched cultural models that portray aging as a form of inertia and Alzheimer's as a process by which one simply fades away into oblivion. Certainly, aging enfeebles us all; but "scarlet letter" disease labels such as AD imply social uselessness and create embarrassment and shame that seal off affected persons from a "normally functioning" culture.

Gerontological literature consistently shows that social integration has a positive correlative effect with mental and physical health in old age. Physical activity in older adults is associated with decreased incidence of mortality, hypertension, cardiovascular disease, depression, falls, and disability (Tinetti et al. 1994, pp. 821–27; Fried et al. 1998, pp. 585–92; Stuck et al. 1999, pp. 445–69; Appel et al. 2003, pp. 2083). And beyond physical benefits, regular participation in structured social and productive activities (Rowe and Kahn 1987, pp. 143–49, 1998, pp. 142–44; Stuck et al. 1999, pp. 445–69) and membership in large social networks have been shown to independently benefit health and functional outcomes, and cognitively stimulating activity such as social interaction may preserve cognition throughout the course of brain aging (Welin et al. 1992, pp. 127–32; Unger et al. 1997, pp. 152–60). Tellingly, social disengagement is a correlative predictor for age-related cognitive decline.

In Cleveland, one of us (Peter) has structured his practice around the belief that changing the label can also remove the social impediments that have for decades blockaded Alzheimer's victims from being contributing members to society. His patients are already being put on a more biopsychosocial trajectory of medical care, and no promises are made about magic-bullet cures. We believe that every psychosocial intervention is also de facto a biological intervention. Telling a story, reading a book, or participating in talk therapy engenders complex but undoubtedly real changes in the brain. In fact, it is not a stretch to refer to reading a book as a multineurotransmitter, neuroprotective, lexical access enhancement device, especially when pills tend to act on only one or just a few primary neurotransmitter systems!

Though the standard cholinesterase-inhibiting pills can be part of their regimen of care, Peter's patients are eating healthy diets; staying physically fit; volunteering in a mentorship program with Cleveland city children who are learning to read; using local resources to learn new skills such as meditation techniques (to maintain mindfulness); staying cognitively vital through art, music, and bibliotherapy; keeping socially engaged; and participating in structured conversations and writing exercises designed to guide families through difficult decision making at the end of life. We need research to better understand the value of such interventions. However, our research agenda must include a broader portfolio of inquiry that goes beyond molecular genetic approaches to include ecological, educational, psychosocial, and public health research. Moreover, we must encourage the wise integration of thoughts and values in our deeper scholarship.

By reimagining the experience of memory loss as an expected part of aging rather than medicalizing it as a "disease process," we can push the range of therapeutic options beyond asking "Do we have a pill for that?" thereby making life easier for persons and families who are coping with the difficulties of cognitive loss. We can honor the suffering caused by cognitive aging and seek efficacious treatments without creating a subspecies of people we call "Alzheimer's disease victims" and relegating them to the fringes of society, where they are expected simply to fade away while waiting for a biological cure that may never arrive. As we have already seen in Cleveland, an individual need not have a fully functioning mind to draw pleasure from social interaction, to enjoy music, art, or storytelling or to teach young schoolchildren how to read. If we engage our moral imaginations and thoughtfully consider brain aging against the problematic backdrop of the last hundred years of AD, we will be compelled to transform Alzheimer's, the so-called disease of the twentieth century, into the disease *no longer* of the twenty-first century, and so enrich the therapeutic possibilities for all of us as we age.

The political climate in the United States today is infused with terrorism. The word *terror* has taken on new meaning and shifted our entire focus to protecting ourselves from outside terrorists, even though terror is an internal state that we create in ourselves. In a similar sense, have we been terrified by AD? Do we depend too much on outside sources (like molecular-oriented doctors) for our conceptions of "dis-ease"? Do some medical models of illness create unnecessary disease categories and hence intensify "dis-ease"? Can we reclaim our abilities to chart our own courses as we face the cognitive challenges of aging? Can we continue to invest in a more honest science and hope for biological interventions? Or if we put too much faith in the magic of science, do we endorse scientism as our dominant modern religion?

The stakes for this debate about MCI and AD are high. How we tell and retell the story of Alzheimer's disease is a key chapter in the story of the human species at this point in its history. Science has and will continue to give us much to be grateful for, but it has limits. All of us die, and it is likely that for various reasons our greatest evolutionary gift, the embodied brain, will suffer the ravages of aging the most. Science cannot cure death, but this should not be reason for consternation. Death and its impending approach can actually be enlightening and, if dealt with properly, awareness of its imminence can enhance our quality of life and imbue our lives with purpose and meaning. So perhaps MCI, rather than being viewed as the beginning of AD in individuals, can be viewed as the end or at least the beginning of the end of AD as a social construct. Any words we use to replace MCI and AD, such as returning to using "senility" or referring to brain aging as presenting us with "age-associated cognitive challenges," are social constructs as well. Our task is to select the terms that lead to optimal use of social resources and human wisdom. It is a tragedy that medicine and science are letting us down in this regard.

ACKNOWLEDGMENTS

A number of colleagues have influenced our thinking about this topic over the years: Atwood Gaines, Department of Anthropology, Case Western Reserve University; Eric Juengst and Melissa Barber, Department of Bioethics, Case Western Reserve University; Marian Patterson, Department of Neurology, Case Western Reserve University; Jesse Ballenger, Penn State University; Jason Karlawish, University of Pennsylvania; Margaret Lock, McGill University; and Rick Moody, AARP. Thank you all. The work was supported by grant AG/HS17511-01A1 Medical Goals in Dementia: Ethics and Quality of Life from the National Institutes of Health / NIA; grant AG10483-13 from the National Institutes of Health / National Institute on Aging and Alzheimer's Disease Cooperative Study—Quality of Lives; and a grant from the Shigeo and Megumi Takayama Foundation, Tokyo, Japan.

NOTES

1. www.alz.org/alzheimers_disease_stages_of_alzheimers.asp.
2. Therapeutics Initiative evidence based drug therapy: Drugs for Alzheimer's disease. *Therapeutics Newsletter* (April–August 2005). Therapeutics Initiative, University of British Columbia Department of Pharmacology and Therapeutics.

REFERENCES

Alzheimer's Association. 2006. Statistics about Alzheimer's disease. www.alz.org/AboutAD/statistics.asp.

American Psychiatric Association. 1952. *Diagnostic and statistical manual of mental disorders.* Washington, D.C.: APA.

———. 1980. *Diagnostic and statistical manual of mental disorders,* 3rd ed. Washington, D.C.: APA.

———. 1987. *Diagnostic and statistical manual of mental disorders,* 3rd ed., revised. Washington, D.C.: APA.

———. 1994. *Diagnostic and statistical manual of mental disorders,* 4th ed. Washington, D.C.: APA.

Appel, L. J., C. M. Champagne, D. W. Harsha, L. S. Cooper, E. Obarzanek, P. J. Elmer, V. J. Stevens et al.; Writing Group of the PREMIER Collaborative Research Group. 2003. Effects of comprehensive lifestyle modification on blood pressure control: Main results of the PREMIER clinical trial. *JAMA* 289 (16): 2083–93.

Ballenger, J. F. 2000. Beyond the characteristic plaques and tangles: Mid-twentieth century U.S. psychiatry and the fight against senility. In *Concepts of Alzheimer disease: Biological, clinical, and cultural perspectives,* ed. P. Whitehouse, K. Maurer, and J. F. Ballenger. Baltimore: Johns Hopkins University Press.

———. 2006. *Self, senility, and Alzheimer's disease in modern America.* Baltimore: Johns Hopkins University Press.

Bick, K. L., L. Amaducci, and G. Pepeu. 1987. *The early story of Alzheimer's disease: Translation of the historical papers by Alois Alzheimer, Oskar Fischer, Francesco Bonfiglio, Emil Kraepelin, Gaetano Perusini*. Padua: Liviana Press.

Butler, R. N., and B. T. Engel. 1978. Editorial: Psychosomatic medicine and aging research. *Psychosomatic Medicine* 40 (5): 365–67.

Canguilhem, G. 1989. *The normal and the pathological*. New York: Zone Books.

Cohen, D., and C. Eisdorfer. 1986. *The loss of self: A family resource for the care of Alzheimer's disease and related disorders*. New York, Norton.

Corner, L., and J. Bond. 2006. The impact of the label of mild cognitive impairment on the individual's sense of self. *Philosophy, Psychiatry, and Psychology* 13 (1): 3–12.

Crook T. H., R. T. Bartus, S. H. Ferris, P. Whitehouse, G. D. Cohen, and S. Gershon. 1986. Age-associated memory impairment: Proposed diagnostic criteria and measures of clinical change—Report of a National Institute of Mental Health work group. *Developmental Neuropsychology* 2:261–76.

Dziegielewski, S. 2002. *DSM-IV-TR in action*. New York: John Wiley & Sons.

Fox, P. 1989. Rise of the Alzheimer's disease movement. *Milbank Quarterly* 67 (1): 58–102.

Fried, L. P., R. A. Kronmal, D. Bild, J. Gardin, M. Mittelmark, A. Newman, J. Polak, and J. Robbins, for the Cardiovascular Health Study Collaborative Research Group. 1998. Risk factors for five-year mortality in older adults: The Cardiovascular Health Study. *JAMA* 279:585–92.

Gaines, A. D., and P. J. Whitehouse. 2006. Building a mystery: Alzheimer disease, mild cognitive impairment, and beyond. *Journal of Philosophy, Psychiatry, and Psychology* 13 (1): 61–74.

Hart, J., and S. Semple. 1990. *Neuropsychology and the dementias*. London: Taylor & Francis.

Katzman, R., and K. Bick. 2000. *Alzheimer's disease: The changing view*. San Diego: Academic Press.

Kleinman, A. 1988. *The illness narratives*. New York: Basic Books.

Kral, V. 1962. Senescent forgetfulness: Benign and malignant. *Canadian Medical Association Journal* 86:257–60.

Levy, R. 1994. Aging-associated cognitive decline. Working Party of the International Psychogeriatric Association in collaboration with the World Health Organization. *International Psychogeriatrics* 6 (1): 63–8.

Mace, N. L. and P. V. Rabins. 1981. *The 36-hour day: A family guide to caring for persons with Alzheimer's disease, related dementing illnesses, and memory loss in later life*. Baltimore, Johns Hopkins University Press.

Maurer, K., and U. Maurer. 2003. *Alzheimer: The life of a physician and the career of a disease*. New York: Columbia University Press.

Maurer, K., S. Volk, and H. Gerbaldo. 2000. Auguste D.: The history of Alois Alzheimer's first case. In *Concepts of Alzheimer disease: Biological, clinical, and cultural perspectives*, ed. P. J. Whitehouse, K. Maurer, and J. F. Ballenger. Baltimore: Johns Hopkins University Press.

McCarthy, J., and M. Zald. 1987. Resource mobilization theory. In *Social movements in organizational society*, ed. C. Estes, R. Newcomer, and associates. Beverly Hills, Calif.: Sage Publications.

Möller, H.-J., and M. B. Graeber. 2000. Johann F.: The historical relevance of the case for the concept of Alzheimer disease. In *Concepts of Alzheimer disease: Biological, clinical, and cultural perspectives*, ed. P. J. Whitehouse, K. Maurer, and J. F. Ballenger. Baltimore: Johns Hopkins University Press.

Morris, J. C. 2006. Mild cognitive impairment *is* early-stage Alzheimer disease. *Archives of Neurology* 63:15–16.

Petersen, R. C., J. C. Stevens, M. Ganguli, E. G. Tangalos, J. L. Cummings, and S. T. DeKosky. 2001. Practice parameter: Early detection of dementia: Mild cognitive impairment (an evidence-based review). Report of the Quality Standards Subcommittee of the American Academy of Neurology. *Neurology* 56:1133–42.

Reagan, R. 1994. Letter to the American people. Available at www.americanpresidents.org/letters/39.asp.

Rothschild, D. 1947. The practical value of research in the psychoses of later life. *Diseases of the Nervous System* 8:123–28.

Rowe, J. W., and R. L. Kahn. 1987. Human aging: Usual and successful. *Science* 237 (4811): 143–49.

———. 1998. Successful aging. *Aging* 10 (2): 142–44.

Stuck, A. E., J. M. Walthert, T. Nikolaus, C. J. Bula, C. Hohmann, and J. C. Beck. 1999. Risk factors for functional status decline in community-living elderly people: A systematic literature review. *Social Science and Medicine* 48:445–69.

Tinetti, M. E., D. I. Baker, G. McAvay, E. B. Claus, P. Garrett, M. Gottschalk, M. L. Koch, K. Trainor, and R. I. Horwitz. 1994. A multifactorial intervention to reduce the risk of falling among elderly people living in the community. *New England Journal of* Medicine 331 (13): 821–27.

Torack, R. M. 1978. *The pathological physiology of dementia.* New York: Springer-Verlag.

Unger, J. B., C. A. Johnson, and G. Marks. 1997. Functional decline in the elderly: Evidence for direct and stress-buffering protective effects of social interactions and physical activity. *Annals of Behavioral Medicine* 19 (2): 152–60.

Welin, L., B. Larsson, K. Svardsudd, B. Tibblin, and G. Tibblin. 1992. Social network and activities in relation to mortality from cardiovascular diseases, cancer and other causes: A 12-year follow up of the study of men born in 1913 and 1923. *Journal of Epidemiology and Community Health* 46 (2): 127–32.

Whitehouse, P. J. 1986. The concept of cortical and subcortical dementia: Another look. *Annals of Neurology* 19:1–6.

———. 2001. The end of Alzheimer disease. *Alzheimer Disease and Associated Disorders* 15 (2): 59–62.

———. 2004a. Mild cognitive impairment: The beginning of the end of AD. *Psychiatric Times* 87–88.

———. 2004b. Regulatory aspects of mild cognitive impairment: Toward a harmonized perspective. *Dialogues in Clinical Neuroscience* 6 (4): 409–14.

Whitehouse, P. J., and AGS Clinical Practice Committee. 2003. Guidelines abstracted from the American Academy of Neurology's dementia guidelines for early detection, diagnosis, and management of dementia, special article. *Journal of the American Geriatrics Society* 51:1417–22.

Whitehouse, P. J., and Juengst, E. T. 2005. Anti-aging medicine and mild cognitive impairment: Practice and policy issues for geriatrics. *Journal of the American Geriatrics Society* 53:1417–22.

CHAPTER 2

Notes toward a Future History of Treatments for Cognitive Failure

DAVID HEALY, M.D., FRCPSYCH

The history of treatments for cognitive failure falls into three broad areas. First, there is an early history, when claims for treatments that would now be termed "cognitive enhancing" and for putative treatments for dementia were much more common than many would now suspect. Second, there is a history determined primarily by events happening in the psychopharmacology of the functional psychoses. The dynamic of developments during this period aimed at conforming the domain of dementia to developments happening in the antidepressant field. Third, there is a more recent period in which both clinical and laboratory-based neuroscientific developments have begun to play more of a part.

The Early Period

The history of treatments for cognitive failure extends back at least as far as does the history of treatments for depression or psychosis. The nineteenth-century medical and lay literature featured advertisements for a range of compounds to treat the infirmities of old age and, in particular, what was termed senility. Indeed, such ads were much more common than ads touting a cure for frank mental illness. In the early twentieth century, a range of compounds including the classical stimulants such as dexamphetamine and methylphenidate crept into use for this purpose alongside a group of drugs termed "analeptics," which included Metrazole and even strychnine in low doses. This use appears to have been on the simple basis that every effort should be made to "stimulate" any remaining cognitive function to its maximum.

In the 1950s and 1960s, against a backdrop of interest in arteriosclerosis, there was an increasing emphasis on the role of brain vascular disease as a cause of cognitive decline in old age. This led to the introduction of a group of treatments aimed at enhancing cerebral blood flow and to claims that drugs already in use had such flow-enhancing properties. Drugs such as dihydroergotamine (Hydergine), nicergoline, cyclandelate, and naftidrofuryl came to be widely advertised and used for this purpose. None came with the kind of clinical trial evidence that would now be needed to introduce a drug on the market.

With the eclipse of the vasodilator theories, in the 1970s, Hydergine was reinvented by Sandoz as a cerebral metabolism enhancer: "The old belief—that mental deterioration in the elderly is caused by impaired blood supply to the brain—has been exploded. A report in the *Lancet* reviewing world wide published evidence concludes that atherosclerosis does not cause mental deterioration and that the term 'cerebral arteriosclerosis' is inaccurate and should not be used in this condition. The only rational way to reverse insidious mental deterioration is to treat the real defect at source. Hydergine does precisely that. Hydergine acts directly to improve cerebral metabolism" (Sandoz 1970).

The vast majority of vasodilator, cerebral metabolism enhancer, and stimulant drugs used for senility were swept away in the 1970s as part of the Drug Efficacy Study Implementation (DESI) program instituted after the 1962 amendment to the Food, Drugs, and Cosmetics Act. Following the 1962 amendment, the U.S. Food and Drug Administration (FDA) was charged with establishing not only whether new drugs worked but also whether drugs currently on the market were effective in addition to being safe. This led to the creation of a number of efficacy panels made up largely of scientists with links to the National Academy of Sciences. These panels ruled on more than 3000 compounds based on the published study data. A majority of the psychotropic compounds reviewed were adjudged by the psychiatry panel not to have a strong evidence base in terms of controlled trial data, but nevertheless to have considerable evidence of efficacy. Companies sponsoring these drugs had the opportunity to undertake further studies, but in the case of drugs off patent, most companies chose not to do so. Unless compounds were determined to have a clear evidence base, the FDA removed them from the market, in many cases despite considerable evidence of efficacy (Shorter 2002).

Retrospectively, the case for Hydergine looks strong (Schneider and Olin 1994). In the case of Metrazole, another drug eliminated, the manufacturers protested and took their action to the Supreme Court, where, in *Weinberger v. Bentex*, which was decided on June 18, 1973, a decision confirmed the authority of the FDA to withdraw such drugs. It seems likely that a number of important therapeutic leads may have been lost as a result of this clearing out of the therapeutic armamentarium.

The Concept of a Nootropic

The consequences of this clearout were felt in the conceptual as well as the therapeutic domain and led to the paradox of a new development that already feels more part of a distant history than some of the notions it sought to replace. In the 1960s, the psychotropic marketplace looked very different from what it looked like at the end of the century. It was dominated by broadly stimulant or sedative compounds that would not readily be classified as anxiolytics, antidepressants, or antipsychotics and by concepts of nervous disorder such as senility and nervous breakdown. The notion of a tranquilizer came into being only in the mid-1950s, and while it was immediately popular, the word "antidepressant" does not feature in popular dictionaries until the 1980s (Healy 1997). A number of neologisms, such as "neuroleptics" and "thymoleptics," were conjured up to account for the effects of drugs like chlorpromazine and imipramine. The pharmacological revolution of the 1950s and 1960s called forth new conceptual developments of this sort, one of which was the concept of a nootropic.

The term "nootropic" was coined by Corneliu Giurgea, a Romanian who had trained in psychophysiology in the Soviet Union and later became director of research at UCB Pharma in the late 1960s on the back of the development of piracetam (2-oxo-pyrrolidone) (Giurgea 1973). Originally developed to combat motion sickness in 1964, piracetam appeared in animal tests to promote learning and prevent hypoxic-induced amnesia. By 1972, there were already 700 papers on various aspects of piracetam's profile. The key features of a nootropic were that it would promote learning as well as enhance resistance of learned behaviors to disruption by stressors like hypoxia, barbiturates, and scopolamine. Such compounds, it was intimated, would increase cerebral "tone" and would be almost completely lacking in conventional psychotropic side effects. These were drugs that would forestall senility rather than agents that would treat an established dementia.

A range of compounds followed piracetam into the nootropic stable—pyritinol, centrophenoxine, aniracetam, pramiracetam, oxiracetam, and idebenone—sparking a great deal of basic animal research in laboratories from Venezuela to Poland. Many of these compounds came on to the market in European countries. Claims have been made that piracetam is effective in alcohol withdrawal (Skondia and Kabes 1985) and in dementia or other cognitive impairments (Chouinard et al. 1983; Croisile et al. 1993; Platt et al. 1993). But no nootropic has ever made it to the U.S. market.

Biochemically, the demonstrated effects of piracetam in the 1970s and 1980s were also exciting; it reduced lipofuscin accumulation in the brain and reversed the effects of both anticholinergics and protein synthesis inhibitors. Demonstrations of enhanced cholinergic function on combinations of piracetam and choline or lecithin in animals (Bartus, Dean, and Beer 1981), and in patients with dementing disorders (Ferris et al. 1982; Smith et al. 1984) helped the emergence of a cholinergic hypothesis of dementia in the 1980s, and this hypothesis in turn helped to maintain interest in piracetam and other drugs in this group. With the emergence of interest in glutamate, a flood of articles demonstrated clear effects of piracetam on glutamatergic systems.

Both piracetam and the very concept of a nootropic have, however, disappeared. A multipotent, side-effect free agent was perhaps too good to be true, but there remain three aspects of interest to the piracetam story. First, piracetam, and the notion of a nootropic, function almost as a Rorschach test for the field of cognitive enhancement in general. Almost every neurotransmitter system, most degenerative disorders, and a variety of conditions unresponsive to other therapies found a home under the nootropic roof at one point—or put another way, were colonized by this conceptual virus (meme). Second, a great deal of solid research on protein disruption, or protein synthesis enhancement, through to research on cholinergic systems in the 1970s and 1980s was done under the nootropic banner. Clinicians and basic researchers saw themselves as working in the nootropic field, in just the way that other researchers saw themselves as working on antidepressants or neuroleptics. And finally, the concept of nootropic arguably survives in the popular notion of a smart drug.

The Middle Period
The Chlorpromazine Watershed

The introduction of chlorpromazine in France in 1952 and in the United States in 1955 changed mindsets regarding the pharmacotherapy of psychiatric disorders. It ultimately led to the introduction of the notion of a lesion that drug treatment might correct. To appreciate the significance of this, one must recall that there was little or no understanding of the possibility of chemical neurotransmission at the time and as such no basis for a lesion that chlorpromazine might rectify. In the case of chlorpromazine, this new understanding was ultimately formulated in the 1970s as the dopamine hypothesis of schizophrenia, which postulated defective dopaminergic neurotransmission that neuroleptic therapy corrected.

It took a great deal of neuroscientific development, however, for such an idea to catch hold. Only in the 1970s did the treatment of schizophrenia, for example, become supposedly rational in this sense. Before that, the use of the antipsychotics or neuroleptics was largely for behavioral disturbances or for symptomatic use. Many advertisements featured the use of the neuroleptics for senile disturbances of behavior, for example.

At the same time that chlorpromazine was introduced, a range of investigators noted the effects of isoniazid and iproniazid on the mental states of tubercular patients (Healy 1997). From this set of observations, the antidepressant class of drugs were developed. Iproniazid in particular was proposed early on to work by virtue of being a monoamine oxidase inhibitor (MAOI), supposedly increasing cerebral monoamines. This notion led directly to the most influential lesion theory—the catecholamine hypothesis of depression (Schildkraut 1965).

This theory, which appeared eminently rational at the time, retrospectively appears no less mythological than the notion that Hydergine might be a cerebral metabolism enhancer (Healy 1997). There were, in fact, always good grounds to doubt the theory. For instance, isoniazid, which appears to be an effective antidepressant (Salzer and Lurie 1955), was known not to be an MAOI. Furthermore, when iproniazid, which was an MAOI, was removed from the market because of liver toxicity and replaced by isocarboxazid, also an MAOI, the new drug simply didn't seem to work well (Kline 1970). Finally, iproniazid, unlike subsequent MAOIs, in high doses appeared to cause psychosis. This indicates that iproniazid may have significant actions on systems other than the monoamine systems. If isoniazid and iproniazid do not have effects in common with other MAOIs on catecholamine or serotonergic systems, it remains entirely possible that they have common effects on glutamatergic or other systems.

There are further lessons to be learned from the MAOI group of drugs. The discovery of their antidepressant effects stemmed essentially from a capitalization upon their side effects. For instance, these drugs caused weight gain when used in tuberculosis, so it seemed like a good idea to try them out on depressed patients, who commonly lost weight. However, the new focus on catecholamines and serotonin, as a result of the supposed biochemical effects of the MAOIs, brought with it the notion that the primary effects of the drugs were biochemical. These new biochemical side effects were unlike any previous side effects of treatment—they were ideological side effects rather than the real thing.

For instance, as depression came to be seen as a disorder involving a monoamine lesion, then the anticholinergic effects of early antidepressants were transformed pretty much by definition into side effects. A generation of textbooks noted that these anticholinergic side effects included blurred vision, urinary retention, and cognitive disturbances, particularly memory disturbances, all of which were problems that would be done away with by the creation of more selective norepinephrine or serotonin reuptake inhibiting drugs. It took thirty years for the established wisdom to be overturned by the example of urinary retention in antidepressants such as reboxetine and duloxetine, which were norepinephrine reuptake inhibitors devoid of effects on cholinergic systems. But arguably such ideas should never have developed in the first instance, as the same clinicians who talked about anticholinergic problems such as urinary retention were regularly treating patients with much more potent anticholinergic antidotes to neuroleptic-induced parkinsonism, without any resulting urinary problems. Neuroscience was beginning to lead rather than follow clinical observation.

As what might be called a "side effect" of this process, a premium was put on the notion that acetylcholine (ACh) might be the neurotransmitter involved in Alzheimer's disease. The proposal that ACh might play a role in dementia stemmed from two sources, one of which was a linkage between anticholinergic drugs and amnestic effects. But a second, and at least as important, source was the fact that few neurotransmitters were known to exist in the body, and as serotonin and noradrenaline had become parceled out among the mood disorders, and dopamine was implicated in schizophrenia, this left only one neurotransmitter, acetylcholine, to play a role in the dementias. By the 1970s, early speculation began to implicate acetylcholine in dementia, and this was supported by findings of cholinergic changes in dementing brains, leading by the early 1980s to a range of articles proposing a cholinergic hypothesis of dementia (Bartus et al. 1982; Davis and Mohs 1986). This development ran counter to centuries of clinical observation in that excessive dosing with drugs—now known to be anticholinergic—had traditionally been linked to delirium rather than dementia.

The Cholinergic Hypothesis of Dementia

The cholinergic hypothesis led to a focusing of efforts on the production of drugs that would enhance cholinergic function, reversing a presumed deficit of cholinergic function in dementia. The first drugs of this sort included agents like choline and lecithin, which were aimed at replacing deficiencies in acetylcholine levels, in much the same way that L-dopa reversed the effects of Parkinson's disease. Some early results suggested beneficial effects of these treatments, especially when combined with nootropic agents such as piracetam. A subsequent generation of drugs aimed at inhibiting the breakdown of acetylcholine by its metabolizing enzyme cholinesterase. These early cholinesterase inhibitors included tetrahydroaminoacridine (tacrine) and later pyridostigmine.

The tacrine story has been outlined in detail elsewhere (Leber 1996). In brief, early reports in 1983 (Summers et al. 1986) suggested that tacrine had an awakening effect on Alzheimer's dementia comparable to the use of agents such as L-dopa for Parkinson's disease. Efforts to replicate this early work proved unsuccessful. However, tacrine quickly ended up being used widely off label, despite the fact that this drug had little toxicity data available to indicate whether such use would be safe. Subsequent efforts to demonstrate the efficacy of tacrine were unsuccessful (Leber 1996), but by this time a clamor for the licensing of tacrine had built up so that it was all but impossible not to license this drug. Once licensed, tacrine failed to have any clear impact clinically other than on the development of a greater number of memory clinics and the creation of an expectation that a new generation of specifically antidementia drugs would emerge in due course.

The development of tacrine spurred interest in the cholinesterase inhibitors, which ultimately led to the licensing of donepezil, a drug developed by Eisai and licensed by Pfizer, followed by rivastigmine and galantamine. The fuss around tacrine also played a key part in the emergence of these drugs and their subsequent marketing in another way. In an effort to cope with the problems of efficacy assessment that tacrine posed, the regulators and a range of interested clinicians set about developing standards by which antidementia drugs might be recognized. The new standards included statements of the size of a treatment effect on instruments such as the Alzheimer's Disease Assessment Scale-cognitive subscale (ADAS-cog). These standards later permitted the licensing of drugs such as donepezil, even though the apparent treatment benefits, at least when judged across groups of patients with dementia, were minimal.

The early years of the rising popularity of the cholinesterase inhibitors were a time of concern for some, who worried that the extensive use of these drugs would potentially bust health care budgets, considering the scale of the clinical problem, the cost of the drugs, and the expectations that had been engendered. However, the actual adoption in most countries has been far more modest. Given indicators of an extensive use of stimulants among elderly people in the 1940s, 1950s, and 1960s, the rate of use of cholinesterase inhibitors may in fact not have been substantially different from the use of stimulants for elderly people in a previous generation.

By the mid- to late 1990s, a further feature of this marketplace was an almost exclusive focus on the treatment of Alzheimer's dementia, where the previous focus had been on the management of cognitive decline or the treatment of cognitive failure. By the late 1980s, most dementing disorders had been subsumed under the heading of Alzheimer's dementia and, aside from the use of aspirin, the notion of managing a cerebrovascular input to the clinical picture had been all but precluded. During this period, multi-infarct dementia had, rhetorically at least, all but ceased to exist.

The Recent Period
Enhancement or Cure?

While the formal selling of selective serotonin reuptake inhibitors (SSRIs) was constrained within a disease and lesion framework—"to correct the chemical imbalance known to be involved in these disorders"—the failure to find a lesion opened up the possibility that aminergic drugs enhanced certain cerebral functions and that this enhancement could be more or less helpful in certain disorders. If this was the case, it was also possible that these drugs might also have an effect in nondiseased states.

The initial conceptual basis for psychotropic drug use in fact included the possibility that these agents might have an effect on nondiseased states. Before chlorpromazine, the potential effects of psychotropic agents were framed within dimensional models of personality such as that put forward by Eysenck (Eysenck 1952; Claridge 1969; Healy 2002). Theories such as Eysenck's proposed that people vary on axes such as introversion and extraversion and that, for example, stimulants and sedatives can affect introverts and extraverts differently and that these differential effects are grounded in genetic/constitutional factors.

The use of the antipsychotics and antidepressants through the 1960s led to a gradual eclipse of this line of dimensional thinking and the emergence of much more categorical views of mental illness, best enshrined perhaps in popular notions that the *Diagnostic and Statistical Manual of Mental Disorders*, 3rd edition (DSM-III) embodied a revival of Kraepelinian thinking, when in fact the new focus on syndromes arguably owed much more to Adolf Meyer than to Kraepelin. Dimensional ideas, though, persisted as a subterranean stream within the modern era. This stream resurfaced at certain points, as, for example, in the suggestions in *Listening to Prozac* (Kramer 1993) that Prozac could make even people who might not be ill better than they had been, that it enhanced functions. Such an action is most parsimoniously viewed in terms of Prozac having effects on a dimensional spectrum so that certain ingrained features of particular personalities change, allowing some people who take it to become better than well.

There is a considerable amount of evidence that selective noradrenaline and selective serotonin reuptake inhibitors indeed have effects on functional aspects of personality and different effects on different personality types (Tranter et al. 2002; Healy 2004). Furthermore, in contrast to the supposed anticholinergic side effects of antidepressants, for centuries anticholinergic agents such as mandragora and henbane, and later hyoscine, had been used to treat nervous problems; they helped calm patients and gave a euphoric sense to many (Healy 2002). Indeed, a series of early controlled clinical trials suggested that atropine might be beneficial in melancholic depression (Hoch and Maus 1932; Herz 1965; Loew and Taeschler 1965; Kasper, Moises, and Beckmann 1981). But for a variety of reasons, probably primarily to do with patents, no modern pharmaceutical company has seen fit to develop agents of this kind, and as popular awareness of the traditional origins of these drugs vanished, it became easier to brand the anticholinergic effects as side effects. As the efficacy of anticholinergic agents in nervous states would not now lead to a cholinergic-deficit theory of depression, these results might best be recon-ceptualized in dimensional or functional terms.

Early research on antidepressants gave rise to an orthodox view of how catecholamine and serotonin systems function. In contrast, through the 1960s, an effort to produce more selective MAOIs led to the development of monoamine oxidase-B inhibitors and the development of drugs such as de-prenyl by Joseph Knoll and colleagues (Varga and Tringer 1967; Knoll 2000). The use of deprenyl in particular led to a recognition that underneath the tra-ditional economy of the catecholamine system lay a group of catecholamine-release-enhancing mechanisms. These appeared to be much more finely tuned physiological mechanisms than reuptake processes; they are the mech-anisms that are called into play, for example, when animals are in situations of extreme stress, such as when a hare finds itself the likely victim of an attack by an eagle. In such situations, the animal must mobilize its resources with extraordinary rapidity and must achieve a superoptimal level of functioning if there is to be any chance of escape.

Considerations of this phenomenon led Knoll to posit a theory of active reflexes (1969), which stood at odds with then dominant Pavlovian theories of conditioning. Hand in hand with the development of this theory, Knoll began to focus on the catecholamine-release mechanism and to develop drugs more selective to it. A combination of drugs selective to this mecha-nism, experiments on these drugs, and an emphasis on active reflexes led ul-timately to the proposal by Knoll among others that Parkinson's disease, Alz-heimer's disease, and other degenerative diseases might be manifestations of an aging process rather than discrete diseases in their own right and that agents active on monoamine-release mechanisms, by enhancing the econ-omy and efficiency of the organism, might forestall aging and minimize risks of developing degenerative disorders (Knoll 2003). There appears to be con-siderable evidence from animal studies that, for example, aspects of aging can be delayed by agents such as deprenyl. Deprenyl in turn became an agent aimed at forestalling the progression of Parkinson's disease. Whether such a drug might have had a comparable effect on Alzheimer's disease remains un-certain in the case of deprenyl and untested in the case of other compounds in this group (Sano et al. 1997).

The prospect of such an effect raises a number of questions. Is forestalling aging an example of enhancement or a treatment of a disease? Drugs that might prevent disease by delaying an aging process furthermore face a critical problem in terms of their development, which is that the structure and regulation of the current marketplace would require a demonstration of a preventative effect on a pathology that might otherwise appear. Such a demonstration would require holding a large number of subjects in a clinical trial program over a long period of time. This would involve a much greater scientific effort and financial outlay than drug companies have been used to hitherto. Current FDA models, which license drugs on the basis of two well-controlled trials, permit the economic development of antidepressants of the type we've had but do not sit readily with the licensing of agents that might be preventative.

A New Neuroscience: Glutamate

At much the same time as the monoamine hypothesis of depression was taking shape in the 1960s, awareness had developed that the brain had components such as glutamate and GABA, and in fact these were present in the brain in much greater quantities than the catecholamines, serotonin, or acetylcholine. This was a time, however, when the notion of chemical neurotransmission itself was first proposed and was not generally accepted. In the 1960s, no one was prepared to concede that glutamate was a neurotransmitter.

The preliminary work, which demonstrated the role of glutamate in the cerebral economy, came from Jeff Watkins, a chemist who had left Australia and done undergraduate and postgraduate work in England and later at Yale. After John Eccles, the famous neurophysiologist, moved back to Melbourne, Watkins applied to join his laboratory. Part of Eccles's fame stemmed from the fact that he was the most celebrated convert from the group of scientists who had espoused an electrical theory of neurotransmission in preference to a chemical theory.

While working in Melbourne, Watkins and a colleague, David Curtis, took a simple approach toward the question of mapping further neurotransmitters in the brain. They began with chemicals that could be found on the laboratory shelf. One of these was glutamate, which applied from the laboratory jar appeared to act as though it were a neurotransmitter (Watkins 1998).

Several difficulties stood in the way of recognizing what had been discovered. One of these was the continuing bias against the notion of chemical neurotransmission. A second was the disbelief that a chemical present in such great quantities in the brain might be a neurotransmitter. A third and perhaps more pressing problem was that there were no apparent drugs that could manipulate this system, and without such agents it was difficult to know whether this discovery had any functional significance.

The following two decades led Watkins, and growing numbers of scientists interested in glutamate, to map out the new system, to discover its receptors, and finally to help isolate drugs that manipulated glutamate functions. It transpired that the glutamate system had a number of receptors, of which the most famous has become the NMDA receptor. This is a hugely complex receptor system that has multiple sites, in particular a site that binds glycine. A variety of agents can act on the different components of the site, both directly on the ionic channel in the receptor and indirectly by modulating entry to the channel or through changes to the channel structure itself. Ions such as magnesium and zinc are needed as co-transmitters. Furthermore, it has become clear that the NMDA receptor comes in a number of different forms. There is a form that would now be thought of as a classical receptor, which is an ionophore that permits a flow of ions through it, and a further group of receptors called metabotropic receptors (Parsons, Wojciech, and Quack 1998).

The first evidence that there might be drugs that could act on glutamate offered a gloomy glimpse of the future. It appeared that such drugs, which included phencyclidine and ketamine, caused psychosis. In short order, drugs acting on the glutamate system became associated with a triggering of both psychosis and convulsions. The incentive to continue research in this area, however, lay in accumulating evidence that the glutamate system is linked to neurodegenerative processes and that most excitotoxic agents appear to act on the glutamate system (Olney 1992).

The key to unlocking a range of drugs that would act more safely on the glutamate systems lay in two sets of developments. One was the recognition of metabotropic receptors, which act to modulate the system rather than acting directly on it. The drugs with problematic effects were ones that acted directly on ion channels. The second was to recognize that a great number of drugs that were then in use, which had not been developed as agents to act on the glutamate system, did in fact act on that system. The mistake had been to attempt to devise agents genetically specific to the receptor system—an approach that might be regarded as a physician's approach to the issues. It was better to take a surgeon's approach it seemed—look for something that did in fact work rather than something that should in principle work (Watkins 1998).

Awareness grew that a number of agents had effects on the glutamate system. Some of these had low affinity effects on the channel, such as the antiviral agent amantadine, or memantine, an agent developed for glucose regulation, or the analgesic dextrophan and the anticholinergic drug orphenadrine (Parsons, Wojciech, and Quack 1998). Haloperidol is a selective NMDA antagonist, and the antitubercular agent d-cycloserine is a glycine partial agonist. Indeed as mentioned above, the original antitubercular psychotropic drug iproniazid, which was known to cause psychosis, may also have effects on this system. The effects of iproniazid and the comparable anxiolytic effects of d-cycloserine open up the question of whether the glutamate system is primarily involved in degenerative disorders or whether it might have a broader psychotropic role.

Memantine, having first been developed as a glucose stabilizer in the 1970s by Lilly, crept into use in Germany primarily as a tonic for older people. Through its use as a tonic, awareness developed that it might potentially have beneficial effects in preventing neurodegeneration. This led to an increasing use of the compound in dementing conditions and sufficient evidence that it had beneficial effects in these conditions to permit its development as a treatment for dementia. However, it remains unclear whether this drug actually interferes with the disease process, and is therefore delaying the progression of the disease, or whether it has some unspecified functional effect that shows up beneficially in patients who have neurodegenerative disorders. Other agents active on the NMDA system, such as cycloserine for example, appear to be effective anxiolytic agents.

Cognitive Rigidity and Other Prodromes

The end of the twentieth century also brought a return of interest in the possible cerebrovascular basis for cognitive failure. There was an increasing awareness that many apparently normal individuals over the age of 50 show extensive lacunar infarcts. There is every reason to believe that "small" vessel disease (Cummings 1994; Kramer et al. 2002) might underpin cognitive failure in a broader sense than Alzheimer's dementia. It seems highly likely, for instance, that such changes underpin the physical rigidity or infirmity of old age. There seems little reason to think that they might not also underpin wider cognitive changes, such as the development of what Shakespeare termed "Crabbed Age," with its associated mental inflexibility and inflexibility and sometimes bitterness of personality.

Shakespeare and the literature of old age remind us that there is a wider set of changes that, whether linked to vascular processes or not, have been eclipsed in the development of our currently prevailing models of dementia. There are likely to be syndromes other than age-associated memory impairment that deserve our attention. Our current models are in fact recent, having originated only in the period 1975 through 2000. We may need to revert to a much broader concept like "lacunatic" if we are to recognize the full range of agents that might have functional effects upon aging.

A more enduring focus of attention has been on mild cognitive impairment, which led to the delineation of syndromes such as age-associated memory impairment and the benign senile forgetfulness first proposed by Kral in 1962. These states have been proposed as prodromes of more serious disease, the treatment of which might forestall the development of full-blown dementias. But would agents effective in states of mild cognitive impairment remain confined to a disease domain, or would they be employed as enhancement agents?

One of the great features of early twenty-first-century medicine has been a focus on enhancement. Agents first introduced for clear-cut organic disorders such as erectile dysfunction, as in the case of Viagra, have been adopted to enhance functioning in much younger populations without convincing evidence of an organic lesion. Similarly, drugs first developed for the narcoleptic syndrome, such as modafinil, have since been explored as agents to "optimize wakefulness."

It is almost certain that if agents showed beneficial effects on memory, there would be a much greater market in the domain of memory enhancement than in traditionally medical domains such as the treatment of dementia. Until the end of the twentieth century, such paramedical uses were constrained within a disease model, and the notion of enhancement would have brought a frown to the face of most physicians. However, by the start of the twenty-first century, medical reserve in these areas was diminishing, and there was far more open advocacy of enhancement models (Elliott 2003; Rothman and Rothman 2004). And it is worth noting that there is probably some middle ground between these medical and nonmedical domains in which it is possible to contemplate a maintenance of functionality in older age (Marshall and Katz 2002).

The question of cognitive enhancement probably has greater political resonance than the notion of enhancement in other domains. For instance, one of the bases on which discrimination is still permissible is intellectual ability. Children and others who perform better intellectually get to go to universities, and indeed are often subsidized to do so, and end up in better-paying jobs than children not so favored. "Smart" drugs, however, are more likely to help those less advantaged in the current educational system or those whose abilities have begun to fail by virtue of age. On this basis those currently most advantaged in society perhaps stand to lose most. Against this background, the question of whether drugs should be widely available or constrained within a disease framework, albeit one that contains expanded concepts such as mild cognitive impairment, is a question with immense ramifications (Healy 2002; Rose 2002; Juengst et al. 2003).

It is highly likely that research on neurodegenerative disorders—for instance, research on glutamate—will lead to more effective agents to treat affective and schizophrenic disorders than will emerge from research programs dedicated to developing new antipsychotics or antidepressants. It is also likely that leads from drugs like haloperidol or orphenadrine that turn out to have unrecognized effects on glutamatergic or other systems will provide breakthroughs in the development of some agents that will enhance cognitive function and others that will arrest the pathological processes that underpin dementia. Should there be developments in either of these domains, our understanding of what the key lines of historical development in the field of psychopharmacology have been is likely to be transformed.

REFERENCES

Bartus, R. T., R. L. Dean, and B. Beer. 1981. An evaluation of drugs for improving memory in aged monkeys: Implications for clinical trials in humans. *Psychopharmacology Bulletin* 19:168–84.

Bartus, R. T., R. L. Dean, B. Beer, and A. S. Lippa. 1982. The cholinergic hypothesis of geriatric memory dysfunction. *Science* 217:408–17

Chouinard, G., L. Annable, A. Ross-Chouinard, M. Olivier, and F. Fontaine. 1983. Piracetam in elderly psychiatric patients with mild diffuse cerebral impairment. *Psychopharmacology* 81: 100–106.

Claridge, G. 1969. *Drugs and human behaviour.* Middlesex, UK: Allen Lane.

Croisile, B., M. Trillet, J. Fondarai, B. Laurent, F. Mauguierre, and F. Billardon. 1993. Long-term and high dose piracetam treatment of Alzheimer's disease. *Neurology* 43:301–5.

Crook, T., R. T. Bartus, S. H. Ferris, P. J. Whitehouse, G. D. Cohen, and S. Gershon. 1986. Age-associated memory impairment: Proposed diagnostic criteria and measures of clinical change—Report of a National Institute of Mental Health Work Group. *Developmental Neuropsychology* 2:261–76.

Cummings, J. L. 1994. Vascular subcortical dementias. *Dementia* 5:77–80.

———. 1995. Anatomic and behavioral aspects of frontal-subcortical circuits. *Annals of the New York Academy of Sciences* 769.

Davis, K. L., and R. C. Mohs. 1986. Cholinergic drugs in Alzheimer's disease. *New England Journal of Medicine* 315 (20): 1286–87.

Elliott, C. 2003. *Better than well: American medicine meets the American dream.* New York: Norton.

Eysenck, H. 1952. *The scientific study of personality.* London: Routledge & Kegan Paul.

Ferris, S. H., B. Reisberg, E. Friedman, M. K. Schneck, K. A. Sherman, P. Mir, and R. T. Bartus. 1982. Combination choline/piracetam treatment of senile dementia. *Psychopharmacology Bulletin* 18:96–98.

Giurgea, C. 1973. The "nootropic" approach to the pharmacology of the integrative activity of the brain. *Conditional Reflex* 8:108–15.

Healy, D. 1997. *The antidepressant era.* Cambridge, Mass.: Harvard University Press.

———. 2002. *The creation of psychopharmacology.* Cambridge, Mass.: Harvard University Press.

———. 2004. *Let them eat Prozac.* New York: New York University Press.

Herz, A. 1965. Central cholinolytic activity and antidepressant effect. In *Neuropsychopharmacology* 4, Proceedings of the 4th Meeting of CINP, ed. D. Bente and P. B. Bradley, 404–7. Amsterdam: Elsevier.

Hoch, P., and W. Mauss. 1932. Atropinbehandlung bei Geisteskrankheiten. *Archives de psychiatrie* 97:546–52.

Juengst, E., R. H. Binstock, M. Mehlman, S. G. Post, and P. J. Whitehouse. 2003. Biogerontology, "anti-aging medicine," and the challenges of human enhancement. *Hastings Center Report* 33 (4): 21–30.

Kaspar, S., H.-W. Moises, and H. Beckmann. 1981. The anticholinergic biperiden in depressive disorders. *Pharmacopsychiatry* 14:195–98.

Kline, N. S. 1970. Monoamine oxidase inhibitors: An unfinished picaresque tale. In *Discoveries in biological psychiatry,* ed. F. J. Ayd and B. Blackwell, 194–204. Philadelphia: Lippincott.

Knoll, J. 1969. *The theory of active reflexes: An analysis of some fundamental mechanisms of higher nervous activity.* Budapest: Publishing House of the Hungarian Academy of Sciences; New York: Hafner Publishing.

———. 2000. The psychopharmacology of life and death. In *The psychopharmacologists,* vol. 3, ed. D. Healy, 81–110. London: Arnold.

———. 2003. Enhancer regulation/endogenous and synthetic enhancer compounds: A neurochemical concept of the innate and acquired drives. *Neurochemical Research* 28:1275–97.

Krall, V. A. 1962. Senescent forgetfulness: Benign and malignant. *Journal of the Canadian Medical Association* 86:257–60.

Kramer, J. H., B. R. Reed, D. Mungas, M. W. Weiner, and H. C. Chui. 2002. Executive dysfunction in subcortical ischaemic vascular disease. *Journal of Neurology, Neurosurgery, and Psychiatry* 72:217–20.

Kramer, P. 1993. *Listening to Prozac.* New York: Viking Press.

Leber, P. 1996. The role of the regulator in the evaluation of the acceptability of new drug products. In *Psychotropic drug development: Social, economic and pharmacological aspects,* ed. D. Healy and D. Doogan. London: Chapman & Hall.

Loew, D., and M. Taeschler. 1965. Central anticholinergic properties of antidepressants. In *Neuropsychopharmacology* 4, Proceedings of the 4th Meeting of CINP, ed. D. Bente and P. B. Bradley, 404–7. Amsterdam: Elsevier.

Marshall, B. L., and S. Katz. 2002. Forever functional: Sexual fitness and the aging male body. *Body and Society* 8:43–70.

Olney, J. 1992. Memoirs of an excitotoxicologist. In *The neurosciences: Paths of discovery,* vol. 2, ed. F. Samson and G. Adelman, 168–87. Boston: Birkhauser.

Parsons, C. G., D. Wojciech, and G. Quack. 1998. Glutamate in CNS disorders as a target for drug development: An update. *Drug News and Perspectives* 11:523–69.

Platt, D., et al. 1993. On the efficacy of piracetam in geriatric patients with acute cerebral ischaemia: A clinically controlled double blind study. *Archives of Gerontology and Geriatrics* 16:149–64.

Rose, S. 2002. Smart drugs: Do they work? Are they ethical? Will they be legal? *Nature Reviews Neuroscience* 3:975–79.

Rothman, S., and D. Rothman. 2004. *The pursuit of perfection: The promise and perils of medical enhancement.* New York: Pantheon Books.

Salzer, H. M., and M. L. Lurie. 1955. Depressive states treated with isonicotinyl hydrazide (Isoniazid): A follow-up study. *Ohio State Medical Journal* 51:437–41.

Sandoz. 1970. Advertising copy for Hydergine in *British Journal of Psychiatry* and other journals.

Sano, M., C. Ernesto, R. G. Thomas, M. R. Klauber, K. Schafer, M. Grundman, P. Woodbury, et al. 1997. A controlled trial of selegiline, alpha-tocopherol, or both as treatment for Alzheimer's disease. *New England Journal of Medicine* 336:1216–22.

Schildkraut, J. J. 1965. The catecholamine hypothesis of affective disorders: A review of supporting evidence. *American Journal of Psychiatry* 122:519–22.

Schneider, L. S., and J. T. Olin. 1994. Overview of clinical trials of hydergine in dementia. *Archives of Neurology* 51:787–98.

Shorter, E. 2002. Looking backwards: A possible new path for drug discovery in psychopharmacology. *Nature Reviews Drug Discovery* 1:1003–6.

Skondia, V., and J. Kabes. 1985. Piracetam in alcoholic psychoses: A double-blind, crossover, placebo controlled study. *Journal of International Medical Research* 13:185–87.

Smith, R. C., G. Vroulis, R. Johnson, R. Morgan. 1984. Comparison of therapeutic response to long-term treatment with lecithin versus piracetam plus lecithin in patients with Alzheimer's disease. *Psychopharmacology Bulletin* 20:542–45.

Summers, W. K., L. V. Majovski, G. M. Marsh, K. Tachiki, and A. Kling. 1986. Oral tetrahydroaminoacridine in long-term treatment of senile dementia, Alzheimer's type. *New England Journal of Medicine* 315:1241–45.

Tranter, R., H. Healy, D. Cattell, and D. Healy. 2002. Functional variations in agents differentially selective to monoaminergic systems. *Psychological Medicine* 32:517–24.

Varga, E., and L. Tringer. 1967. Clinical trial of a new type of promptly acting psychoenergetic agent (phenyl-isopropylmethyl-propinylamine. HCl), E-250. *Acta Medica Academiae Scientiarum Hungaricae* 23:289–95.

Watkins, J. 1998. Excitatory amino acids: From basic science to therapeutic applications. In *The psychopharmacologists*, vol. 2, ed. D. Healy, 351–76. London: Arnold.

CHAPTER 3

Alzheimer's Disease

Pathogenesis, Models, and Experimental Therapeutics

DONALD L. PRICE, M.D.
TONG LI, PH.D.
FIONA M. LAIRD, PH.D.
MOHAMED H. FARAH, PH.D.
ALENA V. SAVONENKO, M.D., PH.D.
VASSILIS E. KOLIATSOS, M.D.
JUAN C. TRONCOSO, M.D.
PHILIP C. WONG, PH.D.

Alzheimer's disease (AD), characterized by progressive loss of memory and cognitive impairments, affects more than four million elderly individuals in the United States (Brookmeyer, Gray, and Kawas 1998; Mayeux 2003; Cummings 2004; Wong, Li, and Price 2005). Due to increased life expectancy and postwar "baby boom" demographics, elderly people are the most rapidly growing segment of our society, and the number of persons with AD is predicted to triple over the next several decades. Prevalence, cost of care, impact on individuals and caregivers, and lack of mechanism-based treatments make AD one of the most challenging diseases of this new century (Price et al. 1998; Wong et al. 2002; Selkoe and Schenk 2003; Citron 2004; Cummings 2004; Walsh and Selkoe 2004; Wong, Li, and Price 2005). The syndrome results from dysfunction and death of neurons in specific regions/circuits, particularly those populations of nerve cells participating in memory and cognitive functions (Whitehouse et al. 1982; Hyman et al. 1984; Braak and Braak 1991, 1994; West et al. 1994, 2000, 2004; Price et al. 1998; Wong, Li, and Price 2005). Characteristics of the neuropathology are accumulations of intracellular and extracellular protein aggregates (for example, phosphory-lated tau assembles into paired helical filaments [PHF] comprising neuro-fibrillary tangles [NFT] and neuritis) and β-pleated assemblies of Aβ peptide oligomers at the core of neuritic amyloid plaques, which represent sites of synaptic disconnection (Lee, Goedert, and Trojanowski 2001; Wong et al. 2002; Walsh et al. 2002).

Inheritance of mutations in several genes cause autosomal dominant fa-milial AD (fAD), while the presence of alleles of other genes are significant risk factors for putative sporadic disease (Price et al. 1998; Tanzi and Bertram 2001; Bertram and Tanzi 2005; Hardy 2006). In familial AD (fAD), mutant genes encoding the amyloid precursor protein (*APP*) or the presenilins (*PS1* and *PS2*) influence the levels and/or character of Aβ peptides, which are gen-erated via *APP* cleavages by the activities of β-secretase 1 (*BACE1*), and γ-secretase (the *PS*, *Nct*, *pen2*, *Aph-1* multi-protein complex).

Over many years, investigators have taken advantage of advances in knowledge of the disease to design symptomatic therapies for AD: the demon-stration of abnormalities of basal forebrain neurons with cholinergic deficits in the cortex and hippocampus led to the introduction of cholinesterase in-hibitors for treatment; and the documentation of involvement of glutama-tergic systems in ventro-medial temporal lobes in AD, coupled with informa-tion about glutamate excitotoxicity (mediated by NMDA receptor [NMDA-R]), led to trials of NMDA-R antagonists. More recently, building on biochemical observations by George Glenner (identification of the Aβ peptide sequence) and on studies of many geneticists (identification of AD-related genes), inves-tigators have generated a variety of in vitro and in vivo models relevant to dis-ease mechanisms. Particularly valuable are transgenic and knockout (KO) mice that recapitulate some of the anatomical and biochemical pathologies of AD or alter the expression of proteins (secretases) critical in pathogenesis of disease. For example, mice overexpressing mutant *APP/PS1* develop age-associated increases in brain levels of Aβ42, Aβ oligomers, neuritic plaques, and deficits in working memory. To gain insights into potential therapeutic targets, genes encoding proteins hypothesized to be critical for proamyloido-genic secretase activities have been targeted: *BACE1* -/- mice are viable and do not produce Aβ; more significantly, regarding potential therapy, *APPswe; PS1ΔE9; BACE1* -/- mice do not form Aβ deposits or plaques, nor do they show memory deficits. Thus, inhibition of *BACE1*, the neuronal β-secretase, is an attractive anti-amyloidogenic treatment strategy. Studies of these models have greatly enhanced understanding of amyloid-related disease mechanisms, led to identification of therapeutic targets, and allowed testing of novel mechanism-based treatments.

Disease-mechanism-based strategies are now being developed to: reduce production of Aβ; modify the nature (length) of Aβ peptides to shorter forms that are less likely to damage neurons; reduce formation of oligomeric species; decrease impact of toxic peptides; enhance clearance of Aβ; and attenuate aberrant conformations of tau leading to NFT.

As background for discussions of therapies of the past and those being developed for the future, we review the clinical syndromes of mild cognitive impairment (MCI) and AD, diagnostic methods, genetics, and pathology and biochemistry of the disease. Subsequently, we describe the ways in which transgenic and gene-targeted animals have been of value in creating disease models (for example, mice expressing mutant transgenes), and in identifying therapeutic opportunities (targeting of genes encoding proteins implicated in disease pathways). The potential efficacies and toxicities of these treatments are being tested in model systems. Careful review of the studies can provide important information regarding benefits as well as the potential for adverse events. As outcomes and safety are defined, some of these therapeutic approaches will enter human trials. These new disease-modifying therapies should have a major impact on the health and care of elderly people.

Clinical Features and Laboratory Studies Syndrome

Initially, the majority of affected individuals exhibit MCI, characterized by a memory complaint and impairments on formal testing associated with intact general cognition and preserved daily activities. This syndrome, particularly the amnestic form of MCI, is usually regarded as a transitional stage between normal aging and early AD or as an initial manifestation of AD (Morris et al. 2001; Petersen et al. 2001, 2006; Petersen 2003; Jicha et al. 2006; Markesbery et al. 2006). Patients with early AD show progressive difficulties with memory and, other cognitive functions (Morris and Price 2001; Morris et al. 2001; Petersen et al. 2001; Cummings 2004; Nestor, Scheltens, and Hodges 2004). In the late stages of AD, individuals experience profound dementia.

For diagnosis, clinicians rely on histories; physical, neurological, and psychiatric examinations; and neuropsychological tests (Albert et al. 2001; Cummings 2004; Nestor, Scheltens, and Hodges 2004). Laboratory studies are of increasing value (Albert et al. 2001; Sunderland et al. 2003; Cummings 2004; Klunk et al. 2004; Nestor, Scheltens, and Hodges 2004). Magnetic resonance imaging (MRI) often discloses atrophy of specific regions of the brain, particularly the hippocampus and entorhinal cortex (Cummings 2004; Nestor, Scheltens, and Hodges 2004); the rates of atrophy may have predictive value for diagnosis (Killiany et al. 2000). Moreover, MRI (accomplished by automated image regression analyses and voxel-based morphometry) can disclose abnormalities of specific populations, for example, reduced signal in the regions of the basal forebrain (the nucleus basalis of Meynert [nbM]) have been correlated with reductions in cortical gray matter (Teipel et al. 2005). Positron emission tomography (PET) using ^{18}F deoxyglucose (FDG) or single photon emission computerized tomography (SPECT) demonstrate decreased use of glucose and early reductions in regional blood flow in the parietal and temporal lobes, respectively (Nestor, Scheltens, and Hodges 2004). These studies, particularly FDG PET, can have high predictive value for development of overt AD. Moreover, the PET patterns of brain labeling following administration of a brain penetrant ^{11}C-labeled thioflavin derivative (Pittsburgh Compound B [PIB]), which binds to Aβ with high affinity, are interpreted to reflect the Aβ burden in the brain (Klunk et al. 2004). In cases of AD, the CSF levels of Aβ peptides are often low, and levels of tau in CSF may be higher than controls (Sunderland et al. 2003). On the basis of studies of transgenic models of amyloidosis in the central nervous system (CNS), it has been suggested that efflux of Aβ from brain to plasma may serve as a measure of Aβ brain burden (DeMattos et al. 2002). More recently, an inverse relationship has been demonstrated to exist between the amyloid load (as assessed by PET amyloid imaging) and levels of Aβ in CSF (Fagan et al. 2005). Combinations of these various laboratory assessments should allow clinicians to make a more accurate diagnosis of AD in early stages (McKhann et al. 1984; Jicha et al. 2006; Markesbery et al. 2006; Petersen et al. 2006) and, presumably, allow demonstration of the efficacies of new antiamyloid therapeutics.

Neuropathology and Biochemistry of Alzheimer's Disease

The clinical manifestations of AD stem from abnormalities involving populations of neurons in neural systems / brain regions essential for memory, learning, and cognitive performance (West et al. 1994, 2000, 2004; Price and Sisodia 1998; Gastard, Troncoso, and Koliatsos 2003). Damaged circuits include: the basal forebrain cholinergic system; amygdala; hippocampus; entorhinal and limbic cortices; and neocortex (Whitehouse et al. 1982; Coyle,

Price, and DeLong 1983; Hyman et al. 1984; Braak and Braak 1991, 1994; Jicha et al. 2006; Markesbery et al. 2006; Petersen et al. 2006). In a recent study (Markesbery et al. 2006), the character, abundance, and distributions of lesions (diffuse plaques, neuritic plaques, and tangles) were correlated with clinical signs in several cognitively characterized cohorts: controls; individuals with amnestic mild cognitve impairment (aMCI); and cases of early onset AD (eAD). No differences were present in the number of diffuse plaques between subject groups, but in cases of aMCI, tangles were significantly increased in the ventral medial temporal lobe regions as compared to controls. Individuals with eAD showed greater numbers of NFT and neuritic plaques in both frontal lobes and temporal regions. Individuals with aMCI exhibited increased numbers of neuritic plaques in neocortical regions as compared to controls, but they were fewer than those documented in cases of eAD. Memory deficits appeared to correlate most closely with the abundance of NFT in CA1 of the hippocampus and in the entorhinal cortex, leading the authors to conclude that tangles are more important than amyloid deposition in the progression from normal to MCI to eAD and that tangles in the medial temporal lobe play a key role in the memory declines in aMCI (Markesbery et al. 2006). Additional studies (Jicha et al. 2006; Petersen et al. 2006) demonstrated that the majority of patients with MCI show pathology, but the severity of lesions did not meet neuropathological criteria for AD; the data were interpreted to indicate that this aMCI reflects a transitional state in the evolution of AD. Because the regional distributions of NFT correlated most closely with the degree of clinical impairment from aged healthy controls to individuals with aMCI to cases of AD, the spread of NFT beyond the medial temporal lobe is hypothesized to be most closely linked to the development of dementia. Postmortem neuropathological examinations of clinically well-characterized older subjects indicate that the lesions of AD (plaques and tangles) precede the clinical onset of MCI or AD dementia by years or decades (Troncoso et al. 1996; Schmitt et al. 2000; Morris et al. 2001).

Cellular abnormalities within these regional neural circuits include: the presence within neurons of conformationally altered isoforms of tau comprising the PHF in NFT; neurites; and neuropil threads (Lee, Goedert, and Trojanowski 2001; Goedert and Spillantini 2006). A variety of axonal pathologies, including varicosities and terminal clubs, also observed in aged, memory-impaired Rhesus monkeys with Aβ deposits (Kitt et al. 1984, 1985; Selkoe et al. 1987; Martin et al. 1994), are present in the brain (Price and Sisodia 1998; Lazarov et al. 2005; Stokin et al. 2005), as are the abundant Aβcontaining neuritic plaques (sites of synaptic disconnection [Martin et al. 1994]) in regions receiving inputs from these populations of neurons. Decrements in generic and transmitter-specific synaptic markers have been found in the target fields of these cells (Whitehouse et al. 1982; Coyle, Price, and DeLong 1983; Sze et al. 1997). Local astroglial and microglial responses are particularly associated with plaques (Akiyama et al. 2000). Thus, the clinical manifestation of aMCI and AD reflects disruption of synaptic communication in subsets of neural circuits associated with degeneration of axon terminals followed by axonal degeneration, a process that ultimately leads to death of neurons (Whitehouse et al. 1982; Coyle, Price, and DeLong 1983; Hyman et al. 1984; Braak and Braak 1991, 1994).

In one hypothetical model that mechanistically links Aβ peptides and phosphorylated tau, Aβ42 species, liberated at terminals, oligomerize to form Aβ assemblies or Aβ-derived diffusible ligands (ADDLs) (Lambert et al. 1998; Hartley et al. 1999; McLean et al. 1999; Walsh et al. 1999; Klein, Krafft, and Finch 2001; Weninger and Yankner 2001; Wang et al. 2002; Gong et al. 2003; Kawarabayashi et al. 2004; Cleary et al. 2005; Lesne et al. 2006) which are associated with synaptic damage and disconnection of terminals from postsynaptic targets (Selkoe 2002; Wong et al. 2002; Wong, Li, and Price 2005). Subsequently, a retrograde signal (of unknown nature) that originates at damaged terminals triggers the activation of kinases (or the inhibition of phosphatases) in cell bodies; subsequent hyperphosphorylation of tau at certain serine and threonine residues leads to conformational changes in tau leading to the formation of PHF, and, eventually, NFT (Lee, Goedert, and Trojanowski 2001; Goedert and Spillantini 2006). Secondary disturbances of the cytoskeleton and alterations in axonal transport (Price and Sisodia 1998; Lazarov et al. 2005; Stokin et al. 2005; Wong et al. 2005) can, in turn, compromise the functions and viability of neurons. Eventually, disconnected nerve cells die (Whitehouse et al. 1982; Hyman et al. 1984; Braak and Braak 1994; Lee, Goedert, and Trojanowski 2001; Goedert and Spillantini 2006) and extracellular tangles remain as "tombstones" of the neurons destroyed by disease.

Familial Alzheimer's Disease and Risk Factors

Genetic factors implicated in AD include mutations in *APP* (chromosome 21), mutations in *presenilin 1* (*PS1*) (chromosome 14) and *PS2* (chromosome 1), and the susceptibility allele of APOE4 (chromosome 19) (Price et al. 1998;

Ghiso and Wisniewski 2004; Bertram and Tanzi 2005; Hardy 2006). Autosomal dominant mutations in *APP, PS1,* or *PS2* usually cause disease earlier than occurs in sporadic cases, with the majority of mutations in *APP, PS1* and *PS2* influencing *BACE1* and γ-secretase cleavages of *APP* to increase the levels of all Aβ species or the relative amounts of toxic Aβ42 (Price et al. 1998; Ghiso and Wisniewski 2004). Individuals with duplications of *APP* (Rovelet-Lecrux et al. 2006) or with trisomy 21 (Down syndrome) (Hardy 2006) have an extra copy of *APP* and develop AD pathology relatively early in life. The presence of APOE4 predisposes to later onset AD and, in some cases, to late-onset familial AD (fAD) (Corder et al. 1994; Mayeux 2003; Bertram and Tanzi 2005).

A member of the *APP* gene family (*APP, APLP1* and *2*), *APP* encodes a type I transmembrane protein whose function is not fully defined (Cao and Sudhof 2001; Wong, Li, and Price 2005); it is abundant in the nervous system, rich in neurons, and transported rapidly anterograde in axons to terminals (Koo et al. 1989; Sisodia et al. 1993; Buxbaum et al. 1998; Lazarov et al. 2005). At a variety of sites (see below), *APP* is cleaved by activities of *BACE1* (β-site *APP* cleaving enzyme 1) of the +1 and +11 sites and by the γ-secretase complex, which generate the N- and C-termini of Aβ peptides, respectively (Vassar et al. 1999; Cai et al. 2001; Li et al. 2003; Selkoe and Kopan 2003; Citron 2004; Iwatsubo 2004; Laird et al. 2005; Ma et al. 2005). The *APPswe* mutation greatly enhances manyfold the *BACE1* cleavage at the N-terminus of Aβ (+1 site), resulting in substantial elevations in levels of all Aβ peptides. APP_{717} mutations promote γ-secretase cleavages to increase secretion of Aβ42, the most toxic peptide. These mutations alter the processing of *APP* and increase the production of Aβ peptides or the amounts of the more toxic Aβ42. Other *APP* mutations enhance local fibril formation and vascular amyloidosis (Ghiso and Wisniewski 2004). Investigators have taken advantage of this information in creating transgenic models of amyloidosis. (See Savonenko et al. 2006 for a recent review of models.)

PS1 and PS2 encode two highly homologous and conserved 43- to 50-kD multipass transmembrane proteins (Sherrington et al. 1995; Price et al. 1998), which are involved in *Notch1* signaling critical for cell fate decisions (Selkoe and Kopan 2003). *PS* are endoproteolytically cleaved by a "presenilinase" to form an N-terminal ~28-kDa fragment and a C-terminal ~18-kDa fragment (Thinakaran et al. 1997), both of which are critical components of the γ-secretase complex (Selkoe and Kopan 2003; Iwatsubo 2004). Nearly 50 percent of early-onset cases of fAD are linked to more than 90 different mutations in *PS1* (Sherrington et al. 1995; Price et al. 1998; Bertram and Tanzi 2005; Hardy 2006). A relatively small number of *PS2* mutations also cause autosomal dominant fAD (Price et al. 1998; Bertram and Tanzi 2005). The majority of abnormalities in *PS* genes are missense mutations that enhance γ-secretase activities to increase the levels of Aβ42 peptides.

APP and Secretases

APP is cleaved by β-and γ-secretases that release the ectodomain of *APP* (*APPs*), liberate a cytosolic fragment termed *APP* intracellular domain (AICD), and generate several species of Aβ peptides. In the CNS (but not the peripheral nervous system, or PNS) (Buxbaum et al. 1998; Lazarov et al. 2005), Aβ peptides are generated by sequential endoproteolytic cleavages by *BACE1* (at the Aβ +1 and +11 sites) to generate *APP-β* carboxyl terminal fragments (*APP-βCTFs*) (Cai et al. 2001; Luo et al. 2001) and by the γ-secretase complex (at several sites varying from Aβ 36,38,40,42,43) to form Aβ species peptides (Li et al. 2003; Citron 2004; Iwatsubo 2004; Ma et al. 2005). The intramembranous cleavages of *APP-βCTF* by γ-secretase releases an AICD (Cao et al. 2001), which can form a complex with Fe65, a nuclear adaptor protein (Cao and Sudhof 2001); Fe65 and Aβ or Fe65 alone (in a novel conformation) can gain access to the nucleus to influence gene transcription (Cao and Sudhof 2001), a signaling mechanism analogous to that occurring in the *Notch1* pathway (Selkoe and Kopan2003; Iwatsubo 2004; Barrick and Kopan 2006). It has been suggested that AICD signaling may play a role in learning and memory, a hypothesis outlined below (Laird et al. 2005). In other cells in other organs, *APP* is cleaved endoproteolytically within the Aβ sequence through alternative, nonamyloidogenic pathways: α-secretase (TNF-alpha converting enzyme or TACE) cleave between 16 and 17 (Sisodia et al. 1990); *BACE2* cleaves between 19 and 20 and between 20 and 21 (Farzan et al. 2000). These cleavages, which occur in nonneural tissues, preclude the formation of Aβ peptides and serve to protect these cells and organs from Aβ amyloidosis (Wong, Price, and Cai 2001).

BACE1, encoded by a gene on chromosome 11, is transmembrane aspartyl protease that is directly involved in the cleavage of *APP* at the +11 > +1 sites of Aβ in *APP* (Vassar et al. 1999; Farzan et al. 2000; Cai et al. 2001; Luo et al. 2001; Laird et al. 2005). Present in the CNS, *BACE1* is demonstrable in a variety of presynaptic terminals (Laird et al. 2005). Brain cells from *BACE1* -/- mice (Cai et al. 2001; Luo et al. 2001; Laird et al. 2005) do not produce Aβ1–40/42 and Aβ11- 40/42, indicating that *BACE1* is the neuronal β secretase (Cai et al. 2001; Luo et al. 2001; Laird et al. 2005). As compared to wild type *APP, APPswe* is cleaved approximately a hundredfold more efficiently at the +1 site, resulting in a greater increase in *BACE1* cleavage products (elevating of all Aβ species).

γ-secretase, essential for the regulated intramembranous proteolysis of a variety of transmembrane proteins, is a multiprotein catalytic complex that includes: *PS1* and *PS2;* Nicastrin (*Nct*), a type I transmembrane glycoprotein; and *Aph-1* and *Pen-2,* two multipass transmembrane proteins (Goutte et al. 2002; Kimberly et al. 2003; Li et al. 2003; Selkoe and Kopan 2003; Iwatsubo 2004; Ma et al. 2005; Serneels et al. 2005). *PS* contains aspartyl residues that play roles in intramembranous cleavage, and substitutions of aspartate residues at D257 in TM 6 and at D385 in TM 7 are reported to reduce secretion of Aβ and cleavage of *Notch1* in vitro (Wolfe et al. 1999; Selkoe and Kopan 2003). The functions of the various γ-secretase proteins and their interactions in the complex are not yet fully defined. It has been suggested that the ectodomain of *Nct* may be important in substrate recognition and binding of amino-terminal stubs (of *APP* and other transmembrane proteins) generated by a sheddases (for example, *BACE1* for *APP*) (Shah et al. 2005); after substrate docking occurs, γ-secretase cleavage takes place. In one model, *Aph-1* and *Nct* form a precomplex that interacts with *PS;* subsequently, *Pen-2* enters the complex, where it is critical for the "presenilinase" cleavage of *PS* into two fragments. In concert, this complex is responsible for γ-secretase cleavages of *APP, Notch,* and a variety of other transmembrane proteins (Wolfe et al. 1999; Li et al. 2003; Selkoe and Kopan 2003; Iwatsubo 2004; Serneels et al. 2005).

Genetic Models of Aβ Amyloidosis

In mice, expression of *APPswe* or APP_{717} (with or without mutant *PS1*) leads to an Aβ amyloidosis in the CNS (Mucke et al. 2000; Savonenko et al. 2005, 2006; Lesne et al. 2006). Mutant *APP; PS1* mice develop accelerated disease secondary to increased levels of Aβ (particularly Aβ42) associated with the presence of diffuse Aβ deposits and neuritic plaques in the hippocampus and cortex. Levels of Aβ peptides, particularly Aβ42, increase in brain with age (Borchelt et al. 1996, 1997; Jankowsky et al. 2004; Savonenko et al. 2006), and oligomeric species, variously termed ADDLs, Aβ*56, etc., appear in the CNS (Hartley et al. 1999; Klein, Krafft, and Finch 2001; Walsh et al. 2002; Wang et al. 2002; Gong et al. 2003; Kawarabayashi et al. 2004; Cleary et al. 2005; Klyubin et al. 2005; Lesne et al. 2006). Over time, mice carrying mutant transgenes exhibit Aβ deposits, and swollen neurites develop in proximity to these deposits; subsequently, neuritic plaques become associated glial responses (Savonenko et al. 2006). Some lines of mice show evidence of amyloid in vessels (Calhoun et al. 1999). In forebrain regions, the density of synaptic terminals and several neurotransmitters (cholinergic, peptidergic, etc.) are reduced (Savonenko et al. 2005). In some settings, there are deficiencies in synaptic transmission (Chapman et al. 1999; Savonenko et al. 2006). Moreover, some lines of mice show evidence of degeneration of subsets of neurons (Calhoun et al. 1998).

Behavioral studies of lines of transgenic mice, including those generated by David Borchelt (Savonenko et al. 2003, 2005, 2006), disclose deficits in spatial reference memory (Morris water maze task) and episodiclike memory (repeated reversal and radial water maze tasks). At six months of age, *APPswe/PS1ΔE9* mice develop plaques, but all genotypes are indistinguishable from nontransgenic animals in these cognitive measures. However, in 18-month-old cohorts, *APPswe/PS1ΔE9* mice perform all cognitive tasks less well than mice of all other genotypes. In the double mutant animals, amyloid burdens are high, and levels of cholinergic markers (cortex and hippocampus) and somatostatin (cortex) are modestly reduced. Relationships exist between deficits in episodiclike memory tasks and total Aβ loads in the brain (Savonenko et al. 2005, 2006). Collectively, these studies suggest that, in *APPswe/PS1ΔE9* mice, some form of Aβ (ultimately associated with amyloid deposition) can disrupt circuits critical for memory, with episodiclike memory more sensitive to the toxic effects of Aβ. Behavioral deficits have been linked to the presence of Aβ oligomers and can be reversed by antibody-mediated reductions of levels of brain Aβ (Cleary et al. 2005; Klyubin et al. 2005; Lesne et al. 2006). Although these transgenic lines do not reproduce the full phenotype of AD, these mice are useful subjects for research designed to correlate behavior and Aβ amyloidosis, to delineate disease mechanisms, and to test novel therapies (Savonenko et al. 2006).

Over the past decade, a variety of Aβ species, oligomers, and structural assemblies, ranging from monomers to amyloid deposits in neuritic plaques, have been suggested to play important roles in impairing synaptic communication (Lambert et al. 1998; Klein, Krafft, and Finch 2001; Walsh et al. 2002; Wang et al. 2002). The pool of insoluble Aβ (or plaques) is believed to exist in equilibrium with peptides in interstitial fluid (Cirrito et al. 2003). Significantly, systemic administration of antibodies increases levels of Aβ in plasma, and the magnitude of this elevation correlates with amyloid burden in the cortex and hippocampus (DeMattos et al. 2002). In one study, a naturally secreted Aβ peptide was injected into the ventricular system of rats and inhibited LTP in the hippocampus (Klyubin et al. 2005); the adverse activity was completely blocked by the injection of a monoclonal Aβ antibody, but active immunization was less effective in rescuing function (Klyubin et al. 2005). These observations are consistent with the concept that oligomers are the toxic entity and that they are both necessary and sufficient to perturb learned behavior (Cleary et al. 2005; Klyubin et al. 2005). More recently, studies of TG2576 mice suggested that extracellular accumulations of a 56KD soluble amyloid assembly, termed Aβ*56 (purified from the brains of memory-impaired mice), interferes with memory in young rats (Lesne et al. 2006).

The paucity of tau abnormalities in various lines of mutant mice with Aβ abnormalities may be related to differences in tau isoforms expressed in this species (Xu, Gonzales, and Borchelt 2002). Early efforts to express mutant tau transgenes in mice did not lead to striking clinical phenotypes or pathology (Goedert and Spillantini 2006). More recently, mice overexpressing tau showed clinical signs attributed to degeneration of motor axons (Lee, Goedert, and Trojanowski 2001). When prion or Thy1 promoters are used to drive tau_{P301L} (a mutation linked to autosomal dominant frontotemporal dementia with parkinsonism), some brain and spinal cord neurons develop tangles (Gotz et al. 2001). Mice expressing $APPswe/tau_{P301L}$ exhibit enhanced tangle-like pathology in limbic system and olfactory cortex (Lewis et al. 2001). Moreover, injection of Aβ42 fibrils into specific brain regions of tau_{P301L} mice increases the number of tangles in those neurons projecting to sites of Aβ injection. A triple transgenic mouse (3×Tg-AD), created by microinjecting $APPswe$ and tau_{P301L} into single cells derived from monozygous $PS1_{M146V}$ knock in mice, develops age-related plaques and tangles as well as deficits in LTP, which appear to antedate overt pathology (Oddo et al. 2003). However, mice bearing both mutant tau and APP (or $APP/PS1$) or mutant tau mice injected with Aβ may not be ideal models of fAD because the presence of the tau mutation alone is associated with the development of tangles and disease.

Targeting of Genes in the Amyloidogenic Pathway

To begin to understand the functions of some of the proteins thought to play roles in AD, investigators have targeted a variety of genes encoding $BACE1$; $PS1$; Nct; and $Aph-1$.

BACE1 -/- Mice

These animals mate successfully and exhibit no overt pathology (Cai et al. 2001; Luo et al. 2001; Laird et al. 2005; Savonenko et al. 2006). *BACE1 -/-* neurons do not cleave at the +1 and +11 sites of Aβ, and the production of Aβ peptides is abolished (Cai et al. 2001; Luo et al. 2001; Laird et al. 2005), establishing that *BACE1* is the neuronal γ-secretase required to generate the N-termini of Aβ. However, *BACE1 -/-* mice show altered performance on some tests of cognition and emotion (Laird et al. 2005; Savonenko et al. 2006); the former deficits can be rescued by overexpression of *APP* transgenes.

PS1 -/- Mice

Embryos develop severe abnormalities of the axial skeleton, ribs and spinal ganglia; a lethal outcome which resembles a partial *Notch1 -/-* phenotype (Shen et al. 1997; Wong et al. 1997). *PS1 -/-* cells show decreased levels of secretion of Aβ (De Strooper et al. 1998; Li et al. 2003) related to the fact that *PS1* (along with *PS2, Nct, Aph-1,* and *Pen-2*) is a component of the γ-secretase complex that carries out the S3 intramembranous cleavage of *Notch1* (De Strooper et al. 1999; Li et al. 2003; Selkoe and Kopan 2003). Without γ-secretase cleavage, NICD is not released from the plasma membrane and cannot reach the nucleus to provide a signal to initiate transcriptional processes essential for cell fate decisions (Selkoe and Kopan 2003; Barrick and Kopan 2006). Significantly, conditional *PS1/2*-targeted mice show impairments in memory and synaptic plasticity in the hippocampus (Saura et al. 2004); raising the question, posed effectively by Jie Shen and colleagues, about the roles of loss of *PS* function in neurodegeneration and AD (Herget et al. 1998; Delacourte et al. 1999). It is important to note that *PS1 -/-* mice whose lethal phenotype is rescued through neuronal expression of *PS1* develop skin cancer; this outcome was interpreted initially to reflect deregulation of the β-catenin pathway (Xia et al. 2001).

Nct -/- Mice

Embryos die early and exhibit several patterning defects (Li et al. 2003), including abnormal segmentation of somites; this phenotype closely resembles that seen in *Notch1 -/-* and *PS1/2 -/-* embryos. *Nct -/-* cells do not secrete Aβ peptides, whereas *NctT +/-* cells show reduction of ~50% (Li et al. 2003). The failure of *NctT -/-* cells to generate Aβ peptides is accompanied by accumulation of *APP* C-terminal fragments. *Nct* +/- mice develop tumors of the skin, a phenotype accelerated by reducing *PS1* and *P53*, both of which exacerbate the tumor phenotype. The tumors appear to be related to decreased levels of signaling via *Notch1*, which acts as a tumor suppressor in the skin (Li et al. 2007). Available evidence links the formation of these tumors to decreased γ-secretase activity and to upregulation of epidermal growth factor receptor (EGFR), an oncogene implicated in head and neck tumors in humans (Li et al. 2007).

Aph-1a -/- Mice

Three murine *Aph-1* alleles (*Aph-1a, Aph-1b,* and *Aph-1c*) encode four distinct *Aph-1* isoforms: *Aph-1aL* and *Aph-1aS* (derived from differential splicing of *Aph-1a*); *Aph-1b*; and *Aph-1c* (Ma et al. 2005; Serneels et al. 2005). *Aph-1a -/-* embryos show patterning defects that resemble, but are not identical to, those of *Notch1, Nct* or *PS -/-* embryos (Ma et al. 2005; Serneels et al. 2005). Moreover, in *Aph-1a -/-* derived cells, the levels of *Nct, PS* fragments, and *Pen-2* are decreased, and there is a concomitant reduction in levels of the high molecular weight γ-secretase complex and a decrease in secretion of Aβ (Ma et al. 2005). In *Aph-1a -/-* cells other mammalian *Aph-1* isoforms can restore the levels of *Nct, PS,* and *Pen-2* (Ma et al. 2005; Serneels et al. 2005).

Experimental Treatments and Therapeutics

Models relevant to amyloidogenesis provide a test of the influence of ablation or knock down of specific genes, the modulation of cleavage patterns influencing peptide neurotoxicity, and the enhancement of clearance and/or degradation of Aβ (Li et al. 2003; Monsonego and Weiner 2003; Citron 2004; Walsh and Selkoe 2004; Cleary et al. 2005; Klyubin et al. 2005; Laird et al. 2005; Lesne et al. 2006; Savonenko et al. 2006). In the section below, we comment on selected studies which illustrate experimental strategies directed at specific therapeutic targets that we predict will provide mechanism-based therapeutic benefits to patients with AD (Savonenko et al. 2006).

Reduction in β-Secretase Activity

Significantly, deletion of *BACE1* in *APPswe;PS1ΔE9* mice prevents both Aβ deposition and age-associated cognitive abnormalities that occur in this model (Laird et al. 2005; Masliah et al. 2005). Significantly, *BACE1 -/-; APP-swe;PS1ΔE9* mice do not develop the Aβ deposits or the age-associated abnormalities in working memory that occur in the *APPswe;PS1ΔE9* model of Aβ amyloidosis (Borchelt et al. 1996; McDonald and Howard 2002; Laird et al. 2005). Similarly, *BACE1 -/- Tg2576* mice appear to be spared age-dependent memory deficits and physiological abnormalities (Ohno et al. 2004; Savonenko et al. 2006). Moreover, Aβ deposits are sensitive to *BACE1* dosage and can be efficiently cleared from regions of the CNS when *BACE1* is silenced at these sites (Laird et al. 2005; Singer et al. 2005). Inhibitors of β-secretase, conjugated to carrier peptides, are effective inhibitors in vitro and in vivo (following intraperitoneal injection of compounds into Tg2576 mice) (Chang et al. 2004). New approaches using conditional expression systems or RNAi silencing will allow investigators to examine the pathogenesis of diseases and to assess the degrees of reversibility of the disease processes (Ohno et al. 2004; Laird et al. 2005; Singer et al. 2005). The results of these approaches will provide a better understanding of the mechanisms that lead to diseases and will aid in the design of new treatments. The above-described data indicate that *BACE1* is an attractive therapeutic target. However, several potential problems exist with this approach. First, the *BACE1* catalytic site is large, and it is uncertain whether it will be possible to achieve adequate brain penetration of a compound of sufficient size that will act in vivo. Second, *BACE1*-null mice manifest alterations in both hippocampal synaptic plasticity and in performance on tests of cognition and emotion (Laird et al. 2005); the memory deficits but not emotional alterations in *BACE1 -/-* mice are prevented by co-expressing *APPswe;PS1ΔE9* transgenes. This discovery indicates that *APP* processing influences cognition/memory and that the other potential substrates of *BACE1* may play roles in neural circuits related to emotion. These results establish that *BACE1* and *APP* processing pathways are critical for cognitive, emotional, and synaptic functions and that inhibition of β-secretase activity is an exciting therapeutic opportunity. However, future studies should be alert to potential mechanism-based side effects that may occur with inhibition of *BACE1* (Chang et al. 2004; Laird et al. 2005; Wong, Li, and Price 2005; Savonenko et al. 2006).

Inhibition of γ-Secretase Activity

Both genetic and pharmaceutical lowering of γ-secretase activity decrease production of Aβ peptides in cell-free and cell-based systems and reduce levels of Aβ in mutant mice with Aβ amyloidosis (Li et al. 2007). Thus, γ-secre-tase activity is a significant target for therapy (Li et al. 2003; Saura et al. 2004; Ma et al. 2005; Wong, Li, and Price 2005). However, γ-secretase activity is also essential for processing of *Notch*, which is critical for lineage specification and cell growth during embryonic development (Shen et al. 1997; Wong et al. 1997, 2004; Li et al. 2003; Selkoe and Kopan 2003; Wolfe and Kopan 2004; Ma et al. 2005). Significantly, one inhibitor of γ-secretase (LY-411,575), re-duced production of Aβ but also had profound effects on T and B cell develop-ment and on the appearance of intestinal mucosa (proliferation of goblet cells, increased mucin in gut lumen, and crypt necrosis) (Milano et al. 2004; Wong et al. 2004; Barten et al. 2005). Moreover, as described above, *Nct +/- APPswe;PS1ΔE9* mice show reduced levels of Aβ and amyloid plaques, but these mice also develop skin tumors (Li et al. 2007), presumably, in part, be-cause of reduced γ-secretase activity, via signaling by *Notch* (a tumor suppres-sor in skin) (Xia et al. 2001; Nicolas et al. 2003). Thus, clinicians carrying out trials of this inhibitor will have to be alert to several potential adverse events associated with inhibition of this enzyme complex.

γ-Secretase Modulation by NSAID Compounds

Retrospective epidemiological studies suggested that significant exposure to NSAIDs reduces risk of AD (Anthony et al. 2000), an outcome initially in-terpreted as related to suppression of the well-documented inflammatory pro-cess occurring in brains of AD cases (Akiyama et al. 2000; Lim et al. 2000; Cummings 2004). However, more recent in vitro studies indicate that a sub-set of NSAID compounds in this class can modulate secretase cleavages to shorter, less toxic Aβ species without altering *Notch* or other *APP* processing (Weggen et al. 2001). Moreover, short-term treatment of mutant mice ap-pears to have some benefit in terms of lowering Aβ and plaque pathology (Lim et al. 2000). This strategy is now being evaluated in clinical trials (Weggen et al. 2001).

Aβ Immunotherapy

Multiple lines of evidence, including lesions of entorhinal cortex or per-forant pathway (Lazarov et al. 2002; Sheng, Price, and Koliatsos 2002, 2003), indicate that removing the source of Aβ (for example, lesioning cell bodies or axons/terminals transporting *APP* to terminals) significantly reduces levels of Aβ and amyloid plaques in target fields. Similarly, increasing local increase in levels of degrading enzymes (IDE and NEP) can facilitate cleavage and can reduce levels of Aβ (Iwata et al. 2000, 2004; Vekrellis et al. 2000; Carson and Turner 2002; Farris et al. 2003; Leissring et al. 2003; Marr et al. 2003; Miller et al. 2003).

However, to date, the most exciting findings regarding clearance of Aβ come from studies using active and passive Aβ immunotherapy (Monsonego and Weiner 2003; Selkoe and Schenk 2003; Federoff and Bowers 2005; Savonenko et al. 2006). In treatment trials in mutant mice, both Aβ immunization (with Freund's adjuvant) and passive transfer of Aβ antibodies reduce levels of Aβ and plaque burden (Schenk et al. 1999; Bard et al. 2000; Morgan et al. 2000; DeMattos et al. 2001, 2002; Dodart et al. 2002; Kotilinek et al. 2002; Monsonego and Weiner 2003; Wilcock et al. 2003, 2004b; Hutton and Mc-Gowan 2004; Oddo et al. 2004; Federoff and Bowers 2005; Klyubin et al. 2005). Although, the mechanisms of enhanced clearance are not certain (Federoff and Bowers 2005; Wong, Li, and Price 2005), at least two not mutually exclusive hypotheses have been suggested: (1) a small amount of Aβ antibody enters the brain, binds to Aβ peptides, promotes the disassembly of fibrils, and, via the Fc-antibody domain, encourages activated microglia to enter the affected regions and remove Aβ (Schenk et al. 1999); and/or (2) serum antibodies serve as "a sink" to draw the amyloid peptides from the brain into the circulation, thus changing the equilibrium of Aβ in different compartments and promoting removal of Aβ from the CNS (Morgan et al. 2000; DeMattos et al. 2002; Dodart et al. 2002; Cirrito et al. 2003). Whatever the mechanism(s), Aβ immunotherapy in mutant mice is successful in partially clearing Aβ, in attenuating learning and behavioral deficits in several cohorts of mutant *APP* or *APP/PS1* mice, and in partially reducing tau abnormalities in the triple transgenic mice (Morgan et al. 2000; Dodart et al. 2002; Kotilinek et al. 2002; Hutton and McGowan 2004; Oddo et al. 2004; Sigurdsson et al. 2004; Wilcock et al. 2004a, 2004b; Savonenko et al. 2006).

However, in the presence of congophilic angiopathy, several problems have been associated with Aβ therapy. Brain hemorrhages may be linked to immunotherapy (Pfeifer et al. 2002; Gandy and Walker 2004). The presence of congophilic angiopathy could weaken vascular walls (Winkler et al. 2001; Herzig et al. 2004), and, potentially, immunotherapeutic removal of some intramural vascular amyloid could contribute to rupture of damaged vessels and bleeding. Significantly, mutant mice who received immunotherapy were not reported to develop evidence of meningoencephalitis, but a subset of patients in a clinical trial did manifest these problems (see below). Thus, trials in mice are useful for testing efficacy but they are not necessarily predictive of adverse events in humans.

Enhanced Degradation of Aβ

Recently, investigators have attempted to influence levels of Aβ degrading enzymes, including neprolysis (NEP) and insulin-degrading enzymes (IDE), to promote degradation and clearance (Hulette et al. 1995; Iwata et al. 2000, 2001, 2004; Vekrellis et al. 2000; Carson and Turner 2002; Farris et al. 2003; Lauritzen and Gold 2003; Marr et al. 2003). Space constraints prevent our reviewing this interesting field of research.

Clinical Approaches to Alzheimer's Disease

Currently available treatments for AD include: cholinesterase inhibitors (Cummings 2004; Winblad et al. 2006); agents that influence the effects of glutamate on specific receptors, including NMDA-R, which plays roles in excitotoxicity (Reisberg et al. 2003; Cummings 2004); and pharmacological agents useful for behavioral disturbances (Cummings 2004).

Cholinesterase Inhibitors

The "cholinergic hypothesis" of AD is based in part on the demonstration that cholinergic markers, including acetylcholinesterase (AChE) and choline acetyltransferase (ChAT), are reduced in the brains of patients (Bowen et al. 1976a, 1976b; Davies and Maloney 1976a, 1976b; E. K. Perry et al. 1977). Cholinergic deficits in the cortexes of patients with AD were reported to correlate with the severity of intellectual impairment and with the regional densities of senile plaques (Blessed Tomlinson, and Roth 1968; E. K. Perry, Perry, et al. 1978; E. K. Perry, Tomlinson, et al. 1978; T. L. Perry et al. 1978; Francis and Bowen 1985; Francis et al. 1985). The cholinergic hypothesis received support by investigations of animals suggesting that acetylcholine plays a role in memory (Deutsch 1971) as well as studies in humans demonstrating that cholinergic antagonists like scopolamine induce memory problems in normal individuals (Drachman and Leavitt 1974). The discovery that basal forebrain cholinergic neurons are the major source of cortical cholinergic innervation (Mesulam and Van Hoesen 1976) directed investigators to reexamine this population of neurons in the context of the cholinergic hypothesis. It should be mentioned that experimental studies of the effects of cholinergic neurons on arousal and attention make it difficult to assess the influences of these cells on learning and memory. In one nonhuman primate study that involved a near complete excitotoxic destruction of the basal nucleus complex, it was demonstrated that these cholinergic neurons play a role in attention rather than learning and memory (Voytko et al. 1994). Significantly, with regard to AD, the index case for AD focused on the basal forebrain (a 72-year-old man with a 14-year history of dementia and brain abnormalities consistent with AD) and showed reductions of the number of neurons in the nucleus basalis (Whitehouse et al. 1981, 1982; Coyle, Price, and DeLong 1983).

Over many years, investigators have examined the effects of direct agonists, AChE inhibitors, and precursor loading with lecithin (for example, the dietary form of choline). The cholinomimetic approach uses anticholinesterases with long half-lives and predilection for central cholinergic synapses and attempts to maximize the amount of available acetylcholine in the postsynaptic receptors (Cummings 2004; Winblad et al. 2006). Postsynaptic cholinergic receptor agonists have also been tried (Bymaster et al. 1994; Nishizaki et al. 2000; Zhao et al. 2001), but many of these drugs, especially muscarinic agonists, have encountered problems because of autonomic, gastrointestinal, and motoric side effects. Among the FDA-approved compounds (tacrine, donepezil, rivastigmine, and galantamine), donepezil and rivastigmine have been shown to have some efficacy. It has been suggested that anticholinesterases may slow in the progressive cognitive deterioration compared to placebo (Cummings 2004).

NMDA Antagonists

More recently, memantine, a noncompetitive, low-affinity, open-channel NMDA receptor antagonist (Lipton 2004), has been used to treat patients with AD (Reisberg et al. 2003; Cummings 2004). This drug enters the open receptor channel and because it does not accumulate at the site, it does not interfere with synaptic transmission. The drug is thought to affect excitotoxicity mediated by excessive glutamate stimulation of NMDA-R (increased Ca++ influx through the channel). The benefits on clinical disease have been modest (Cummings 2004).

Aβ Immunotherapy

Individuals receiving vaccinations with preaggregated Aβ and an adjuvant (followed by a booster), develop antibodies that recognize Aβ in the brain and vessels (Hock et al. 2002; Selkoe and Schenk 2003; Schenk, Hagen, and Seubert 2004; Federoff and Bowers 2005). Unfortunately, although phase 1 trials with Aβ peptide and adjuvant vaccination were not associated with any adverse events, phase 2 trials detected complications (meningoencephalitis) in a subset of patients and were suspended (Hock et al. 2003; Monsonego and Weiner 2003; Nicoll et al. 2003; Schenk, Hagen, and Seubert 2004; Bayer et al. 2005; Masliah et al. 2005). The pathology in the index case, consistent with T-cell meningitis (Nicoll et al. 2003), was interpreted to show some clearance of Aβ deposits, but some regions contained a relatively high density of tangles, neuropil threads, and vascular amyloid (Nicoll et al. 2003). Aβ immunoreactivity was sometimes associated with microglia, and T-cells were conspicuous in subarachnoid space and around some vessels (Nicoll et al. 2003). In another case, there was significant reduction in amyloid deposits in the absence of clinical evidence of encephalitis (Masliah et al. 2005). Although the trial was stopped, assessment of cognitive functions in a small subset of patients (30) who received vaccination and booster immunizations disclosed that patients who generated Aβ antibodies (as measured by a new assay) had a slower decline in several functional measures (Hock et al. 2003). The events occurring in this subset of patients illustrate the challenges of extrapolating outcomes in mutant mice to human trials. Investigators continue to pursue the passive immunization approaches and are attempting to make new antigens/adjuvant formulations that do not stimulate T-cell mediated immunologic attack (Monsonego and Weiner 2003; Selkoe and Schenk 2003; Schenk, Hagen, and Seubert 2004; Federoff and Bowers 2005; Zamora et al. 2006).

Over many years, investigators have more accurately defined MCI and early AD, developed diagnostic approaches, and clarified the character and stages of pathology, correlating these findings to clinical features. Parallel studies of AD and of genetically engineered models of Aβ amyloidosis (and the tauopathies) have greatly increased our understanding of pathogenic mechanisms, therapeutic targets, and potential mechanism-based treatments designed to benefit patients with AD. Following leads from human autopsy studies and from investigations of in vitro and in vivo models, investigators are now on the threshold of implementing novel treatments based on an understanding of the neurobiology, neuropathology, biochemistry, and genetics of this illness. Moreover, a variety of tools, including amyloid imaging and measure of Aβ flux between compartments, have the potential to assess efficacies of treatment. It is anticipated that discoveries over the next few years will lead to the design of new mechanism-based therapies that can be tested in animal models, and, eventually, these approaches will be introduced into the clinic for the benefit of patients with this devastating illness.

ACKNOWLEDGMENTS

We wish to thank the many colleagues who have worked at the Johns Hopkins Medical Institutions as well as those at other institutions for their contributions to some of the original work cited in this review and for their helpful discussions. Aspects of this work were supported by grants from the U.S. Public Health Service (AGO05146, NS41438, NS45150, NS049088, AG14248, NS1058017) as well funds from the Metropolitan Life Foundation, Adler Foundation, Alzheimer's Association, CART Foundation, Merck Research Laboratories, and Bristol-Myers Squibb Foundation.

REFERENCES

Because of space constraints, the citations are limited. Additional references relevant to the research can be found in Wong, Li, and Price (2005); Wong et al. (2002); Laird et al. (2005); Savonenko et al. (2006); and Price et al. (2006).

Akiyama, H., S. W. Barger, S. Barnum, B. Bradt, J. Bauer, G. M. Cole, N. R. Cooper, et al. 2000. Inflammation and Alzheimer's disease. *Neurobiology of Aging* 21 (3): 383–421.

Albert, M. S., M. B. Moss, R. Tanzi, and K. Jones. 2001. Preclinical prediction of AD using neuropsychological tests. *Journal of the International Neuropsychological Society* 7 (5): 631–39.

Anthony, J. C., J. C. Breitner, P. P. Zandi, M. R. Meyer, I. Jurasova, M. C. Norton, and S. V. Stone. 2000. Reduced prevalence of AD in users of NSAIDs and H2 receptors antagonists: The Cache County study. *Neurology* 54:2066–71.

Bard, F., C. Cannon, R. Barbour, R. L. Burke, D. Games, H. Grajeda, T. Guido, et al. 2000. Peripherally administered antibodies against amyloid beta-peptide enter the central nervous system and reduce pathology in a mouse model of Alzheimer disease. *Nature Medicine* 6 (8): 916–19.

Barrick, D., and R. Kopan. 2006. The notch transcription activation complex makes its move. *Cell* 124 (5): 883–85.

Barten, D. M., V. L. Guss, J. A. Corsa, A. Loo, S. B. Hansel, M. Zheng, B. Munoz, et al. 2005. Dynamics of beta-amyloid reductions in brain, cerebrospinal fluid, and plasma of beta-amyloid precursor protein transgenic mice treated with a gamma-secretase inhibitor. *Journal of Pharmacology and Experimental Therapeutics* 312 (2): 635–43.

Bayer, A. J., R. Bullock, R. W. Jones, D. Wilkinson, K. R. Paterson, L. Jenkins, S. B. Millais, and S. Donoghue. 2005. Evaluation of the safety and immunogenicity of synthetic Abeta42 (AN1792) in patients with AD. *Neurology* 64 (1): 94–101.

Bertram, L., and R. E. Tanzi. 2005. The genetic epidemiology of neurodegenerative disease. *Journal of Clinical Investigation* 115 (6): 1449–57.

Blessed, G., B. E. Tomlinson, and M. Roth. 1968. The association between quantitative measures of dementia and of senile change in the cerebral grey matter of elderly subjects. *British Journal of Psychiatry* 114:797–811.

Borchelt, D. R., T. Ratovitski, J. Van Lare, M. K. Lee, V. Gonzales, N. A. Jenkins, N. G. Copeland, D. L. Price, and S. S. Sisodia. 1997. Accelerated amyloid deposition in the brains of transgenic mice coexpressing mutant presenilin 1 and amyloid precursor proteins. *Neuron* 19 (4): 939–45.

Borchelt, D. R., G. Thinakaran, C. B. Eckman, M. K. Lee, F. Davenport, T. Ratovitsky, C. M. Prada, et al. 1996. Familial Alzheimer's disease-linked presenilin 1 variants elevate Abeta1-42/1-40 ratio in vitro and in vivo. *Neuron* 17 (5): 1005–13.

Bowen, D. M., C. B. Smith, P. White, and A. N. Davison. 1976a. Neurotransmitter-related enzymes and indices of hypoxia in senile dementia and other abiotrophies. *Brain* 99:459–96.

Bowen, D. M., C. B. Smith, P. White, and A. N. Davison. 1976b. Senile dementia and related abiotrophies: Biochemical studies on historically evaluated human postmortem specimens. In *Neurobiology of Aging,* ed. R. D. Terry and S. Gershon, vol. 3: *Aging.* New York: Raven Press.

Braak, H., and E. Braak. 1991. Neuropathological staging of Alzheimer-related changes. *Acta Neuropathologica* 82:239–59.

———. 1994. Pathology of Alzheimer's disease. In *Neurodegenerative diseases,* ed. D. B. Calne. Philadelphia: W. B. Saunders.

Brookmeyer, R., S. Gray, and C. Kawas. 1998. Projections of Alzheimer's disease in the United States and the public health impact of delaying disease onset. *American Journal of Public Health* 88 (9): 1337–42.

Buxbaum, J. D., G. Thinakaran, V. Koliatsos, J. O'Callahan, H. H. Slunt, D. L. Price, and S. S. Sisodia. 1998. Alzheimer amyloid protein precursor in the rat hippocampus: Transport and processing through the perforant path. *Journal of Neuroscience* 18 (23): 9629–37.

Bymaster, F. P., D. T. Wong, C. H. Mitch, J. S. Ward, D. O. Calligaro, D. D. Schoepp, H. E. Shannon, M. J. Sheardown, P. H. Olesen, and P. D. Suzdak. 1994. Neurochemical effects of the M1 muscarinic agonist xanomeline. *Journal of Pharmacology and Experimental Therapeutics* 269:282–89.

Cai, H., Y. Wang, D. McCarthy, H. Wen, D. R. Borchelt, D. L. Price, and P. C. Wong. 2001. BACE1 is the major beta-secretase for generation of Abeta peptides by neurons. *Nature Neuroscience* 4 (3): 233–34.

Calhoun, M. E., P. Burgermeister, A. L. Phinney, M. Stalder, M. Tolnay, K.-H. Wiederhold, D. Abramowski, et al. 1999. Neuronal overexpression of mutant amyloid precursor protein results in prominent deposition of cerebrovascula amyloid. *Proceedings of the National Academy of Sciences* 96:14088–93.

Calhoun, M. E., K. H. Wiederhold, D. Abramowski, A. L. Phinney, A. Probst, C. Stuchler-Pierrat, M. Staufenbiel, B. Sommer, and M. Jucker. 1998. Neuron loss in APP transgenic mice. *Nature* 395:755–56.

Cao, X., and T. C. Sudhof. 2001. A transcriptionally [correction of transcriptively] active complex of APP with Fe65 and histone acetyltransferase Tip60. *Science* 293 (5527): 115–20.

Carson, J. A., and A. J. Turner. 2002. Beta-amyloid catabolism: Roles for neprilysin (NEP) and other metallopeptidases? *Journal of Neurochemistry* 81 (1): 1–8.

Chang, W. P., G. Koelsch, S. Wong, D. Downs, H. Da, V. Weerasena, B. Gordon, et al. 2004. In vivo inhibition of Abeta production by memapsin 2 (beta-secretase) inhibitors. *Journal of Neurochemistry* 89 (6): 1409–16.

Chapman, P. F., G. L. White, M. W. Jones, D. Cooper-Blacketer, V. J. Marshall, M. Irizarry, L. Younkin, et al. 1999. Impaired synaptic plasticity and learning in aged amyloid precursor protein transgenic mice. *Nature Neuroscience* 2:271–76.

Cirrito, J. R., P. C. May, M. A. O'Dell, J. W. Taylor, M. Parsadanian, J. W. Cramer, J. E. Audia, et al. 2003. In vivo assessment of brain interstitial fluid with microdialysis reveals plaque-associated changes in amyloid-beta metabolism and half-life. *Journal of Neuroscience* 23 (26): 8844–53.

Citron, M. 2004. Strategies for disease modification in Alzheimer's disease. *Nature Reviews Neuroscience* 5 (9): 677–85.

Cleary, J. P., D. M. Walsh, J. J. Hofmeister, G. M. Shankar, M. A. Kuskowski, D. J. Selkoe, and K. H. Ashe. 2005. Natural oligomers of the amyloid-beta protein specifically disrupt cognitive function. *Nature Neuroscience* 8 (1): 79–84.

Corder, E. H., A. M. Saunders, N. J. Risch, W. J. Strittmatter, D. E. Schmechel, P. C. Gaskell Jr., J. B. Rimmler, et al. 1994. Protective effect of apolipoprotein E type 2 allele for late onset Alzheimer disease. *Nature Genetics* 7:180–84.

Coyle, J. T., D. L. Price, and M. R. DeLong. 1983. Alzheimer's disease: A disorder of cortical cholinergic innervation. *Science* 219:1184–90.

Cummings, J. L. 2004. Alzheimer's disease. *New England Journal of Medicine* 351 (1): 56–67.

Davies, P., and A. J. F. Maloney. 1976a. Selective loss of central cholinergic neurons in Alzheimer senile dementia. *Nature* 288:279–80.

———. 1976b. Selective loss of central cholinergic neurons in Alzheimer's disease. *Lancet* 2: 1403.

Delacourte, A., J. P. David, N. Sergeant, L. Buee, A. Wattez, P. Vermersch, F. Ghozali, et al. 1999. The biochemical pathway of neurofibrillary degeneration in aging and Alzheimer's disease. *American Academy of Neurology* 52:1158–65.

DeMattos, R. B., K. R. Bales, D. J. Cummins, J. C. Dodart, S. M. Paul, and D. M. Holtzman. 2001. Peripheral anti-Ab antibody alters CNS and plasma Ab clearance and decreases brain Ab burden in a mouse model of Alzheimer's disease. *Proceedings of the National Academy of Sciences* 98:8850–55.

DeMattos, R. B., K. R. Bales, D. J. Cummins, S. M. Paul, and D. M. Holtzman. 2002. Brain to plasma amyloid-beta efflux: A measure of brain amyloid burden in a mouse model of Alzheimer's disease. *Science* 295:2264–67.

De Strooper, B., P. Saftig, K. Craessaerts, H. Vanderstichele, G. Guhde, W. G. Annaert, K. Von

Figura, and F. Van Leuven. 1998. Deficiency of presenilin-1 inhibits the normal cleavage of amyloid precursor protein. *Nature* 391 (6665): 387–90.

De Strooper, B., W. G. Annaert, P. Cupers, P. Saftig, K. Craessaerts, J. S. Mumm, E. H. Schroeter, et al. 1999. A presenilin-1-dependent gamma-secretase-like protease mediates release of notch intracellular domain. *Nature* 398 (6727): 518–22.

Deutsch, J. A. 1971. The cholinergic synapse and the site of memory. *Science* 174:788–94.

Dodart, J. C., K. R. Bales, K. S. Gannon, S. J. Greene, R. B. DeMattos, C. Mathis, C. A. DeLong, et al. 2002. Immunization reverses memory deficits without reducing brain Abeta burden in Alzheimer's disease model. *Nature Neuroscience* 5 (5): 452–7.

Drachman, D. A., and J. L. Leavitt. 1974. Human memory and the cholinergic system: A relationship to aging? *Archives of Neurology* 30:113–21.

Fagan, A. M., M. A. Mintun, R. H. Mach, S-Y Lee, C. S. Dence, A. R. Shah, G. N. LaRossa, et al. 2005. Inverse relation between in vivo amyloid imaging load and cerebrospinal fluid AV42 in humans. *Annals of Neurology* 59 (3): 512–19.

Farris, W., S. Mansourian, Y. Chang, L. Lindsley, E. A. Eckman, M. P. Frosch, C. B. Eckman, R. E. Tanzi, D. J. Selkoe, and S. Guenette. 2003. Insulin-degrading enzyme regulates the levels of insulin, amyloid beta-protein, and the beta-amyloid precursor protein intracellular domain in vivo. *Proceedings of the National Academy of Sciences USA* 100 (7): 4162–67.

Farzan, M., C. E. Schnitzler, N. Vasilieva, D. Leung, and H. Choe. 2000. BACE2, a b-secretase homolog, cleaves at the b site and within the amyloid-b region of the amyloid-b precursor protein. *Proceedings of the National Academy of Sciences* 97:9712–17.

Federoff, H. J., and W. J. Bowers. 2005. Immune shaping and the development of Alzheimer's disease vaccines. *Science of Aging Knowledge Environment* 2005 (46): e35.

Francis, P. T., and D. M. Bowen. 1985. Relevance of reduced concentrations of somatostatin in Alzheimer's disease. *Biochemical Society Transactions* 13:170–71.

Francis, P. T., A. M. Palmer, N. R. Sims, D. M. Bowen, A. N. Davison, M. M. Esiri, D. Neary, J. S. Snowden, and G. K. Wilcock. 1985. Neurochemical studies of early-onset Alzheimer's disease. Possible influence on treatment. *New England Journal of Medicine* 313:7–11.

Gandy, S., and L. Walker. 2004. Toward modeling hemorrhagic and encephalitic complications of Alzheimer amyloid-beta vaccination in nonhuman primates. *Current Opinion in Immunology* 16 (5): 607–15.

Gastard, M. C., J. C. Troncoso, and V. E. Koliatsos. 2003. Caspase activation in the limbic cortex of subjects with early Alzheimer's disease. *Annals of Neurology* 54 (3): 393–98.

Ghiso, J. and T. Wisniewski. 2004. An animal model of vascular amyloidosis. *Nature Neuroscience* 7 (9): 902–4.

Goedert, M., and M.-G. Spillantini. 2006. Neurodegenerative alpha-Synucleinopathies and Tauopathies. In *Basic neurochemistry: Molecular, cellular, and medical aspects,* 7th ed., ed. G. Siegel, R. Albers, S. Brady, and D. Price. Burlington, Mass.: Elsevier.

Gong, Y., L. Chang, K. L. Viola, P. N. Lacor, M. P. Lambert, C. E. Finch, G. A. Krafft, and W. L. Klein. 2003. Alzheimer's disease-affected brain: Presence of oligomeric A beta ligands (ADDLs) suggests a molecular basis for reversible memory loss. *Proceedings of the National Academy of Sciences USA* 100 (18): 10417–22.

Gotz, J., F. Chen, J. Van Dorpe, and R. M. Nitsch. 2001. Formation of neurofibrillary tangles in P301l tau transgenic mice induced by Abeta fibrils. *Science* 293:1491–95.

Goutte, C., M. Tsunozaki, V. A. Hale, and J. R. Priess. 2002. APH-1 is a multipass membrane protein essential for the Notch signaling pathway in *Caenorhabditis elegans* embryos. *Proceedings of the National Academy of Sciences USA* 99 (2): 775–79.

Hardy, John. 2006. Amyloid double trouble. *Nature Genetics* 38 (1): 11–12.

Hartley, D. M., D. M. Walsh, C. P. Ye, T. Diehl, S. Vasquez, P. M. Vassilev, D. B. Teplow, and D. J. Selkoe. 1999. Protofibrillar intermediates of amyloid beta-protein induce acute electrophysiological changes and progressive neurotoxicity in cortical neurons. *Journal of Neuroscience* 19 (20): 8876–84.

Herget, T., H. Specht, C. Esdar, S. A. Oehrlein, and A. Maelicke. 1998. Retinoic acid induces apoptosis-associated neural differentiation of a murine teratocarcinoma cell line. *Journal of Neurochemistry* 70 (1): 47–58.

Herzig, M. C., D. T. Winkler, P. Burgermeister, M. Pfeifer, E. Kohler, S. D. Schmidt, S. Danner, et al. 2004. Abeta is targeted to the vasculature in a mouse model of hereditary cerebral hemorrhage with amyloidosis. *Nature Neuroscience* 7 (9): 954–60.

Hock, C., U. Konietzko, A. Papassotiropoulos, A. Wollmer, J. Streffer, R. C. von Rotz, G. Davey, E. Moritz, and R. M. Nitsch. 2002. Generation of antibodies specific for beta-amyloid by vaccination of patients with Alzheimer disease. *Nature Medicine* 8 (11): 1270–75.

Hock, C., U. Konietzko, J. R. Streffer, J. Tracy, A. Signorell, B. Muller-Tillmanns, U. Lemke, et al. 2003. Antibodies against beta-amyloid slow cognitive decline in Alzheimer's disease. *Neuron* 38 (4): 547–54.

Hulette, C., S. Mirra, W. Wilkinson, A. Heyman, G. Fillenbaum, and C. Clark. 1995. The consortium to establish a registry for Alzheimer's disease (CERAD). Part IX. A prospective cliniconeuropathologic study of Parkinson's features in Alzheimer's disease. *Neurology* 45:1991–95.

Hutton, M., and E. McGowan. 2004. Clearing tau pathology with abeta immunotherapy: Reversible and irreversible stages revealed. *Neuron* 43 (3): 293–94.

Hyman, B. T., G. W. Van Hoesen, A. R. Damasio, and C. L. Barnes. 1984. Alzheimer's disease: Cell-specific pathology isolates the hippocampal formation. *Science* 225:1168–70.

Iwata, N., H. Mizukami, K. Shirotani, Y. Takaki, S. Muramatsu, B. Lu, N. P. Gerard, C. Gerard, K. Ozawa, and T. C. Saido. 2004. Presynaptic localization of neprilysin contributes to efficient clearance of amyloid-beta peptide in mouse brain. *Journal of Neuroscience* 24 (4): 991–98.

Iwata, N., S. Tsubuki, Y. Takaki, K. Shirotani, B. Lu, N. P. Gerard, C. Gerard, E. Hama, H. J. Lee, and T. C. Saido. 2001. Metabolic regulation of brain Aβ by neprilysin. *Science* 292:1550–52.

Iwata, N., S. Tsubuki, Y. Takaki, K. Watanabe, M. Sekiguchi, E. Hosoki, M. Kawashima-Morishima, et al. 2000. Identification of the major Aβ1–42-degrading catabolic pathway in brain parenchyma: Suppression leads to biochemical and pathological deposition. *Nature Medicine* 2:143–50.

Iwatsubo, T. 2004. The gamma-secretase complex: Machinery for intramembrane proteolysis. *Current Opinion in Neurobiology* 14 (3): 379–83.

Jankowsky, J. L., D. J. Fadale, J. Anderson, G. M. Xu, V. Gonzales, N. A. Jenkins, N. G. Copeland, et al. 2004. Mutant presenilins specifically elevate the levels of the 42 residue beta-amyloid peptide in vivo: Evidence for augmentation of a 42-specific gamma secretase. *Humam Molecular Genetics* 13 (2): 159–70.

Jicha, G. A., J. E. Parisi, D. W. Dickson, K. Johnson, R. Cha, R. J. Ivnik, E. G. Tangalos, et al. 2006.

Neuropathologic outcome of mild cognitive impairment following progression to clinical dementia. *Archives of Neurology* 63 (5): 674–81.

Kawarabayashi, T., M. Shoji, L. H. Younkin, L. Wen-Lang, D. W. Dickson, T. Murakami, E. Matsubara, K. Abe, K. H. Ashe, and S. G. Younkin. 2004. Dimeric amyloid beta protein rapidly accumulates in lipid rafts followed by apolipoprotein E and phosphorylated tau accumulation in the Tg2576 mouse model of Alzheimer's disease. *Journal of Neuroscience* 24 (15): 3801–9.

Killiany, R. J., T. Gomez-Isla, M. Moss, R. Kikinis, T. Sandor, F. Jolesz, R. Tanzi, K. Jones, B. T. Hyman, and M. S. Albert. 2000. Use of structural magnetic resonance imaging to predict who will get Alzheimer's disease. *Annals of Neurology* 47:430–39.

Kimberly, W. T., M. J. LaVoie, B. L. Ostaszewski, W. Ye, M. S. Wolfe, and D. J. Selkoe. 2003. Gammasecretase is a membrane protein complex comprised of presenilin, nicastrin, Aph-1, and Pen-2. *Proceedings of the National Academy of Sciences USA* 100 (11): 6382–87.

Kitt, C. A., D. L. Price, R. G. Struble, L. C. Cork, B. H. Wainer, M. W. Becher, and W. C. Mobley. 1984. Evidence for cholinergic neurites in senile plaques. *Science* 226 (4681): 1443–45.

Kitt, C. A., R. G. Struble, L. C. Cork, W. C. Mobley, L. C. Walker, T. H. Joh, and D. L. Price. 1985. Catecholaminergic neurites in senile plaques in prefrontal cortex of aged nonhuman primates. *Neuroscience* 16:691–99.

Klein, W. L., G. A. Krafft, and C. E. Finch. 2001. Targeting small Ab oligomers: The solution to an Alzheimer's disease conundrum? *Trends in Neuroscience* 24:219–23.

Klunk, W. E., H. Engler, A. Nordberg, Y. Wang, G. Blomstrand, D. P. Holt, M. Bergstrom, et al. 2004. Imaging brain amyloid in Alzheimer's disease using the novel positron emission tomography tracer, Pittsburgh compound-B. *Annals of Neurology* 55:1–14.

Klyubin, I., D. M. Walsh, C. A. Lemere, W. K. Cullen, G. M. Shankar, V. Betts, E. T. Spooner, et al. 2005. Amyloid beta protein immunotherapy neutralizes Abeta oligomers that disrupt synaptic plasticity in vivo. *Nature Medicine* 11 (5): 556–61.

Koo, E. H., S. S. Sisodia, D. R. Archer, L. J. Martin, K. T. Beyreuther, A. Weidemann, and D. L. Price. 1989. Amyloid precursor protein (APP) undergoes fast anterograde transport. *Society for Neuroscience Abstracts* 15:23.

Kotilinek, L. A., B. J. Bacskai, M. Westerman, T. Kawarabayashi, L. Younkin, B. T. Hyman, S. Younkin, and K. H. Ashe. 2002. Reversible memory loss in a mouse transgenic model of Alzheimer's disease. *Journal of Neuroscience* 22 (15): 6331–35.

Laird, F. M., H. Savonenko, A. V. Cai, M. H. Farah, K. He, T. Wen, H. Melnikova, et al. 2005. BACE1, a major determinant of selective vulnerability of the brain to Ab amyloidogenesis, is essential for cognitive, emotional and synaptic functions. *Journal of Neuroscience* 25 (50): 11693–709.

Lambert, M. P., A. K. Barlow, B. A. Chromy, C. Edwards, R. Freed, M. Liosatos, T. E. Morgan, et al. 1998. Diffusible, nonfibrillar ligands derived from Abeta1–42 are potent central nervous system neurotoxins. *Proceedings of the National Academy of Sciences USA* 95 (11): 6448–53.

Lauritzen, M., and L. Gold. 2003. Brain function and neurophysiological correlates of signals used in functional neuroimaging. *Journal of Neuroscience* 23 (10): 3972–80.

Lazarov, O., M. Lee, D. A. Peterson, and S. S. Sisodia. 2002. Evidence that synaptically released beta-amyloid accumulates as extracellular deposits in the hippocampus of transgenic mice. *Journal of Neuroscience* 22 (22): 9785–93.

Lazarov, O., G. A. Morfini, E. B. Lee, M. H. Farah, A. Szodorai, S. R. Deboer, V. E. Koliatsos, et al.

2005. Axonal transport, amyloid precursor protein, kinesin-1, and the processing apparatus: Revisited. *Journal of Neuroscience* 25 (9): 2386–95.

Lee, V. M., M. Goedert, and J. Q. Trojanowski. 2001. Neurodegenerative tauopathies. *Annual Review of Neuroscience* 24:1121–59.

Leissring, M. A., W. Farris, A. Y. Chang, D. M. Walsh, X. Wu, X. Sun, M. P. Frosch, and D. J. Selkoe. 2003. Enhanced proteolysis of beta-amyloid in APP transgenic mice prevents plaque formation, secondary pathology, and premature death. *Neuron* 40 (6): 1087–93.

Lesne, S., M. T. Koh, L. Kotilinek, R. Kayed, C. G. Glabe, A. Yang, M. Gallagher, and K. H. Ashe. 2006. A specific amyloid-beta protein assembly in the brain impairs memory. *Nature* 440 (7082): 352–57.

Lewis, J., D. W. Dickson, W.-L. Lin, L. Chisholm, A. Corral, G. Jones, S.-H. Yen, et al. 2001. Enhanced neurofibrillary degeneration in transgenic mice expressing mutat tau and APP. *Science* 293:1487–91.

Li, T., G. Ma, H. Cai, D. L. Price, and P. C. Wong. 2003. Nicastrin is required for assembly of presenilin/gamma-secretase complexes to mediate notch signaling and for processing and trafficking of beta-amyloid precursor protein in mammals. *Journal of Neuroscience* 23 (8): 3272–77.

Li, T., H. Wen, C. Brayton, P. Das, L. A. Smithson, A. Fauq, X. Fan, et al. 2007. Epidermal growth factor receptor and notch pathways participate in the tumor suppressor function of gamma-secretase. *Journal of Biological Chemistry* 282 (44): 32264–73.

Lim, G. P., F. Yang, T. Chu, P. Chen, W. Beech, B. Teter, T. Tran, et al. 2000. Ibuprofen suppresses plaque pathology and inflammation in a mouse model for Alzheimer's disease. *Journal of Neuroscience* 20:5709–14.

Lipton, Stuart. 2004. Paradigm shift in NMDA receptor antagonist drug development: Molecular mechanism of uncompetitive inhibition by memantine in the treatment of Alzheimer's disease and other neurologic disorders. *Journal of Alzheimer's Disease* 6 (6 suppl.): S61–74.

Luo, Y., B. Bolon, S. Kahn, B. D. Bennett, S. Babu-Khan, P. Denis, W. Fan, et al. 2001. Mice deficient in BACE1, the Alzheimer's beta-secretase, have normal phenotype and abolished beta-amyloid generation. *Nature Neuroscience* 4 (3): 231–32.

Ma, G., T. Li, D. L. Price, and P. C. Wong. 2005. APH-1a is the principal mammalian APH-1 isoform present in gamma-secretase complexes during embryonic development. *Journal of Neuroscience* 25 (1): 192–98.

Markesbery, W. R., F. A. Schmitt, R. J. Kryscio, D. G. Davis, C. D. Smith, and D. R. Wekstein. 2006. Neuropathologic substrate of mild cognitive impairment. *Archives of Neurology* 63 (1): 38–46.

Marr, R. A., E. Rockenstein, A. Mukherjee, M. S. Kindy, L. B. Hersh, F. H. Gage, I. M. Verma, and E. Masliah. 2003. Neprilysin gene transfer reduces human amyloid pathology in transgenic mice. *Journal of Neuroscience* 23 (6): 1992–96.

Martin, L. J., C. A. Pardo, L. C. Cork, and D. L. Price. 1994. Synaptic pathology and glial responses to neuronal injury precede the formation of senile plaques and amyloid deposits in the aging cerebral cortex. *American Journal of Pathology* 145 (6): 1358–81.

Masliah, E., L. Hansen, A. Adame, L. Crews, F. Bard, C. Lee, P. Seubert, D. Games, L. Kirby, and D. Schenk. 2005. A{beta} vaccination effects on plaque pathology in the absence of encephalitis in Alzheimer disease. *Neurology* 64 (1): 129–31.

Mayeux, R. 2003. Epidemiology of neurodegeneration. *Annual Review of Neuroscience* 26:81–104.

McDonald, J. W., and M. J. Howard. 2002. Repairing the damaged spinal cord: A summary of our early success with embryonic stem cell transplantation and remyelination. *Progress in Brain Research* 137:299–309.

McKhann, G., D. Drachman, M. Folstein, R. Katzman, D. Price, and E. M. Stadlan. 1984. Clinical diagnosis of Alzheimer's disease: Report of the NINCDS-ADRDA Work Group under the auspices of the Department of Health and Human Services Task Force on Alzheimer's Disease. *Neurology* 34:939–44.

McLean, C. A., R. A. Cherny, F. W. Fraser, S. J. Fuller, M. J. Smith, K. T. Beyreuther, A. I. Bush, and C. L. Masters. 1999. Soluble pool of Abeta amyloid as a determinant of severity of neurodegeneration in Alzheimer's disease. *Annals of Neurology* 46 (6): 860–66.

Mesulam, M.-M., and G. W. Van Hoesen. 1976. Acetylcholinesterase-rich projections from the basal forebrain of the rhesus monkey to neocortex. *Brain Research* 109:152–57.

Milano, J., J. McKay, C. Dagenais, L. Foster-Brown, F. Pognan, R. Gadient, R. T. Jacobs, A. Zacco, B. Greenberg, and P. J. Ciaccio. 2004. Modulation of notch processing by gamma-secretase inhibitors causes intestinal goblet cell metaplasia and induction of genes known to specify gut secretory lineage differentiation. *Toxicological Sciences* 82 (1): 341–58.

Miller, B. C., E. A. Eckman, K. Sambamurti, N. Dobbs, K. M. Chow, C. B. Eckman, L. B. Hersh, and D. L. Thiele. 2003. Amyloid-beta peptide levels in brain are inversely correlated with insulysin activity levels in vivo. *Proceedings of the National Academy of Sciences USA* 100 (10): 6221–26.

Monsonego, A., and H. L. Weiner. 2003. Immunotherapeutic approaches to Alzheimer's disease. *Science* 302 (5646): 834–38.

Morgan, D., D. M. Diamond, P. E. Gottschall, K. E. Ugen, C. Dickey, J. Hardy, K. Duff, et al. 2000. Ab peptide vaccination prevents memory loss in an animal model of Alzheimer's disease. *Nature* 408:982–85.

Morris, J. C., and J. L. Price. 2001. Pathologic correlates of nondemented aging, mild cognitive impairment, and early-stage Alzheimer's disease. *Journal of Molecular Neuroscience* 17 (2): 101–18.

Morris, J. C., M. Storandt, J. P. Miller, D. W. McKeel, J. L. Price, E. H. Rubin, and L. Berg. 2001. Mild cognitive impairment represents early-stage Alzheimer disease. *Archives of Neurology* 58 (3): 397–405.

Mucke, L., E. Masliah, G. Q. Yu, M. Mallory, E. M. Rockenstein, G. Tatsuno, K. Hu, D. Kholodenko, K. Johnson-Wood, and L. McConlogue. 2000. High-level neuronal expression of Ab1–42 in wild-type human amyloid protein precursor transgenic mice: Synaptotoxicity without plaque formation. *Journal of Neuroscience* 20:4050–58.

Nestor, P. J., P. Scheltens, and J. R. Hodges. 2004. Advances in the early detection of Alzheimer's disease. *Nature Medicine* 10 (suppl.): S34–41.

Nicolas, M., A. Wolfer, K. Raj, J. A. Kummer, P. Mill, M. van Noort, C. C. Hui, et al. 2003. Notch1 functions as a tumor suppressor in mouse skin. *Nature Genetics* 33 (3): 416–21.

Nicoll, J. A., D. Wilkinson, C. Holmes, P. Steart, H. Markham, and R. O. Weller. 2003. Neuropathology of human Alzheimer disease after immunization with amyloid-beta peptide: A case report. *Nature Medicine* 9 (4): 448–52.

Nishizaki, T., T. Matsuoka, T. Nomura, T. Kondoh, S. Watabe, T. Shiotani, and M. Yoshii. 2000.

Presynaptic nicotinic acetylcholine receptors as a functional target of nefiracetam in inducing a long-lasting facilitation of hippocampal neurotransmission. *Alzheimer Disease and Associated Disorders* 14:S82–94.

Oddo, S., L. Billings, J. P. Kesslak, D. H. Cribbs, and F. M. LaFerla. 2004. Abeta immunotherapy leads to clearance of early, but not late, hyperphosphorylated tau aggregates via the proteasome. *Neuron* 43 (3): 321–32.

Oddo, S., A. Caccamo, J. D. Shepherd, M. P. Murphy, T. E. Golde, R. Kayed, R. Metherate, M. P. Mattson, Y. Akbari, and F. M. LaFerla. 2003. Triple-transgenic model of Alzheimer's disease with plaques and tangles: Intracellular Abeta and synaptic dysfunction. *Neuron* 39 (3): 409–21.

Ohno, M., E. A. Sametsky, L. H. Younkin, H. Oakley, S. G. Younkin, M. Citron, R. Vassar, and J. F. Disterhoft. 2004. BACE1 Deficiency rescues memory deficits and cholinergic dysfunction in a mouse model of Alzheimer's disease. *Neuron* 41 (1): 27–33.

Perry, E. K., P. H. Gibson, G. Blessed, R. H. Perry, and B. E. Tomlinson. 1977. Neurotransmitter enzyme abnormalities in senile dementia. *Journal of the Neurological Sciences* 34:247–65.

Perry, E. K., R. H. Perry, G. Blessed, and B. E. Tomlinson. 1978. Changes in brain cholinesterases in senile dementia of Alzheimer type. *Neuropathology and Applied Neurobiology* 4:273–77.

Perry, E. K., B. E. Tomlinson, G. Blessed, K. Bergmann, P. H. Gibson, and R. H. Perry. 1978. Correlation of cholinergic abnormalities with senile plaques and mental test scores in senile dementia. *British Medical Journal* 2:1457–59.

Perry, T. L., S. Hansen, R. D. Currier, and K. Berry. 1978. Abnormalities in neurotransmitter amino acids in dominantly inherited cerebellar disorders. In *The inherited ataxias: Biochemical, viral, and pathological studies*, ed. R. A. P. Kark, R. N. Rosenberg, and L. J. Schut, vol. 21: *Advances in neurology*. New York: Raven Press.

Petersen, R. C. 2003. Mild cognitive impairment clinical trials. *Nature Reviews Drug Discovery* 2 (8): 646–53.

Petersen, R. C., R. Doody, A. Kurz, R. C. Mohs, J. C. Morris, P. V. Rabins, K. Ritchie, M. Rossor, L. Thal, and B. Winblad. 2001. Current concepts in mild cognitive impairment. *Archives of Neurology* 58 (12): 1985–92.

Petersen, R. C., J. E. Parisi, D. W. Dickson, K. A. Johnson, D. S. Knopman, B. F. Boeve, G. A. Jicha, et al. 2006. Neuropathologic features of amnestic mild cognitive impairment. *Archives of Neurology* 63 (5): 665–72.

Pfeifer, M., S. Boncristiano, L. Bondolfi, A. Stalder, T. Deller, M. Staufenbiel, P. M. Mathews, and M. Jucker. 2002. Cerebral hemorrhage after passive anti-Abeta immunotherapy. *Science* 298 (5597): 1379.

Price, D. L., and S. S. Sisodia. 1998. Mutant genes in familial Alzheimer's disease and transgenic models. *Annual Review of Neuroscience* 21:479–505.

Price, D. L., R. E. Tanzi, D. R. Borchelt, and S. S. Sisodia. 1998. Alzheimer's disease: Genetic studies and transgenic models. *Annual Review of Genetics* 32:461–93.

Reisberg, B., R. Doody, A. Stoffler, F. Schmitt, S. Ferris, and H. J. Mobius. 2003. Memantine in moderate-to-severe Alzheimer's disease. *New England Journal of Medicine* 348 (14): 1333–41.

Rovelet-Lecrux, A., D. Hannequin, G. Raux, N. Le Meur, A. Laquerriere, A. Vital, C. Dumanchin, et al. 2006. APP locus duplication causes autosomal dominant early-onset Alzheimer disease with cerebral amyloid angiopathy. *Nature Genetics* 38 (1): 24–26.

Saura, C. A., S. Y. Choi, V. Beglopoulos, S. Malkani, D. Zhang, B. S. Rao, S. Chattarji, et al. 2004.

Loss of presenilin function causes impairments of memory and synaptic plasticity followed by age-dependent neurodegeneration. *Neuron* 42 (1): 23–36.

Savonenko, A. V., F. M. Laird, J. C. Troncoso, P. C. Wong, and D. L. Price. 2006. Role of Alzheimer's disease models in designing and testing experimental therapeutics. *Drug Discovery Today* 17 (2): 233–57.

Savonenko, A. V., G. M. Xu, T. Melnikova, J. L. Morton, V. Gonzales, M. P. F. Wong, D. L. Price, F. Tang, A. L. Markowska, and D. R. Borchelt. 2005. Episodic-like memory deficits in the APP-swe/PS1dE9 mouse model of Alzheimer's disease: Relationships to beta-amyloid deposition and neurotransmitter abnormalities. *Neurobiology of Disease* 18 (3): 602–17.

Savonenko, A. V., G. M. Xu, D. L. Price, D. R. Borchelt, and A. L. Markowska. 2003. Normal cognitive behavior in two distinct congenic lines of transgenic mice hyperexpressing mutant APPswe. *Neurobiology of Disease* 12 (3): 194–211.

Schenk, D., R. Barbour, W. Dunn, G. Gordon, H. Grajeda, T. Guido, K. Hu, et al. 1999. Immunization with amyloid-beta attenuates Alzheimer disease-like pathology in the PDAPP mouse. *Nature* 400 (6740): 173–77.

Schenk, D., M. Hagen, and P. Seubert. 2004. Current progress in beta-amyloid immunotherapy. *Current Opinion in Immunology* 16 (5): 599–606.

Schmitt, F. A., D. G. Davis, D. R. Wekstein, C. D. Smith, J. W. Ashford, and W. R. Markesbery. 2000. "Preclinical" AD revisited. *Neurology* 55:370–76.

Selkoe, D. J. 2002. Alzheimer's disease is a synaptic failure. *Science* 298 (5594): 789–91.

Selkoe, D. J., D. Bell, M. Podlisny, D. Price, and L. Cork. 1987. Recognition of senile plaque and microvascular amyloid in aged animals by antibodies to amyloid proteins in Alzheimer's disease (AD). *Journal of Neuropathology and Experimental Neurology* 46:395.

Selkoe, D. J., and R. Kopan. 2003. Notch and presenilin: Regulated intramembrane proteolysis links development and degeneration. *Annual Review of Neuroscience* 26:565–97.

Selkoe, D. J., and D. Schenk. 2003. Alzheimer's disease: Molecular understanding predicts amyloid-based therapeutics. *Annual Review of Pharmacology and Toxicology* 43:545–84.

Serneels, L., T. Dejaegere, K. Craessaerts, K. Horre, E. Jorissen, T. Tousseyn, S. Hebert, et al. 2005. Differential contribution of the three Aph1 genes to gamma-secretase activity in vivo. *Proceedings of the National Academy of Sciences USA* 102 (5): 1719–24.

Shah, S., S. F. Lee, K. Tabuchi, Y. H. Hao, C. Yu, Q. LaPlant, H. Ball, C. E. Dann III, T. Sudhof, and G. Yu. 2005. Nicastrin functions as a γ-secretase-substrate receptor. *Cell* 122 (3): 435–47.

Shen, J., R. T. Bronson, D. F. Chen, W. Xia, D. J. Selkoe, and S. Tonegawa. 1997. Skeletal and CNS defects in presenilin-1-deficient mice. *Cell* 89 (4): 629–39.

Sheng, J. G., D. L. Price, and V. E. Koliatsos. 2002. Disruption of corticocortical connections ameliorates amyloid burden in terminal fields in a transgenic model of Abeta amyloidosis. *Journal of Neuroscience* 22 (22): 9794–99.

———. 2003. The beta-amyloid-related proteins presenilin 1 and BACE1 are axonally transported to nerve terminals in the brain. *Experimental Neurology* 184 (2): 1053–57.

Sherrington, R., E. I. Rogaev, Y. Liang, E. A. Rogaeva, G. Levesque, M. Ikeda, H. Chi, et al. 1995. Cloning of a gene bearing missense mutations in early-onset familial Alzheimer's disease. *Nature* 375:754–60.

Sigurdsson, E. M., E. Knudsen, A. Asuni, C. Fitzer-Attas, D. Sage, D. Quartermain, F. Goni, B. Frangione, and T. Wisniewski. 2004. An attenuated immune response is sufficient to enhance cognition in an Alzheimer's disease mouse model immunized with amyloid-beta derivatives. *Journal of Neuroscience* 24 (28): 6277–82.

Sisodia, S. S., E. H. Koo, K. T. Beyreuther, A. Unterbeck, and D. L. Price. 1990. Evidence that b-amyloid protein in Alzheimer's disease is not derived by normal processing. *Science* 248:492–95.

Sisodia, S. S., E. H. Koo, P. N. Hoffman, G. Perry, and D. L. Price. 1993. Identification and transport of full-length amyloid precursor proteins in rat peripheral nervous system. *Journal of Neuroscience* 13:3136–42.

Stokin, G. B., C. Lillo, T. L. Falzone, R. G. Brusch, E. Rockenstein, S. L. Mount, R. Raman, et al. 2005. Axonapathy and transport deficits early in the pathogenesis of Alzheimer's disease. *Science* 307 (5713): 1282–88.

Sunderland, T., G. Linker, N. Mirza, K. T. Putnam, D. L. Friedman, L. H. Kimmel, J. Bergeson, et al. 2003. Decreased beta-amyloid 1–42 and increased tau levels in cerebrospinal fluid of patients with Alzheimer disease. *JAMA* 289 (16): 2094–2103.

Sze, C.-I., J. C. Troncoso, C. H. Kawas, P. R. Mouton, D. L. Price, and L. J. Martin. 1997. Loss of the presynaptic vesicle protein synaptophysin in hippocampus correlates with early cognitive decline in aged humans. *Journal of Neuropathology and Experimental Neurology* 56:933–44.

Tanzi, R. E., and L. Bertram. 2001. New frontiers in Alzheimer's disease genetics. *Neuron* 32 (2): 181–84.

Teipel, S. J., W. H. Flatz, H. Heinsen, A. L. Bokde, S. O. Schoenberg, S. Stockel, O. Dietrich, M. F. Reiser, H. J. Moller, and H. Hampel. 2005. Measurement of basal forebrain atrophy in Alzheimer's disease using MRI. *Brain* 128 (pt 11): 2626–44.

Thinakaran, G., C. L. Harris, T. Ratovitski, F. Davenport, H. H. Slunt, D. L. Price, D. R. Borchelt, and S. S. Sisodia. 1997. Evidence that levels of presenilins (PS1 and PS2) are coordinately regulated by competition for limiting cellular factors. *Journal of Biological Chemistry* 272:28415–22.

Troncoso, J. C., L. J. Martin, G. Dal Forno, and C. H. Kawas. 1996. Neuropathology in controls and demented subjects from the Baltimore Longitudinal Study of Aging. *Neurobiology of Aging* 17: 365–71.

Vassar, R., B. D. Bennett, S. Babu-Khan, S. Kahn, E. A. Mendiaz, P. Denis, D. B. Teplow, et al. 1999. B-secretase cleavage of Alzheimer's amyloid precursor protein by the transmembrane aspartic protease BACE. *Science* 286:735–41.

Vekrellis, K., Z. Ye, W. Q. Qiu, D. Walsh, D. Hartley, V. Chesneau, M. R. Rosner, and D. J. Selkoe. 2000. Neurons regulate extracellular levels of amyloid á-protein via proteolysis by insulin-degrading enzyme. *Journal of Neuroscience* 20:1657–65.

Voytko, M. L., D. S. Olton, R. T. Richardson, L. K. Gorman, J. R. Tobin, and D. L. Price. 1994. Basal forebrain lesions in monkeys disrupt attention but not learning and memory. *Journal of Neuroscience* 14 (1): 167–86.

Walsh, D. M., D. M. Hartley, Y. Kusumoto, Y. Fezoui, M. M. Condron, A. Lomakin, G. B. Benedek, D. J. Selkoe, and D. B. Teplow. 1999. Amyloid beta-protein fibrillogenesis. Structure and biological activity of protofibrillar intermediates. *Journal of Biological Chemistry* 274 (36): 25945–52.

Walsh, D. M., I. Klyubin, A. I. Faden, J. V. Fadeeva, W. K. Cullen, R. Anwyl, M. S. Wolfe, M. J. Rowan, and D. J. Selkoe. 2002. Naturally secreted oligomers of amyloid b-protein potently inhibit hippocampal LTP in vivo. *Nature* 416 (6880): 535–9.

Walsh, D. M., and D. J. Selkoe. 2004. Deciphering the molecular basis of memory failure in Alzheimer's disease. *Neuron* 44 (1): 181–93.

Wang, H. W., J. F. Pasternak, H. Kuo, H. Ristic, M. P. Lambert, B. Chromy, K. L. Viola, et al. 2002. Soluble oligomers of beta amyloid (1–42) inhibit long-term potentiation but not long-term depression in rat dentate gyrus. *Brain Research* 924 (2): 133–40.

Weggen, S., J. L. Eriksen, P. Das, S. A. Sagl, R. Wang, C. U. Pietrzik, K. A. Findlay, et al. 2001. A subset of NSAIDs lower amyloidogenic Ab42 independently of cyclooxygenase activity. *Nature* 414:212–16.

Weninger, S. C., and B. A. Yankner. 2001. Inflammation and Alzheimer disease: The good, the bad, and the ugly. *Nature Medicine* 7 (5): 527–28.

West, M. J., P. D. Coleman, D. G. Flood, and J. C. Troncoso. 1994. Differences in the pattern of hippocampal neuronal loss in normal ageing and Alzheimer's disease. *Lancet* 344 (8925): 769–72.

West, M. J., C. H. Kawas, L. J. Martin, and J. C. Troncoso. 2000. The CA1 region of the human hippocampus is a hot spot in Alzheimer's disease. *Annals of the New York Academy of Sciences* 908:255–59.

West, M. J., C. H. Kawas, W. F. Stewart, G. Rudow, and J. C. Troncoso. 2004. Hippocampal neurons in pre-clinical Alzheimer's Disease. *Neurobiology of Disease* 25 (9): 1205–12.

Whitehouse, P. J., D. L. Price, A. W. Clark, J. T. Coyle, and M. R. DeLong. 1981. Alzheimer disease: Evidence for selective loss of cholinergic neurons in the nucleus basalis. *Annals of Neurology* 10:122–26.

Whitehouse, P. J., D. L. Price, R. G. Struble, A. W. Clark, J. T. Coyle, and M. R. Delon. 1982. Alzheimer's disease and senile dementia: Loss of neurons in the basal forebrain. *Science* 215 (4537): 1237–39.

Wilcock, D. M., G. DiCarlo, D. Henderson, J. Jackson, K. Clarke, K. E. Ugen, M. N. Gordon, and D. Morgan. 2003. Intracranially administered anti-Abeta antibodies reduce beta-amyloid deposition by mechanisms both independent of and associated with microglial activation. *Journal of Neuroscience* 23 (9): 3745–51.

Wilcock, D. M., S. K. Munireddy, A. Rosenthal, K. E. Ugen, M. N. Gordon, and D. Morgan. 2004. Microglial activation facilitates Abeta plaque removal following intracranial anti-Abeta antibody administration. *Neurobiology of Disease* 15 (1): 11–20.

Wilcock, D. M., A. Rojiani, A. Rosenthal, G. Levkowitz, S. Subbarao, J. Alamed, D. Wilson, et al. 2004. Passive amyloid immunotherapy clears amyloid and transiently activates microglia in a transgenic mouse model of amyloid deposition. *Journal of Neuroscience* 24 (27): 6144–51.

Winblad, B., L. Kilander, S. Eriksson, L. Minthon, S. Batsman, A. L. Wetterholm, C. Jansson-Blixt, and A. Haglund. 2006. Donepezil in patients with severe Alzheimer's disease: Double-blind, parallel-group, placebo-controlled study. *Lancet* 367 (9516): 1057–65.

Winkler, D. T., L. Bondolfi, M. C. Herzig, L. Jann, M. E. Calhoun, K. H. Wiederhold, M. Tolnay, M. Staufenbiel, and M. Jucker. 2001. Spontaneous hemorrhagic stroke in a mouse model of cerebral amyloid angiopathy. *Journal of Neuroscience* 21 (5): 1619–27.

Wolfe, M. S., and R. Kopan. 2004. Intramembrane proteolysis: Theme and variations. *Science* 305 (5687): 1119–23.

Wolfe, M. S., W. Xia, B. L. Ostaszewski, T. S. Diehl, W. T. Kimberly, and D. J. Selkoe. 1999. Two transmembrane aspartates in presenilin-1 required for presenilin endoproteolysis and gamma-secretase activity. *Nature* 398 (6727): 513–17.

Wong, P. C., T. Li, and D. L. Price. 2005. Neurobiology of Alzheimer's disease. In *Basic neurochemistry*, 7th ed., Burlington, Mass: Elsevier.

Wong, G. T., D. Manfra, F. M. Poulet, Q. Zhang, H. Josien, T. Bara, L. Engstrom, et al. 2004. Chronic treatment with the gamma-secretase inhibitor LY-411,575 inhibits beta-amyloid peptide production and alters lymphopoiesis and intestinal cell differentiation. *Journal of Biological Chemistry* 279 (13): 12876–82.

Wong, P. C., H. Cai, D. R. Borchelt, and D. L. Price. 2002. Genetically engineered mouse models of neurodegenerative diseases. *Nature Neuroscience* 5 (7): 633–39.

Wong, P. C., D. L. Price, and H. Cai. 2001. The brain's susceptibility to amyloid plaques. *Science* 293: 1434–35.

Wong, P. C., H. Zheng, H. Chen, M. W. Becher, D. J. Sirinathsinghji, M. E. Trumbauer, H. Y. Chen, D. L. Price, L. H. Van der Ploeg, and S. S. Sisodia. 1997. Presenilin 1 is required for Notch1 and DII1 expression in the paraxial mesoderm. *Nature* 387 (6630): 288–92.

Xia, X., S. Qian, S. Soriano, Y. Wu, A. M. Fletcher, X. J. Wang, E. H. Koo, X. Wu, and H. Zheng. 2001. Loss of presenilin 1 is associated with enhanced beta-catenin signaling and skin tumorigenesis. *Proceedings of the National Academy of Sciences USA* 98 (19): 10863–68.

Xu, G., V. Gonzales, and D. R. Borchelt. 2002. Abeta deposition does not cause the aggregation of endogenous tau in transgenic mice. *Alzheimer Disease and Associated Disorders* 16 (3): 196–201.

Zamora, E., A. Handisurya, S. Shafti-Keramat, D. Borchelt, G. Rudow, K. Conant, C. Cox, J. C. Troncoso, and R. Kirnbauer. 2006. Papillomavirus-like particles are an effective platform for amyloid-beta immunization in rabbits and transgenic mice. *Journal of Immunology* 177 (4): 2662–70.

Zhao, X., A. Kuryatov, J. M. Lindstrom, J. Z. Yeh, and T. Natahashi. 2001. Nootropic drug modulation of neuronal nicotinic acetylcholine receptors in rat cortical neurons. *Molecular Pharmacology* 59:674–83.

CHAPTER 4

From the Periphery to the Center

Treating Noncognitive, Especially Behavioral and Psychological, Symptoms of Dementia

ANNETTE LEIBING, PH.D.

Medications have social as well as pharmacological histories that are part of an extensive matrix of ever-changing relations between humans and objects (Reynolds Whyte, van der Geest, and Hardon 2002; Kopytoff 2003). By following some of the entangled paths within such a matrix, one can catch a partial view of a biography of certain drugs. This chapter focuses on medications for Alzheimer's disease (AD), specifically the subset comprised of the *medications for noncognitive symptoms,* or what recently have been called behavioral and psychological symptoms of dementia (BPSD). This subset of Alzheimer medications has recently received considerable professional attention. I argue that the biography of a medication is deeply interwoven with the history of the symptoms and syndromes it is supposed to treat.

What happens when a shift occurs within such a biography—a shift that challenges former notions of classification, diagnosis, and pharmacological efficacy? How does this shift affect people, as well as the medication itself? Swallowing a pill *matters* in the sense that Judith Butler (1993) used the term—as "a process of materialization that stabilizes over time to produce the effect of boundary, fixity, and surface we call matter" (9). Taking a medication, then, entails the incorporation of not only its pharmacological ingredients but also its changing cultural narratives and truth claims. This, what one might call "cultural chemistry,"[1] affects people's lives—it matters. This kind of approach acknowledges the complex interplay of culture and biology as well as the unsteady boundaries between people and things.

To gloss, in the early 1990s, a person diagnosed with dementia who took a medication for highly troubling symptoms such as hallucinations or sleeping problems would have been thought to be treated for symptoms but not for the syndrome itself; the syndrome was largely considered a hopeless situation. At the time, hope lay in the development of future medications intervening in the *real* mechanism of dementia: the brain abnormalities linked to memory impairment.[2] By the year 2000, taking a pill for the same symptoms could mean, at least for some, treating dementia itself. This shift in the understanding of dementia, one could argue, detaches dementia from death—at least for a moment[3]—and at the same time acknowledges the importance of noncognitive symptoms in AD and related dementias. These latter symptoms had not previously received much attention from health professionals, largely due to the preponderance of the cognitive paradigm in dementia research. Clearly, there were, and are, a number of scholars who address the importance of studying and treating noncognitive symptoms (for example, Mace and Rabins 1999; Lawlor 1995); although some of these scholars are involved with biomedicine, more often than not this scholarship is associated with other health professions or the caregiving milieu—persons who generally spend more time with an Alzheimer's patient and/or are trained to acknowledge the context of their care as well as intrapsychic factors in mental health. Nevertheless, until about 2000, most official definitions of dementia, for example the *International Statistical Classification of Diseases and Related Health Problems*, 10th revision's (ICD-10) definition of the disease as the "deteriorization in both memory and thinking which is sufficient to impair personal activities of daily living" (quoted in Cummings and Khachaturian 1996), did not acknowledge the centrality of noncognitive symptoms.

Initially, my interest in this topic was piqued some years ago by a paradox revealed during interviews and participant observation in two psychogeriatric public health units, both located in university hospitals—one in Rio de Janeiro, Brazil (Leibing 2002, 2006), the other in Montreal, Canada. Some doctors conceived dementia as a disease of cognition, to which psychological and behavioral symptoms were peripheral. However, those peripheral symptoms were at the center of treatment, because only through them could clinicians intervene. Medicating cognition was and still is an issue of contention.[4]

Cognitive symptoms have been targeted by a specific pharmacological treatment since 1993, when tacrine (Cognex) entered the market. Tacrine offered a limited improvement (for some but not all persons with dementia),[5] at a high cost, and often with severe side effects. Today other, better-tolerated drugs for dementia are available, but some researchers deny both the efficacy and cost-effectiveness of even these drugs (for example, Trinh et al. 2003; *Harvard Mental Health Letter* 2004; NICE 2005; Royall 2005). Other researchers, many of whom are sponsored by the pharmaceutical industry (see *Harvard Mental Health Letter* 2004),[6] confirm the opposite—a statistically relevant improvement for patients with dementia.

In view of these contradictory opinions, doctors frequently continue to prescribe two classes of medication: those for certain psychiatric comorbidities and those meant to improve cognition, with the latter considered the "real dementia drugs."[7] That does not mean that both are viewed as "efficacious" by all doctors. As one prominent North American Alzheimer's researcher—someone who promotes these drugs—remarked at the beginning of 2000 (and after asking me to turn off the tape recorder): "I would give these [nootropic] pills to my mother, they don't hurt. But they don't help, either."

The drugs used for *behavioral and psychological symptoms* were originally put on the market for adult psychiatric morbidities. Although depression in dementia seems to have a relatively good outcome when treated with pharmaceuticals (see, for example, Petrovic et al. 2005), drug treatment of other behavioral or psychological symptoms often entails severe side effects such as increased confusion or apathy, and in some cases is simply ineffective (Treloar, Beck, and Patton 2001; Sink, Holden, and Yaffe 2005). An intensely discussed related example pertains to the side effects of the traditional antipsychotics[8]—the main reason for the marketing of the newer, pricier, atypical antipsychotics. These, however, have also recently come under attack, because atypical antipsychotics have "their 'own' adverse effects" (van Melick 2004) and, according to a recent study, are not more effective than *some* of the older ones (Lieberman et al. 2005). For example, the risk for ischemic stroke seems to be identical for older and newer antipsychotics (Gill et al. 2005).

Several generalizations made in this controversy are problematic. For example, two articles mentioned in the previous paragraph come to the conclusions that "the overall evidence base for the use of *psychotropic medication* remains poor" (Treloar, Beck, and Patton 2001, p. 445; emphasis added) and that "*pharmacological therapies* are not particularly effective for the management of neuropsychiatric symptoms of dementia" (Sink, Holden, and Yaffe

2005, p. 596; emphasis added). These statements gloss over the differences within the heterogeneous groups of symptoms and medications. This contrasts, for example, with the authors' differentiation with respect to another disorder and treatment: they explain that pharmaceutical treatments of depression are not only underutilized in elderly people with dementia but also "effective in treating multiple pathologies in frail elderly people" (Treloar et al. 2001, p. 445). A great part of the controversy over the use of psychotropics for dementia and BPSD is linked more specifically to antipsychotic drugs. Nevertheless, I argue below that the conceptual merging of all symptoms (as "BPSD") and all medications (as "psychotropics") does not help to elucidate the complexity of the problem of noncognitive symptoms of dementia.[9]

The recent focus on treating behavioral and psychological symptoms is tied to the growing evidence of the inefficacy of nootropic Alzheimer's drugs as well as to the longstanding need to address noncognitive symptoms more effectively. It also means a major, though not complete, break with the predominant understanding of dementia: that dementia is a disease that primarily affects memory and cognition. The marginalization of noncognitive symptoms within the "paradigm of memory" makes the new attention to these symptoms and their treatment into a topic of reflection on "cultural chemistry."

To tell the story of this partial break and its implications, I will first give a short overview of BPSD before discussing selected scientific and media texts that reflect the changing focus in dementia research.

Behavioral and Psychological Symptoms of Dementia

The historian of medicine Edward Shorter (1994) coined the term "symptom pool." This concept is useful for our discussion when understood as a tool for indicating that for certain syndromes, symptoms can be variously grouped together and may be experienced and explained differently in different historical times and places. Further, a syndrome can continue to be made up of the same symptoms, but the salience of one or several of the symptoms in a symptom pool may change, as in the case of BPSD in AD.

As G. E. Berrios (1986) observed, the nineteenth-century concept of "presbyophrenia," conceived of as a subtype of dementia, facilitated the inclusion of noncognitive symptoms such as confabulations, hyperactivity, disorientation, and elevated mood. Dementia was a much broader concept—an exogenous psychosis, a final pathway common to different psychiatric and neurological disorders and therefore one that included a number of noncognitive symptoms (Berrios 1990). But this older concept was abandoned by 1900, "and mania, depression, delusions, and hallucinations were increasingly given a psychodynamic interpretation" that separated them from dementia (Berrios 1989, p. 13).

The change from an organization based on psychosis to one based on cognition can be explained by a number of factors. First of all, by the 1860s, the clinical boundaries of dementia became narrower, restricted to the senile and arteriosclerotic dementias (Berrios 1989). The observation of institutionalized (and therefore more advanced) dementia patients led to an increased recognition of cognitive symptoms. (Berrios [1990] argues that in early stage dementia, symptoms are most commonly noncognitive.) Madness in general was increasingly defined in terms of intellect. And while "intellectual degeneration" such as memory loss could be measured by the 1890s through psychometric testing (Hacking 1999), other symptoms were not so easily quantifiable in the conceptions of the day. Hacking argues that medicine, to this day, "can easily define quantitative tests for memory loss" (1999, p. 237) but does not have scales to measure aggression or irrational jealousy (which were evident in AD as far back as Alois Alzheimer's first famous patient, Auguste D.).

It is impossible to follow here the changes in the different groupings of dementia's cognitive and noncognitive symptoms over the twentieth century; it can, however, be generalized that, at least since the 1970s, noncognitive symptoms were relegated to the periphery of syndromes like AD. As a consequence, and although biomedical research addresses some specific symptoms (depression, sleeping problems, sexual disinhibition, etc.), the treatment of noncognitive symptoms has often been addressed by nonpharmacological interventions such as pet therapy, light therapy, validation therapy, music, massage, therapeutic touch, aromatherapy, and multisensory stimulation (see, for example, Brack 2002; Forbes, Peacock, and Morgan 2005; Leibing 2005, 2006). And although these interventions were treating exactly those symptoms that in everyday life were much harder to deal with for family caregivers and health professionals than the cognitive ones, nonpharmacological interventions were often considered secondary for treating a medical condition such as dementia and received much less funding.[10]

Today these symptoms are often grouped together under the abbreviation BPSD. Following the International Psychogeriatric Association (IPA) Consensus Group, behavioral and psychological symptoms of dementia[11] can be described as the following:

- *Behavioral symptoms*: Usually identified on the basis of observation of the patient, including physical aggression, screaming, restlessness, agitation, wandering, culturally inappropriate behaviors, sexual disinhibition, hoarding, cursing, and shadowing.
- *Psychological symptoms*: Usually and mainly assessed on the basis of interviews with patients and relatives, these symptoms include anxiety, depressive mood, hallucinations, and delusions. (IPA 2002, p. 5)

The Consensus Group stated that up to 90 percent of patients with AD show BPSD-related symptoms (IPA 2002). In the majority of studies, these particular symptoms are responsible for an especially high burden to caregivers (and, one might add, for the suffering of the person experiencing those symptoms), leading to an earlier institutionalization of the person with dementia (Haupt 1999). It is therefore interesting to look at the recent history—or materialization—of BPSD and ask why it was only in the 1990s that BPSD became the focus of scientific attention despite the symptoms long being an important part of the symptom pool of AD and other dementias.

Shifting Boundaries

Part of the answer to this question lies not with AD in particular; a more general dynamic within the recent history of pharmaceuticals is that medications once delimited to specific applications are being more widely applied. On one hand, one can observe a focus on (and sometimes splitting off of) part of a disease category. On the other hand, this focus accompanies a broader, more inclusive notion of the effectiveness of certain drugs—or even a complete reworking of its relation to new disease categories.[12]

An example of this is found in the work of Jonathan Metzl and Joni Angel (2004). They show how selective serotonin reuptake inhibitor (SSRI) antidepressants were used for increasingly general distress. In 1987 SSRIs were approved by the FDA for the treatment of depression. Soon they were also prescribed for the treatment of obsessive-compulsive disorder, post-traumatic stress disorder, general anxiety disorder, and premenopausal dysphoric disorder. In addition to being prescribed for disorders found in the *Diagnostic and Statistical Manual of Mental Disorders* (APA 1994), SSRIs increasingly were defining "normative women's life events such as menstruation or child birth" (Metzl and Angel 2004, p. 577) and even problems with marriage as depressive illness. Other gender-related prescriptions included the use of SSRIs in men to deal with symptoms like aggression or hostility. While the SSRIs' target is on the one hand specific—serotonin neurotransmission—on the other hand it is general, through its amalgamation of previously separated disease categories and behaviors.

Likewise, Andrew Lakoff, writing about pharmaceuticals in the neoliberal Argentina of the 1990s, states that "rather than a precipitous increase in overall psychopharmaceutical consumption due to the economic crisis, the increase in antidepressant revenue could best be explained in terms of a specific tactic: the work by sales reps and opinion leaders to convince doctors to prescribe the newer antidepressants instead of tranquilizers for symptoms of stress, anxiety and depression" (Lakoff 2005, p. 211). The assumed increase in consumption of antidepressants as a reaction to crisis was in reality predominantly a shift to a more inclusive disease category.

In this article, noncognitive symptoms, and especially BPSD-related symptoms, will be followed from their role as a secondary symptom complex to a primary one, sometimes even relegating cognition into "the shadow"—although not without contestations. At the same time as this refocusing on noncognitive symptoms, there is an attempt to widen the applicability of certain dementia drugs: those conceived for cognition are now also effective for BPSD, and those developed for other psychiatric morbidities become redefined for certain BPSD symptoms when prescribed in a novel way.

The (Quasi)Materialization of BPSD

"Cognition and behaviour are independent and heterogeneous dimensions in Alzheimer's disease," states an Italian research group (Spaletta et al. 2004). And a *New York Times* article with the title "Alzheimer's Steals More than Memory" (Grady 2004) describes the same discovery. In this latter article we read the story of Mr. Rapport, a "kind and gentle" 71-year-old man who, because of AD, became "cunning, nasty, aggressive, [and] menacing." "Though memory loss is the best-known Alzheimer's symptom," observes the journalist, "the disease can also cause psychiatric problems that lead to profound changes in personality, mood and behavior." The argument continues, stating that "*only recently* has it become clear that emotional and behavioral troubles are nearly universal among people with Alzheimer's disease, and the problems are frequently intractable and *more upsetting to families than the mental slowing*" (emphasis added). Why has interest among biomedical researchers in these symptoms emerged only recently? The answer in the *New York*

Times article is shame: "Many families hide such symptoms, and perhaps as a result, psychiatric problems were long thought to affect only a minority of people with Alzheimer's disease or other types of dementia."

In this article, the use of medication is a more complex topic. Different views are presented by quoting four psychogeriatricians/geriatricians and adding vignettes from Mr. Rapport and his wife as well as from two other couples. The views can be summarized as follows:

1 No specific drug is approved for psychiatric problems in AD, and emotional disorders can be "difficult or impossible to treat." Many doctors use drugs originally designed for other pathologies (antipsychotics, for example).

2 With the exception of the major part of depressive disorders, "there is 'substantial and increasing controversy' about the use of antipsychotics and other drugs to treat behavioral problems in people with dementia."

3 Medications to slow memory loss (not specified) do not seem to have any effect (case report).

4 BPSD can be reduced via a new antipsychotic medication, Seroquel, produced by AstraZeneca,[13] and, in another case, by adding Ritalin to an Alzheimer's medication, Aricept, plus an antidepressant.

What was decisive in getting someone "out of her shell and get[ting] a spark out of her" (according to a quoted caregiver), was treating behavioral and emotional symptoms through a *novel* use of drugs formerly applied to other psychiatric disorders (especially recommended: atypical antipsychotics) and distrusting those medications developed for cognitive symptoms. In this narrative it is not the treatment of cognition but rather the treatment of BPSD that makes the difference.

This focus on medications targeting BPSD is not as clear-cut as it might appear in the *New York Times* article. In recent scientific texts about AD, one can find three major, coexisting positions on the treatment of symptoms in dementia: (a) medications conceived as acting on cognition are the principal treatment, and the treatment of behavioral and psychological symptoms is thought of as secondary, sometimes left to nonmedical interventions (Greve and O'Connor 2005)—the *conservative position;* (b) medications originally developed to act on cognition can be applied in a novel way to improve activities of daily living, quality of life, or BPSD[14] (Bullock 2005)—*new position 1;* and (c) psychotropic medications, especially atypical antipsychotics, are currently

treated. It may also be possible, especially in the early stages of dementia, to improve someone's memory with medication."[18]

But ADI's website also warns against traditional psychiatric drugs: "Other kinds of drugs [meaning other than nootropics] are sometimes useful for controlling some of the symptoms of Alzheimer's disease, such as sleeplessness and agitation. In general, however, the use of drugs such as sleeping pills or tranquillizers should be kept to a minimum if someone has Alzheimer's disease, as they can cause increased confusion." ADI nevertheless added to its website a factsheet on BPSD, presenting IPA data by quoting its principal authors.

Like ADI, the AA on its website defines AD as a disease of cognition with additional problems of personality and behavior: "Alzheimer's (*AHLZ-high-merz*) disease is a progressive brain disorder that gradually destroys a person's memory and ability to learn, reason, make judgments, communicate, and carry out daily activities. As Alzheimer's progresses, individuals may also experience changes in personality and behavior, such as anxiety, suspiciousness or agitation, as well as delusions or hallucinations." Treatment is conservatively described: no treatment exists for the core symptoms (memory impairment), but some interventions are recommended for the peripheral ones: "Although there is *currently no cure* for Alzheimer's, new treatments are on the horizon as a result of accelerating insight into the biology of the disease. Research has also shown that effective care and support can improve quality of life for individuals and their caregivers over the course of the disease from diagnosis to the end of life" (emphasis added).[19] Here "symptom management" is not linked to a concept like BPSD and, it seems, is also relatively separated from medical interventions—the choice of quoted articles suggests that "symptom management" is more of a topic for nonpharmacological interventions. Environmental interventions are preferred to psychotropic medications, which, following the AA, should be avoided, if possible.

Pushing for Materialization

At the beginning of the twentieth century, behavioral and psychological symptoms held a central position in the treatment plan for dementia. In Alois Alzheimer's first descriptions of his (presenile) dementia patients (see Maurer and Maurer 1998; Jürgs 1999) with their sometimes bizarre and sometimes sadly desperate behaviors, we see many behavioral and psychological symptoms addressed in his treatment plan. Alzheimer treats Auguste D., his first famous patient, with warm baths for her agitation ("balneology"), as well as outdoor physical activities, dietetic measures, gymnastics, and massage for sleeping problems. Hypnosis and "galvanization" (treatment of the head with light electric currencies) are further recommended. Sleeping pills are declared useful, but to be taken with care. By the end of the last century, this had definitely changed: pharmacological interventions were and are the predominant treatments for behavioral and psychological symptoms of dementia, despite a general consensus that nonpharmacological treatments should be employed before drugs are prescribed. This happened due to new scientific developments resulting in better choice and efficacy of medications, one might argue, or because of other reasons regarding the materialization of BPSD; some of them discussed in the following.

In 1998, for example, psychiatrist Alexander Kurz noted that the emergence of interest in BPSD could be attributed to the limited usefulness of cholinergic agents and nootropics in treating memory problems (Kurz 1998). However, five years later, he expressed his astonishment about the exclusive focus, in dementia research and treatment, on cognition. He warned that "considering Alzheimer disease only as a problem of memory and cognitive capacities ignores *the real dimensions of dementias.* Alzheimer has a second, dark and *still unknown side*: the dramatic changes in personality and character . . . For the relatives, these sudden behavior changes are much more scaring than the loss of memory" (Kurz 2003; trans. A. L.; emphasis added).

In 1998, Alexander Kurz wrote that BPSD was in large part a product of the pharmaceutical industry's needs but nonetheless had an important underlying cause. Five years later Kurz described BPSD as a discovery in need of pharmacological treatment. In the 2003 article, he recommended risperidone (an atypical antipsychotic) as effective against behavioral problems, as restoring activities of daily living, and as well tolerated. Kurz, who today works tightly with the drug enterprises, also argues that rivastigmine with its proven "efficacy and tolerability" shows "statistically significant benefits" for activities of daily living (Kurz et al. 2004). However, others, like Ballard et al. (2005), come to the conclusion that "neither quetiapine [atypical antipsychotic] nor rivastigmine [nootropic] are effective in the treatment of agitation in people with dementia in institutional care. Compared with placebo, quetiapine is associated with significantly greater cognitive decline" (p. 874). This kind of contradiction among dementia researchers—and many other examples could be given—reveals at least partly the struggle for the truths of dementia medications. Of course, the Ballard et al. study focused on one symptom, agitation, which nevertheless is one of the most important symptoms in BPSD (Gauthier 2005), and Kurz et al. (2004) talked about activities of daily living, a much more general notion within BPSD. Nonetheless, it is astonishing that some studies clearly recommend this kind of medication when others do not and even warn against dangers associated with them.

These examples demonstrate, once again, that arguments made in the controversy over using medications for BPSD merge concepts. The polemics tend to not specify the many symptoms subsumed under BPSD. This means that the following things become blurry: positive and negative outcomes, heterogeneous concepts such as "quality of life" and "functionality," and cognitive, behavioral, and psychological dimensions of AD.

The pharmaceutical industry most clearly advocated for the new concepts and medications, advocacy that required not only a new understanding of dementia but also a new way of defining effectiveness. While cognition is not being written out of the definition of dementia, the focus on the noncognitive elements of the disease sometimes overshadows that on cognition because the measured noncognitive outcomes are often nonspecific. To follow this shift, I will provide some specific examples to illustrate the redefinition of part of the dementia syndrome and an increasing nonspecific understanding of effectiveness, generally subsumed under labels as "activities of daily living," "functionality," or "quality of life."

While the first drug to treat AD, tacrine, was described as improving memory,[20] newer drugs are linked to the improvement of activities of daily living and psychological and behavioral problems. For example, Pfizer's Aricept website prominently displays the claim that the drug can help with behavior problems in mild to moderate Alzheimer's: "Some caregivers may experience problems with their loved one's behavior, caused by Alzheimer's. One study of mild to moderate patients showed that ARICEPT improved patient behavior compared to a placebo. Caregivers with a loved one on ARICEPT experienced less distress dealing with those behaviors."[21]

Likewise, Janssen-Cilag defines dementia by emphasizing the patient's daily activities as well as noting the patients' caregivers: "Dementia, a progressive brain dysfunction, leads to a gradually increasing restriction *of daily activities*. The most well-known type of dementia is Alzheimer's disease. Dementia not only affects patients but also those surrounding them, as most patients require care in the long-term" (emphasis added).[22]

Janssen-Cilag has marketed the most recent cholinesterase inhibitor, Reminyl (galantamine), as helping to maintain the performance of activities of daily living, although the substance was previously conceived as enhancing memory and cognition:

> Data published in the July issue of the *Journal of the American Geriatrics Society* suggest that treatment with Reminyl® (galantamine hydrobromide) may help to maintain the ability of patients with mild to moderate Alzheimer's disease to perform certain activities of daily living (ADLs), such as grooming, walking and being aware of current events . . .
>
> "Clinical trials most often focus on cognitive testing to assess the progression of the disease," explained Douglas Galasko, M.D., professor, Department of Neurosciences, University of California at San Diego. "However, loss of functional abilities is associated with increased caregiver burden, and once lost, these abilities rarely are recovered. Maintaining a patient's ability to carry out daily activities has the potential to benefit both patients and caregivers."[23]

Janssen also marketed risperidone, the atypical antipsychotic that was originally conceived to treat schizophrenia. Sales of atypical antipsychotics doubled in the United States between 2000 and 2003 to $8.08 billion, according to IMS Health, an agency providing market analysis on the pharmaceutical industry. It should also be noted that these atypical antipsychotics, which quickly became blockbuster drugs (see Lenzer 2005), are expensive—the costs for a month's supply range from $100 to $300, while older antipsychotics cost less than a quarter per pill (Petersen 2004).

Resistances

While some knowledge producers such as the Alzheimer's Association are not opposed to BPSD, they also do not embrace the idea as wholeheartedly as some other groups—most notably some researchers,[24] the IPA, and part of the pharmaceutical industry. There are others, though, who express clear resistances to the concept of BPSD, some of them already mentioned above (for example, Lenzer 2005). Two further examples of resistances are taken from letters to the editor of medical journals. These examples illustrate different instances of the debate on BPSD, as one example dates from 1999 and the other from 2004.

The first letter, to the *British Medical Journal,* is written by four English Alzheimer's researchers (Bentham et al. 1999). The letter comments on two previously published articles[25] that added further evidence to the limited usefulness of Exelon (rivastigmine, a nootropic) in treating cognition. In these articles, however, a new era of treating noncognitive symptoms as core symptoms is heralded, along with claims for improved *functionality* with the use of Exelon. The authors of the letter questioned what had actually been measured in these previous studies, asserting that it was not functionality but, rather, quality of life. The authors called attention to the fuzzy category of "functionality." "Moreover," the authors continued, "Rösler et al. misrepresent the small improvement in progressive deteriorization score seen with rivastigmine . . . by citing in the discussion that one third of patients taking higher dose rivastigmine attained at least 10% improvement in score without noting that 20% of placebo patients also improved to this extent." Bentham et al. came to the conclusion that "it remains unclear whether cholinesterase inhibitors produce sufficient benefit in Alzheimer's disease to justify their widespread use." In a subsequent letter, the first of the criticized authors, Michael Rösler, denied the critiques. Rösler, like three of his coauthors, was employed by Novartis, the producer of the drug in question.

The second example is a letter written by a Dutch research team (van Iersel et al. 2004) to the editor of the *International Journal of Geriatric Psychiatry*. This team called BPSD a marketing tool: "The term 'BPSD' served its goal by marketing the relevant problem of psychiatric co-morbidity and behavioural problems in dementia among scientists, clinicians and industry." The article was especially preoccupied by the increasing merging of the heterogeneous dementia symptoms into "BPSD." The authors listed a number of psychiatric comorbidities that cannot be addressed in its specificity by a category like BPSD and recommended avoiding this label altogether. Also, Ballard and Cream (2005) wrote that "the results [of studies on treating BPSD] are almost impossible to interpret, as the studies group together a range of dissimilar behavioral and psychiatric symptoms, which probably have different etiologies" (6).

> What matters most should never be at the mercy of what matters least.
> —*Johann Wolfgang von Goethe*

The history of BPSD could be interpreted as a history of the search for effectiveness. As in the quote from Goethe above, effectiveness can be considered as being at the mercy of what matters least (for some)—primarily economic interests and bad faith. In this interpretation, the emergence of BPSD and the widening of certain drugs' applications are "marketing goals," separate from a humanistic search for the patient's well-being.[26] But this interpretation reflects only part of the history. Before reaching a final conclusion, let us revisit two other strands of the story.[27]

First, many studies demonstrated that the treatment of noncognitive symptoms entails a better outcome. Can all these studies be reduced to the economic interests of the pharmaceutical industry (and its academic helpers)? The positive personal experiences of a great number of patients and their families with these drugs are difficult to elide. Many studies pointed out the high number of placebo responses in Alzheimer's medications (for example, Brodaty 1996; McShane and Gormley 2002). Shall we reduce these experiences to a mere placebo effect, or would the concept of "mattering" be more appropriate, because it includes what I initially called "cultural chemistry"? The reduction of these experiences to the placebo effect, as traditionally understood,[28] would deny reality. The experiences and reality of the body, in its historical and contextualized manifestations, is perhaps better recognized using the trope of cultural chemistry.

A second point is that the history of noncognitive symptoms has been less visible than other aspects of dementia and needs to be studied more thoroughly to better trace this social biography. How does the treatment of noncognitive symptoms and their transformation into BPSD matter to people? This chapter provides only an introduction into this topic, and more phenomenological research is needed.

Finally, I am not aware of studies that critically trace the social history of concepts such as "quality of life" or "functionality." While BPSD is a controversial category in part because of the danger of merging many heterogenous symptoms, "quality of life" and "functionality"—both increasingly the outcome criteria for Alzheimer's medications—can be criticized for merging effect, improvement, and outcome of such studies: "Improvements in BPSD were commonly seen with atypical antipsychotics and with placebo. In the clinical course of BPSD, symptoms often persist over periods as long as a year, and the improvements with placebo may result from nonpharmacological cointerventions received by all trial participants. Further research is needed to identify effective nonpharmacological interventions for BPSD. Regression to the mean may also contribute to the apparent placebo effect (that is, patients are enrolled into trials when BPSD symptoms are most severe)" (Lee et al. 2004).

The astonishing part of the history of BPSD is not that it has been "discovered" only in the 1990s, but that its antecedents and their treatments—most notably nonpharmacological interventions—are rarely mentioned (see chapter 11 in this volume). However, less biomedically oriented health professionals have often protested the definition of personhood in exclusively cognitive terms (see, for example, Kitwood 1997; Basting 2003) and suggested nonpharmacological interventions. These treatments might be marginalized if BPSD becomes further linked to pharmacological interventions. The official history of BPSD tells the story of a dark period of ignorance, although this period is variously characterized by shame (as in the *New York Times* article) or by the use of generally harmful medications such as the older antipsychotics. But the need to pay more attention to noncognitive symptoms has a long history, which dates at least to Alois Alzheimer. BPSD can be seen as an end product addressing a real need in mental health care—the treatment of noncognitive symptoms, which cause great suffering, and which had been increasingly deemphasized in the biomedical discussions of dementia care. But if one acknowledges the real need to pay more attention to noncognitive symptoms in dementia (for example, Cohen-Mansfield and Mintzer 2005)—which would mean that the marketing of BPSD was positive—one of the possible consequences of this new way of clustering symptoms as BPSD is a possible foggy notion of these symptoms due to merging instead of putting them more into the light. As McShane and Gormley (2002) warn, "Drugs are widely and often excessively used to manage BPSD. The placebo response rate is high in randomized studies. This may be because of the increased attention of triallists and the natural tendency of BPSD to resolve" (241). But if BPSD stands increasingly for dementia itself, what has been resolved may continue nonetheless to be "treated."

NOTES

1. The merging of a material entity with its environment has been discussed by others. For instance, Andrew Barry (2005) talks about "informed materials" and gives the example of molecules produced by pharmaceutical laboratories. These "informed materials" are "rich in information about their (global) legal and economic, as well as their chemical relations to other molecules" (64). Barry argues that a molecule embodies information, with, for example, a different identity in the laboratory than in a body.

2. This attitude of mitigating a hopeless situation is explicitly and implicitly stated, up to the present day, in numerous texts dealing with the treatment of Alzheimer's disease. It is generally stated that nothing can be done, except for bettering the quality of life of dementia patients (see, for instance, the examples given below).

3. Zygmunt Bauman observed that, recently, life-threatening diseases have been "split into small-scale worries, each one separately removable . . . Each particular case of death . . . can be resisted, postponed or avoided altogether . . . I can do nothing to defy mortality. But I can do quite a lot to avoid a blood clot or a lung cancer" (1992, p. 5).

4. Alzheimer's drugs can be roughly divided into three groups:
    1. those conceived as enhancing cognition:
        a. cholinesterase inhibitors
            i. Reminyl (galantamine), released in 2001 by Janssen
            ii. Exelon (rivastigmine), released in 2000 by Novartis
            iii. Aricept (donepezil hydrochloride), released in 1996 by Eisai and Pfizer
            iv. Cognex (tacrine), released in 1993 by Warner-Lambert (not used anymore)
        b. NMDA receptor antagonist: Namenda (memantine), released in 2003 by Merz/Lundbeck
    2. newer psychiatric medications
        a. atypical antipsychotics
            i. Risperdal (risperidone; Janssen, 1993)
            ii. Zyprexa (olanzapine; Eli Lilly, 1996)
            iii. Seroquel (quetiapine; AstraZeneca, 1997)
        b. anticonvulsant
        c. antidepressants
        d. benzodiazepan
    3. so-called alternative medications: vitamin E, ginkgo biloba, and others.

5. See, for example, Adam Hedgecoe's (2004) discussion of the APOE-Tacrine hypothesis.

6. See the strong reactions to the British NICE guidelines that no longer recommended dementia (nootropic) drugs because of their low cost-effectiveness (for example, Jackson 2005). Some Alzheimer's groups, working directly with families, support the continued use of Alzheimer's medications.

7. In Brazil, these nootropics were available to only the elite who could afford them or to those families who took part in clinical trials. In the following I shall call "nootropics" those drugs developed to act on memory and cognition (number 1 in note 4 of this chapter).

8. Some side effects of traditional antipsychotics are called "extrapyramidal symptoms" (EPS), which can involve tremors, involuntary movements, rigidity, body restlessness, muscle contractions, and changes in heart rate. These symptoms are highly disturbing and can even be fatal if untreated (neuroleptic malignant syndrome). Atypical antipsychotics, which were first developed for schizophrenia, are called "atypical" because they do not have the typical adverse effects of the first-generation antipsychotics (but see Lieberman et al. 2005).

9. But see, for example, Lyketsos, Breitner, and Rabins (2001), who suggest to specify BPSD by dividing it into affective and psychotic symptoms. Also, nonpharmacological interventions are generally applied to more specific symptoms.

10. The growing importance of behavioral pharmacology, which had its beginnings in the 1950s with the work of Harvard scientists Dews, Kelleher, and Morse and was influenced by the thinking of I. Pavlov and B. F. Skinner (see Barrett 2002), might have had an influence on the separation of behavioral symptoms from other symptoms and the importance given to pharmacological treatment.

11. Earlier abbreviations were BDD (behavioral disturbances of dementia), followed by BPSSD (behavioral and psychological signs and symptoms of dementia) and then BPSD. In this chapter, the use of the expression "BPSD-related symptoms" will sound redundant. But because BPSD has become something like a syndrome itself (see below), it makes sense to talk about symptoms related to this new category in which the symptoms *are* the syndrome.

12. One could read in the Montreal newspaper *La Presse* an article about the awareness of new "polyvalent medications," effective for a variety of apparently unrelated diseases (*La Presse*, January 23, 2005). The German weekly newspaper *Die Zeit* published an article about "off-label-users"—those patients who had medications prescribed for a disease for which the drug was not (yet) approved. This practice became an issue not necessarily because of the ethical dilemma of untested prescribing practices but because health insurance companies, with increasingly tight budgets, started to refuse to pay for these off-label uses (Wagner and Albrecht 2005).

13. Seroquel was the only drug directly recommended in this article. It seems to be the mildest of the new atypical antipsychotics, avoiding the highly disturbing side effects of conventional antipsychotics. Pierre Tariot's widely quoted study on Seroquel was financed by Astra-Zeneca, the producers of Seroquel.

14. It should be stated that BPSD should not be conflated with activities of daily living or quality of life, which can be affected by cognitive symptoms as well. However, all these concepts change the focus from predominantly cognition toward noncognitive symptoms. Regarding quality of life, for example, the influential study by Lawton (1991, quoted in Ettema et al. 2005), links quality of life (QOL) to "behavioral symptoms, agitation, depression, self-care abilities, meaningful time-use, social engagement, and emotional expression" (Ettema et al. 2005, p. 358).

15. It should be emphasized that Landsdowne stands for the beginning of the specific constellation of symptoms in dementia called BPSD, of its perceptions as a less peripheral phenomenon, and of BPSD as a new category—not as the beginning of the perception of behavioral and psychological symptoms of dementia in general.

16. BEHAVE-AD, the Behavioral Pathology in Alzheimer's Disease Rating Scale, was developed by Barry Reisberg and his research group.

17. "Alzheimer's disease . . . destroys brain cells and nerves disrupting the transmitters that carry messages in the brain, particularly those responsible for storing memories . . . During the course of Alzheimer's disease, nerve cells die in particular regions of the brain. The brain shrinks as gaps develop in the temporal lobe and hippocampus, which are responsible for storing and retrieving new information. This in turn affects people's ability to remember, speak, think and make decisions" (ADI website, www.alz.co.uk/alzheimers/alzheimers.html).

18. ADI website, "Treatments," www.alz.co.uk/alzheimers/treatment.html.

19. AA website, www.alz.org/AboutAD/WhatIsAD.asp.

20. "Tacrine (TAK-reen) is used to treat the symptoms of mild to moderate Alzheimer's disease. Tacrine will not cure Alzheimer's disease, and it will not stop the disease from getting worse. However, tacrine can improve *thinking ability* in some patients with Alzheimer's disease" (www.drugs.com/cons/tacrine.html [1998]; emphasis added).

21. Pfizer, Inc., "On Aricept: What to Expect" (2008). www.aricept.com/expect_aricept.html.

22. Janssen-Cilag, "What Is Dementia?" (2008). www.janssen-cilag.com/disease/detail.jhtml?itemname=dementia_about.

23. Janssen Pharmaceutica, "Reminyl (Galantamine) May Help Patients with Alzheimer's Disease to Maintain Activities of Daily Living" (2004). www.pslgroup.com/dg/244C9E.htm.

24. Attention needs to be paid to diversity within various groups: researchers sponsored by industry, the industry itself, and the IPA, for example. For instance, one may want to distinguish among (1) researchers paid by the pharmacological industry to defend certain medications, as described in the *Harvard Mental Health Letter* (2004), (2) researchers who are paid by the industry and do impartial research, and (3) researchers supporting the BPSD concept because of their (sometimes longstanding) preoccupation with noncognitive symptoms in dementia. The same diversity needs to be acknowledged as existing in the IPA and "the" pharmacological industry.

25. The two articles are Rösler et al. (1999) and Corey-Bloom et al. (1998).

26. A typical example of this kind of thinking is manifest in an article in the *Senior Journal* (2004). The article starts with the statement "There is no effective treatment that can stop the progression of Alzheimer's disease," and continues by quoting Frost and Sullivan (a health care marketing research company), which calculated that the Alzheimer's medication market nevertheless generated "revenues of $514 million in 2000," and that $2.4 billion of profit were expected for 2006.

27. While I address the concerns of the anonymous referees (whom I thank herewith for their suggestions), a discussion has been published in the IPA journal *International Psychogeriatrics* (Osvaldo et al. 2005) that includes a good documentation of the controversy in two articles with opposing sympathies.

28. But see the more critical discussions in *The Placebo Effect* (Harrington 1997).

REFERENCES

Alzheimer, A 1907. Über eine eigenartige Erkrankung der Hirnrinde. *Allg. Z. f. Psychiatrie und Psychisch-Gerichtliche Medizin* 64:146–48.

American Psychiatric Association. 1994. *Diagnostic and statistical manual of mental disorders,* 4th ed. Washington, DC: APA.

Ballard C., and J. Cream. 2005. Drugs used to relieve behavioral symptoms in people with dementia or an unacceptable chemical cosh? Argument. *International Psychogeriatrics* 17 (1): 4–12

Ballard, C., M. Margallo-Lana, E. Juszczak, S. Douglas, A. Swann, A. Thomas, and J. O'Brien, et al. 2005. Quetiapine and rivastigmine and cognitive decline in Alzheimer's disease: Randomized double blind placebo controlled trial. *British Medical Journal* 330:874.

Barrett, J. E. 2002. The emergence of behavioral pharmacology. *Molecular Interventions* 2 (8): 470–75.

Barry, A. 2005. Pharmaceutical matters: The invention of informed material. *Theory, Culture and Society* 22 (1): 51–69.

Basting, A. D. 2003. Looking back from loss: Views of the self in Alzheimer's disease. *Journal of Aging Studies* 17:87–99.

Baumann, Z. 1992. *Morality, immorality and other life strategies.* Cambridge: Polity Press.

Bentham, P., R. Gray, E. Sellwood, and J. Raftery 1999. Effectiveness of rivastigmine in Alzheimer's disease. *British Medical Journal* 319 (7210): 640–41.

Berrios, G. E. 1986. Presbyophrenia: The rise and fall of a concept. *Psychological Medicine* 16: 267–75.

———. 1989. Non-cognitive symptoms and the diagnosis of dementia: Historical and clinical aspects. *British Journal of Psychiatry* 154 (suppl. 4): 11–16.

———. 1990. Memory and the cognitive paradigm of dementia during the nineteenth century: A conceptual history. In *Lectures on the history of psychiatry, the Squibb series*, ed. R. M. Murray and T. H. Turner, 194–211. London: Gaskell.

Brack, H. 2002. A person-centered approach to dementia care. In *The diversity of Alzheimer's disease: Different approaches and contexts*, ed. A. Leibing and L. Scheinkman, 211–30. Rio de Janeiro: CUCA-IPUB.

Brodaty, H. 1996. Tacrine in the treatment of Alzheimer's disease. *Australian Prescriber* 19:14–7.

Bullock, R. 2005. Treatment of behavioural and psychiatric symptoms in dementia: Implications of recent safety warnings. *Current Medical Research Opinion* 21 (1): 1–10.

Butler, J. 1993. *Bodies that matter: On the discursive limits of "sex."* New York: Routledge.

Cohen-Mansfield, J., and J. Mintzer. 2005. Time for change: The role of nonpharmacological interventions in treating behavior problems in nursing home residents with dementia. *Alzheimer Disease and Associated Disorders* 19 (1): 37–40.

Corey-Bloom, J., et al., for the ENA 713 B352 Study. 1998. A randomised trial evaluating the efficacy and safety of ENA 713 (rivastigmine tartrate), a new acetylcholinesterase inhibitor, in patients with mild to moderately severe Alzheimer's disease. *International Journal of Geriatric Psychopharmacology* 1:55–65.

Cummings, J., and Z. Khachaturian. 1996. Definitions and diagnostic criteria. In *Clinical Diagnosis and Management of Alzheimer's Disease*, ed. S. Gauthier. London: Martin Dunitz.

Ekelin, A., and P. Elovaara. 2001. Discourses and cracks: A case study of information technology and writing women in a regional context. In: *Heterogeneous Hybrids, Information Technology in Texts and Practices*, ed. P. Elovaara, 17–36. Malmö: Blekinge Institute of Technology.

Ettema, Teake P., R.-M. Dröes, J. de Lange, M. E. Ooms, G. J. Mellenbergh, and M. J. Ribbe. 2005. The concept of quality of life in dementia in the different stages of the disease. *International Psychogeriatrics* 17 (3): 353–70.

Finkel, S. I. 1996. New focus on behavioral and psychological signs and symptoms of dementia. *International Psychogeriatrics* 8 (suppl. 3): 215–18.

Forbes, D. A., S. Peacock, and D. Morgan 2005. Nonpharmacological management of agitated behaviours associated with dementia. *Geriatrics Aging* 8 (4): 26–30.

Gauthier, S. 2005. Drugs for Alzheimer's disease and related dementias *British Medical Journal* 330:857–58.

Gill, S., et al. 2005. Atypical antipsychotic drugs and risk of ischaemic stroke: Population based retrospective cohort study. *British Medical Journal* 330 (7489): 445.

Grady, D. 2004. Alzheimer's steals more than memory. *New York Times*, November 2.

Greve, M., and D. O'Connor. 2005. A survey of Australian and New Zealand old age psychiatrists' preferred medications to treat behavioral and psychological symptoms of dementia (BPSD). *International Psychogeriatrics* 17 (2): 195–205.

Hacking, I. 1999. *The Social construction of what?* Cambridge, Mass.: Harvard University Press.

Harrington, A., ed. 1997. *The placebo effect: An interdisciplinary exploration.* Cambridge, Mass.: Harvard University Press.

Hartikainen, S., T. Rahkonen, H. Kautiainen, and R. Sulkava. 2003. Use of psychotropics among home-dwelling nondemented and demented elderly. *International Journal of Geriatric Psychiatry* 18 (12): 1135–41.

Harvard Mental Health Letter. 2004. Alzheimer's Drugs: Are they worth it? (November). www .health.harvard.edu.

Haupt, M. 1999. Der Verlauf von Verhaltensstörungen und ihre psychosoziale Behandlung bei Demenzkranken. *Zeitschrift für Gerontologie und Geriatrie* 32 (3): 159–66.

Hedgecoe, A. M. 2004. *The politics of personalised medicine: Pharmacogenetics in the clinic.* Cambridge: Cambridge University Press.

International Psychogeriatric Association. T. S. Radebaugh, N. Buckholtz, and Z. Khachaturian, guest eds. 1996a. Behavioral approaches to the treatment of Alzheimer's disease: Research strategies. *International Psychogeriatrics* 8 (suppl. 1).

———. S. I. Finkel, guest ed. 1996b. Research methodologic issues in evaluating behavioral disturbances of dementia. *International Psychogeriatrics* 8 (suppl. 2).

———. S. I. Finkel, guest ed. 1996c. Behavioral and psychological signs and symptoms of dementia: Implications for research and treatment. *International Psychogeriatrics* 8 (suppl. 3).

———. S. I. Finkel, E. M. Richter ,and C. M. Clary, guest eds. 1999. Comparative efficacy and safety of sertraline versus nortriptyline in major depression in patients 70 and older. *International Psychogeriatrics* 11 (1): 85–99.

———. S. I. Finkel and A. Burns, guest eds. 2000. Behavioral and psychological symptoms of dementia (BPSD): A clinical and research update. *International Psychogeriatrics* 12 (suppl.1).

———. 2002. *Behavioral and psychological symptoms of dementia (BPSD): Educational pack.* Skokie, Ill.: International Psychogeriatric Association.

———. O. P. Almeida, L. Flicker, and N. T. Lautenschlager, guest eds. 2005. Uncommon causes of dementia. *International Psychogeriatrics.* 17 (suppl 1).

Jackson, J. 2005. Dementia Disaster. Alzheimer Scotland publications online. www.alzscot.org/ media/demdisaster.html.

Jürgs, M. 1999. *Alzheimer, Spurensuche im Niemandsland.* München: List.

Kilian, R., M. C. Angermeyer, and T. Becker. 2004. Methodische Grundlagen naturalistischer Beobachtungsstudien zur ökonomischen Evaluation der Neuroleptikabehandlung bei schizophrenen Erkrankungen (Methodolocical Issues of Naturalistic Observational Studies on the Economic Evaluation of Schizophrenia Drug Treatment). *Das Gesundheitswesen* 66 (8–9): 180–85.

Kitwood, T. 1997. *Dementia Reconsidered: The person comes first.* Buckingham: Open University Press.

Kopytoff, I. 2003 [1986]. The cultural biography of things: Commodization as process. In *The Social Life of Things, Commodities in cultural perspective,* ed. A. Appadurai, 64–94. Cambridge: Cambridge University Press.

Kurz, A. 1998. "BPSSD": Verhaltensstörungen bei Demenz, Ein neues diagnostisches und therapeutisches Konzept. *Nervenarzt* 69 (3): 269–73.

———. 2003. Altern in Würde. www.altern-in-wuerde.de/web/aiw_inhalte/de/sonderpresse dienstalzheimer-demenzapril2003.htm.

Kurz, A., M. Farlow, P. Quarg, and R. Spiegel. 2004. Disease stage in Alzheimer disease and treatment effect of rivastigmine. *Alzheimer Disease and Associated Disorders* 18 (3): 123–28.

Lakoff, A. 2005. The private life of numbers: Pharmaceutical marketing in post-welfare Argentina. In *Global assemblages, technology, politics, and ethics as anthropological problems*, ed. A. Ong and S. J. Collier, 194–213. Malden, Mass.: Blackwell Publications.

La Presse. 2005. Des médicaments polyvalents. Cahier "Actuel," January 23, p. 3.

Latour, B. 1999. *Pandora's hope: Essays on the reality of science studies.* Cambridge, Mass.: Harvard University Press.

Lawlor, B. A., ed. 1995. *Behavioral complications in Alzheimer's disease.* Washington, D.C.: American Psychiatric Press.

Lee, P. E., S. Gill, M. Freedman, S. E. Bronskill, M. P. Hillmer, and P. A. Rochon. 2004. Atypical antipsychotic drugs in the treatment of behavioural and psychological symptoms of dementia: systematic review. *British Medical Journal* 329 (7457; July 10): 75.

Leibing, A. 2002. Flexible hips? On Alzheimer's disease and aging in Brazil. *Journal of Cross-Cultural Gerontology* 17:213–32.

———. 2005. La maladie d'Alzheimer et "la personne intérieure." *Cahiers de recherche sociologiques,* "Nouveau malaise dans la civilisation: Regards sociologique sur la santé mentale, la souffrance psychique et la psychologisation," 41/42 (4): 147–68.

———. 2006. Divided gazes: Alzheimer disease, the person within, and death in life. In *Thinking about senility: Culture, loss, and the anthropology of senility,* ed. A. Leibing and L. Cohen. New Brunswick, N.J.: Rutgers University Press.

Lenzer, J. 2005. FDA warns about using antipsychotic drugs for dementia. *British Medical Journal* 330:922 (23 April).

Lieberman, J. A., T. S. Stroup, J. P. McEvoy, M. S. Swartz, R. A. Rosenheck, D. O. Perkins, R. S. E. Keefe, et al. 2005. Effectiveness of antipsychotic drugs in patients with chronic schizophrenia. *New England Journal of Medicine* 353:1209–23.

Lyketsos, C. G., J. C. S. Breitner, and P. V. Rabins. 2001. An evidence-based proposal for the classification of neuropsychiatric disturbance in Alzheimer's disease. *International Journal of Geriatric Psychiatry* 16 (11): 1037–42.

Mace, N. L., and P. V. Rabins. 1999. *The 36-hour day: A family guide to caring for persons with Alzheimer disease, related dementing illnesses, and memory loss in later life.* Baltimore: Johns Hopkins University Press.

Maurer, K., and U. Maurer. 1998. *Alzheimer, das Leben eines Arztes und die Karriere einer Krankheit.* Munich: Piper.

McShane, J. R., and N. Gormley. 2002. Assessment and management of behavioural and psychological symptoms of dementia (BPSD). In *Principles and practice of geriatric psychiatry,* 2nd ed., ed. J. R. M. Copeland, D. Blazer, and M. T. Abou-Saleh. London: John Wiley & Sons.

Metzl, J. M., and J. Angel. 2004. Assessing the impact of SSRI antidepressants on popular notions of women's depressive illness. *Social Science and Medicine* 58:577–84.

NICE. 2005. NICE appraisal of Alzheimer's drugs. www.nice.org.uk/page.aspx?o=248137.

Petersen, A. 2004. New treatments for Alzheimer's symptoms: To curb aggression, paranoia in dementia patients, doctors turn to schizophrenia drugs. *Wall Street Journal,* August 26.

Petrovic, M., B. De Paepe, and L. van Bortel. 2005. Pharmacotherapy of depression in old age. *Acta Clinica Belgica* 60 (3): 150–56.

Potkin, S. G. 2002. The ABC of Alzheimer's disease: ADL and improving day-to-day functioning of patients. *International Psychogeriatrics* 14 (suppl. 1): 7–26.

Rabins, P. V., and C. G. Lyketsos. 2005. Antipsychotic drugs in dementia: What should be made of the risks? *JAMA* 294 (15): 1963–65.

Reisberg, B., I. Monteiro, I. Boksay, S. Auer, C. Torossian, and S. Kenowsky. 2000. Do many of the behavioral and psychological symptoms of dementia constitute a distinct clinical syndrome? Current evidence using the BEHAVE-AD. *International Psychogeriatrics* 12 (suppl. 1): 155–64.

Reynolds Whyte, S., S. van der Geest, and A. Hardon. 2002. *Social Lives of Medicines.* Cambridge: Cambridge University Press.

Rösler, M., et al., on behalf of the B303 Exelon study group. 1999. Efficacy and safety of rivastigmine in patients with Alzheimer's disease: International randomised controlled trial. *British Medical Journal* 318 (7184): 633–39.

Royall, D. R. 2005. The emperor has no clothes: Dementia treatment on the eve of the aging era. *Journal of the American Geriatrics Society* 53 (1): 163–64.

Senior Journal. 2004. Alzheimer's disease drug revenues headed to $2.4 billion in 2006. http://seniorjournal.com/NEWS/Alzheimers/03–05–01AlzMedicine.htm.

Shorter, E. 1994. *Moderne Leiden, Zur Geschichte der psychosomatischen Krankheiten,* trans. Kurt Neff. Frankfurt: Rowohlt. Originally published as *From paralysis to fatigue* (New York: Free Press, 1992).

Sink, K. M., K. F. Holden, and K. Yaffe. 2005. Pharmacological treatment of neuropsychiatric symptoms of dementia: A review of the evidence. *JAMA* 293 (5): 596–608.

Spaletta, G., F. Baldinetta, I. Buccione, L. Fadda, R. Perri, S. Sclamana, L. Serra, and C. Caltagirone. 2004. Cognition and behaviour are independent and heterogeneous dimensions in Alzheimer's disease. *Journal of Neurology* 251:688–95.

Taylor, M., M. Turner, L. Watt, D. Brown, M. Martin, and K. Fraser. 2005. Atypical antipsychotics in the real world: A naturalistic comparative outcome study. *Scottish Medical Journal* 50 (3): 102–6.

Treloar, A., S. Beck, and C. Paton. 2001. Administering medicines to patients with dementia and other organic cognitive syndromes. *Advances in Psychiatric Treatment* 7:444–52.

Trinh, N. H., J. Hoblyn, S. Mohanty, and K. Yaffe. 2003. Efficacy of cholinesterase inhibitors in the treatment of neuropsychiatric symptoms and functional impairment in Alzheimer disease: A meta-analysis. *JAMA* 289 (2): 210–16.

Van Iersel, M., R. Koopmans, S. Zuidema, and M. O. Rikkert. 2004. Do not use "BPSD" if you want to be cited. *International Psychogeriatrics* 19 (8): 803–4.

Van Melick, E. J. 2004. Atypical antipsychotics in the elderly. *Tijdschrift voor Gerontologie en Geriatrie* 35 (6): 240–45 (abstract).

Wagner, B., and H. Albrecht. 2005. Einnahme nur nach Genehmigung. *Die Zeit* 10 (March 3): "Wissen," 1.

Wancata, J. 2004. Efficacy of risperidone for treating patients with behavioral and psychological symptoms of dementia. *International Psychogeriatrics* 16 (1): 107–15.

PART II

THE USE AND EVALUATION
OF DRUGS FOR DEMENTIA

The impact of Alzheimer's disease (AD), it is often noted, extends far beyond the person with dementia. Family members facing the significant emotional and physical challenges of being with and caring for loved ones with dementia are typically characterized as second victims of the disease. But clinicians, professional caregivers, and the institutions in which they work face their own set of challenges in struggling to manage the problems of patients with dementia and their families, and society faces the economic and social challenges of a rising tide of dementia as the baby boom generation ages.

Much less attention has been paid to what this broad circle of impact means for how drugs for dementia have been used and evaluated. If dementia affects not only the person directly experiencing it but also family members, health care professionals, and society as a whole, should drugs for dementia in some sense "treat" the problems dementia poses for all those affected? Absent a "magic bullet" that would completely eradicate the phenomena of age-associated progressive dementia without generating significant side effects—not even a remote possibility in the foreseeable future—shouldn't any medicine prescribed for dementia somehow address this complex web of overlapping but far from identical needs and desires? Because drugs for dementia must selectively target some aspects of the problem while risking side effects that can create new problems, it seems clear that their use and evaluation cannot work equally well in meeting the needs of all those affected.

In light of these difficulties, controversy seems inevitable. This book could not hope to end the controversy surrounding these drugs. But we do hope it can stimulate a broader discussion that will help us understand what we are disagreeing about and why. Our aim is to enhance the ability of different kinds of people to talk to each other about these drugs and to make the process of individual and collective decision making about them more transparent and fair. The first two chapters in this section contribute to this process by presenting different perspectives on drug treatment for dementia—one by an experienced clinician and the other by a layperson whose father has dementia. The third chapter discusses the problem in more theoretical terms and describes what must happen if we are to create a language to meaningfully evaluate drugs for dementia across these different perspectives.

Allan Anderson's description of his use of the acetylcholinesterase inhibitors (AChEIs) and memantine in daily clinical practice seems surprisingly free of doubt. Indeed, he suggests that clinicians have a much more difficult time knowing when to take patients off of these drugs than whether to start them. Anderson is clearly grateful for the drugs that are available now and frames his chapter with a narrative of progress. Twenty years ago, he suggests, clinicians had no effective treatments. (However, as Ballenger points out in chapter 11 of this volume, the drugs available 20 and more years ago certainly had partisans who trumpeted their efficacy within a similar progress narrative.) Anderson acknowledges the limitations of the currently available drugs in terms of their high cost and modest efficacy, particularly for patients in the later stages of dementia, and the difficulty in measuring outcomes. He longs for the day when continued progress will make these drugs look primitive. But from his perspective of a clinician deeply committed to helping his patients deal with the problems of dementia *now*, Anderson clearly believes, as he states in conclusion, that for patients and their families struggling with dementia "any treatment benefit, no matter how trivial or how short acting, is a blessing." Anderson's chapter suggests that until something better comes along, the currently available drugs are likely to find favor with most clinicians.

In contrast, Judith Levine's description of the role of drug treatment in managing her father's dementia suggests why many family members may continue to be ambivalent about these drugs and whatever antidementia drugs are developed in the future. Levine is not so much concerned with quantifiable outcomes like ADAS-cog scores and improved activities of daily living but with the existential problem of balancing the practical need of caregivers and family members in managing her father's dementia against the need to preserve as much as possible the integrity of his identity and her relationship to him. Her chapter is framed by a narrative of medicalization in which the meanings and goals of medicine increasingly dominate and define the lives of patients. When her father is given drugs for his depression and anger, she acknowledges that they provide very real help to the workers in the nursing home who are struggling to "manage" him, but she also worries that they suppress his ability to express legitimate feelings he has about his life. She believes that everyone involved with the care of her father tries hard to act with his interests at heart but worries about how easy it is for them to conflate his interests with their own, turning his feelings into "behaviors" and "symptoms" to be "managed" with a pill. Whatever the efficacy of drugs for dementia, she concludes that preserving the integrity of her father's identity will be accomplished not by chemicals but by relationships and communities.

Anderson and Levine may not represent "typical" clinicians and family members; but their chapters do suggest that these roles can generate very different perspectives on the problem of dementia and strategies to treat it. In the final chapter in this section, Jason Karlawish explains why these differences are so problematic in the case of dementia. Discourse on dementia, he argues, lacks a "coherent language of benefit"—a set of measures defining the diagnosis and development of the disease that make sense across the communities of researchers, clinicians, caregivers, patients, and policy makers. In the case of diabetes, for example, there is a general consensus among researchers, clinicians, and patients on elevated blood glucose as a proper measure of the disease, and drug treatments can be evaluated in terms of whether they properly lower blood glucose. In the case of dementia, no such consensus has been established. While diagnostic criteria like those proposed by the National Institute of Neurological and Communicative Disorders and Stroke and the Alzheimer's Disease and Related Disorders Association (NINCDS-ADRDA) in 1984 have established a coherent definition of AD, they do not prescribe what tests should be used to measure the disease. Without such measures, researchers have and will continue to haggle over whether drugs are truly effective, clinicians will disagree about whether and how to use them, family members will wonder if the drugs work, and policy makers will debate whether they are worth the cost. Karlawish suggests that progress in understanding the basic biological mechanisms of the disease will likely allow us to eventually forge a coherent language of benefit for dementia, because biological phenomena are easier to quantify and measure in the laboratory, and he notes that clinical trials now routinely include "biomarkers" for AD. (For a contrast to Karlawish's view that medical science will eventually produce a clear language of benefit, see Peter Whitehouse's argument in chapter 10 of this volume that a real consideration of quality of life in dementia should lead us *away* from the medical concept of dementia.) But until one or more of these biomarkers is sufficiently validated, controversy over drug treatments for dementia remains inevitable.

CHAPTER 5

Pharmacologic Treatment of Dementia

A Clinician's View

ALLAN A. ANDERSON, M.D.

The clinical evaluation and treatment of dementia have dramatically changed over the last twenty years. Before this time, we had no effective pharmacologic treatment for the disease. Clinicians tried medications like Hydergine and others that were available at that time. However, clinical experience as well as clinical trials of such medications demonstrated their ineffectiveness in the treatment of Alzheimer's disease (AD) (Hollister and Yesavage 1984).

Even the treatment of depression and behavioral problems often associated with the illness had its limits. This was the era of the tricyclic antidepressants and typical or first-generation antipsychotics, before the introduction of the newer serotonergic antidepressants and atypical or second-generation antipsychotics.

Use of tricyclic antidepressants often led to problematic side effects, including anticholinergic side effects. At times, this added to the cognitive deficits already present from the disease. In addition, many patients experienced significant constipation and dry mouth. More significant medical problems might arise, such as worsening of glaucoma, bowel obstruction, urinary retention, and cardiac side effects. Use of the first-generation antipsychotics often led to unwanted anticholinergic, sedative, or neurologic side effects. Currently, with the use of newer medications, we can often avoid these unwanted side effects and safely treat the depression and behavioral problems frequently associated with dementia.

Over the past 15 years, we have seen the emergence of two classes of medication specifically indicated for the treatment of the cognitive deficits in dementia: the acetylcholinesterase inhibitors (tacrine, donepezil, rivastigmine, and galantamine) and the NMDA (N-methyl-D-aspartate) receptor antagonists (memantine). Short-term studies have demonstrated these medications to be efficacious in treating the disease by improving cognition or, more often, slowing the cognitive decline in patients with dementia (Parnetti, Senin, and Mcocci 1977; Farlow 2002; Reisberg et al. 2003; Cummings 2004).

Additional studies have shown efficacy in improving activities of daily living and reducing or ameliorating behavioral symptoms, including severe symptoms such as hallucinations, delusions, agitation, and aggression (Dejong, Osterlund, and Roy 1989; Feldman et al. 2001; Potkin et al. 2002; Cummings et al. 2004). By better managing such symptoms, patients have been able to remain in community settings longer, as shown in studies that demonstrate delay of nursing home placement (Mohs et al. 2001; Geldmacher et al. 2003).

It has been clear from the time these medications were introduced that they did not treat the core etiology of dementia. The disease continued to progress, with all patients eventually having further deterioration. There have been conflicting studies concerning their long-term usefulness. Clearly studies have documented effectiveness over the short term, with most "short-term" studies being 24–38 weeks in duration (Parnetti, Senin, and Mcocci 1977; Farlow 2002; Cummings 2004). More recent studies, often supported by the pharmaceutical industry, have demonstrated benefits of extended treatment from one to five years (AD 2000 Collaborative Group 2004; Bullock et al. 2004; Small et al. 2004). Only one study, a two-year study of donepezil, demonstrated improvement compared to a placebo group (AD 2000 Collaborative Group 2004). The remainder of the longer-term studies compared the treatment group against a projected placebo response, at least in the United States, where many now consider a placebo trial unethical given the proven benefit of medication.

The first of the acetylcholinesterase medications to be released was tacrine (Cognex). It proved difficult to use, with four times daily dosing, significant side effects in a majority of patients, and the potential for serious liver toxicity necessitating baseline and follow-up liver function tests (Watkins et al. 1994). Many clinicians treating patients with dementia held a negative view of this medication, often downplaying its use when asked about it by patients or their family members. However, it became evident that this medication indeed did work in producing cognitive improvement in many patients with AD or by slowing the cognitive decline in others. Despite its side-effect profile, some patients managed to take the medication without side effects or hepatic toxicity. In retrospect, it appears that clinicians tended to underuse tacrine in the treatment of AD.

Fortunately, tacrine was shortly followed by the introduction of donepezil (Aricept). We now had an alternative that was more user friendly, with once-daily dosing, minimal titration, and fewer side effects, and many patients were soon placed on this medication. Fortunately, fewer patients ceased use of it as a result of side effects. Rivastigmine (Exelon) and galantamine (Reminyl/Razodyne) soon followed, and we were off to the races treating patients with AD. Memantine (Namenda) was introduced in 2004, providing an additional option for treatment, for use either in combination with an acetylcholinesterase inhibitor or alone.

How do clinicians use these medication options as they treat AD today? Most clinicians are aware of the clinical benefits of medication in short-term studies. Many clinicians have seen continued, long-term clinical benefits in some of their patients. Significant treatment benefits may continue for years, as indicated in the following case vignette.

FS was a 74-year-old man who moved with his wife to live with their daughter and her family. The daughter had an addition built onto their house to accommodate FS and his wife. The move was based on FS's continued cognitive decline. After living in the new setting for several months, FS began to have problems recognizing this as his new home and at times would even have difficulty recognizing his wife. She would react to this by becoming angry with him. She had significant problems controlling her emotions around his loss of memory and misrecognition. When this occurred, she would often yell explicatives at him, attempting to force on him the reality that she was his wife. She would try to block his way when he attempted to leave their new home. The result was that FS became violent toward her. The family took FS to his internist, who placed him on risperidone for the treatment of his agitation. This helped initially, but after a few weeks the agitation and violence returned.

The internist then referred FS to a geriatric psychiatrist. It was clear that he had a moderate level of dementia. A workup for reversible causes led to no significant findings. The course of cognitive decline had been gradual over the past four years. He struggled with problems recognizing his new home as well as family members. When interviewed alone, he was pleasant and engaging and did not demonstrate any significant psychotic symptoms. He felt perplexed by all the "hoopla" that had occurred and could not remember any of the violent episodes toward his wife. The wife was also interviewed both with the patient and alone. She appeared to be depressed and was struggling greatly to contain her emotions.

Two specific treatments were offered. FS was treated with an acetylcholinesterase inhibitor, initially starting on 5 mg daily of donepezil with an increase to 10 mg after four weeks. The other treatment was targeted toward his wife. She was started on a selective serotonin reuptake inhibitor, as she met the clinical criteria for major depression. She was also engaged in supportive and interpersonal psychotherapy by a therapist working in the psychiatrist's office. The therapist helped her deal with the stress of her husband's decline and the change in their relationship and to shape her responses to him, supporting alternative verbal responses when he became more confused and would not recognize her or the new home.

After approximately two months of taking the combination of donepezil and risperidone, FS showed improvements in behavior, which allowed the elimination of the use of the antipsychotic medication. FS now had no difficulty recognizing his wife and the new home. He also demonstrated improvement in short-term memory. He was able to tolerate the medication without any side effects and was able to remain in the community. In fact, he did not require institutional placement for three years following this. His disease did progress with increased physical problems, including gait instability. By the time he was placed in a nursing home, he had entered the final stage of dementia with little remaining functioning. The acetylcholinesterase was stopped at this time.

As we reflect on this man's improvements, several thoughts come to mind. One is what his course would have been like had he been a patient treated 20 years earlier, a time when no effective pharmacologic treatments were available for AD and neither were any of the newer, second-generation antipsychotic medications. He would likely have been prescribed a medication such as haloperidol, with or without a benzodiazepine. He probably would have required admission to a long-term-care facility much earlier and declined steadily from the progression of his dementia. This would have robbed him and his family of years of life at home.

Many clinicians have difficulty deciding when to stop any of the dementia medications, whether one of the acetylcholinesterase medications or memantine. One aggressive practice is to continue treating until there is no significant function left to preserve. This would assume that patients benefit from medication use throughout the course of their disease up to the final stage of dementia, until the end of their life.

There are now studies that indicate some benefit for one to several years (Mohs et al. 2001; AD 2000 Collaborative Group 2004; Bullock et al. 2004; Small et al. 2004). Many clinicians treating such patients have had patients who had been on the medications for some time, were at a more advanced stage of the disease, and then stopped the medications, after which their condition took a turn for the worse. Perhaps the patient lost some basic function like the ability to use utensils or to recognize a close family member such as a spouse. In retrospect, we might not have discontinued the use of the medication had we known the outcome. In such scenarios, when the medication is restarted, the patient often never regains what was lost. The following case demonstrates how a patient might suddenly deteriorate once medication is discontinued.

CG was a 70-year-old man who had a moderate level of dementia. He had been treated with the acetylcholinesterase inhibitor donepezil and tolerated this medication without any side effects. Both he and his wife saw some improvements in his cognitive abilities and activities of daily living. It was the opinion of the treating physician that there was benefit in continuing the medication, as there was evidence of a slower progression of the disease than would be expected without medication.

CG had been taking the medication for approximately a year when his wife sustained a hip fracture that required surgery and rehabilitation. As she was his sole caretaker, a decision was made to have him placed in a nursing home for respite care until she recuperated and could bring him home. Several weeks after her surgery, she was able to visit him at the nursing home. She was amazed at how different he appeared. While able to recognize her, he was unable to recognize other family members, a distinct change from before. In addition, he had lost some of the ability to fully feed himself, struggling to use utensils properly. Initially she was willing to view such changes as an effect of the placement. She had heard others talk about such "regression" when patients with dementia entered nursing homes or other institutional settings.

As she thought more about it, she questioned her blind acceptance of his changes. She did some investigation and learned that upon CG's admission to the nursing home, the admitting physician decided to stop the Alzheimer's medication, specifically the donepezil CG had taken for more than a year before the nursing home admission. This medication was discontinued without consulting her. She called the psychiatrist who had treated her husband before nursing home placement. He advised that she ask the attending physician to restart the use of donepezil. The medication was once again given, and CG's functioning did improve, but never to the level of before the withdrawal of the medication.

This is a familiar scene to many clinicians who treat patients with these medications. The falling off of function with the inability to regain prior level of function has been replicated in clinical trials.

When pharmacologic treatments for AD were first introduced, their use was primarily for patients with mild disease. Most of these patients were living in the community. Soon studies demonstrated that acetylcholinesterase medications provided a benefit to patients with more moderate and severe dementia (Feldman et al. 2001; Burns, Spiegel, and Quarg 2004). Studies demonstrated that there could be improvements in activities of daily living (ADLs) as well as with some of the behavioral manifestations of the disease (Dejong, Osterlund, and Roy 1989; Feldman et al. 2001; Mohs et al. 2001; Potkin et al. 2002; Cummings et al. 2004). This information led to the prescription of medications to patients with more severe levels of dementia. This occurred with patients living in the community as well as patients in long-term care settings such as nursing homes, domiciliary homes, and assisted-living facilities. We presumed that the benefit seen in community studies would transfer to benefits in the nursing home setting. Unfortunately, few studies have been done that evaluate benefits in function and behavior of patients residing in long-term care settings.

In January 2004, memantine was released for use by patients with moderate or severe AD, expanding the treatment options for persons with dementia (Reisberg et al. 2003). This included patients with more severe levels of disease such as those in nursing home settings (Winblad and Portis 1999). It seemed prudent to use these medications in the various long-term-care settings as it might help improve their quality of life. Clinicians noted that patients treated with medications were better able to assist in their ADLs. Some patients demonstrated significant improvement in problematic behaviors, including wandering, agitation, aggression, apathy, depression, and even at times improvement in psychotic symptoms. Patients in long-term care might benefit from being better able to interact with staff, other residents, and their environment. An example follows.

> TJ was a 75-year-old widowed woman. She had been residing in a nursing home for several years and carried the diagnosis of probable AD. Before treatment, she had an estimated Mini-Mental State Examination (MMSE) score of 5–10. TJ often aimlessly walked the halls of the nursing home. She would wander into others' rooms, though she fortunately did not leave the building. At times her entering others' rooms led to troubling interactions, with residents becoming angry and occasionally physically aggressive to her. Before treatment, she mumbled softly and incomprehensively. She could identify herself but was unable to participate in any formal mental status evaluation. She could follow simple commands. The family was approached about a trial of memantine. They heard about potential benefits and agreed to a trial on the medication.
>
> TJ was given the typical titration of medication and had no problem tolerating the final 20 mg daily dose (given as 10 mg twice daily). A review of her case after two months of treatment showed some benefit in her speech and interactions with others. Family and staff both felt that there were two significant changes. One had to do with her focus in interpersonal relationships. Previously TJ would stop, acknowledge you with her eyes when you called her name, then begin mumbling and move on after a second or two. Now staff and family identified that she would stop and engage for some time. She would answer some simple questions with appropriate responses. She smiled more often. She was noted by staff to be more pleasant and more willing to participate in activities as opposed to wandering aimlessly. There were fewer altercations with other residents, as she was not wandering into their rooms and seemed to respect their privacy. After TJ had been on the medication for five months, staff and family continued to report that it was helpful.

The following case demonstrates how at times use of medication can lead to improvements extensive enough that the patient might be able to be discharged from the facility. This case is of a man who has Lewy body dementia with studies demonstrating at times significant treatments of this subtype of dementia (McKeith et al. 2000).

DM was a 72-year-old married man with a diagnosis of Lewy body dementia. He had the core features of this illness with prominent parkinsonian features (except for tremor), prominent visual hallucinations early in the course of his disease, and some degree of waxing and waning of symptoms. He had been treated with rivastigmine for several years, with some improvement noted, but now seemed to have reached a plateau. He began to have worsening memory, misrecognizing his home and family. At times he would become quite agitated to the point of physical aggression towards others. There was further deterioration in his activities of daily living. He needed more assistance with dressing, grooming, toileting, and bathing. Despite additional psychotropic medication use (atypical antipsychotics and valproic acid) he continued to show significant agitation, and nursing home placement was sought.

In the nursing home, psychiatric care was provided by a new psychiatrist, as DM's previous psychiatrist did not attend at that particular home. After being there for a month, DM was started on memantine, which had just become available on the U.S. market. This was combined with rivastigmine 4.5 mg twice daily and quetiapine increasing to a dose of 25 mg in the morning and 50 mg in the evening. DM made a robust improvement in areas of ADLs, memory, recognition, and behavior. He had fewer hallucinations. In fact the family decided to try caring for him at home, and he was discharged from the nursing home.

He returned to the office of the psychiatrist who originally treated him. During the first visit he demonstrated improved speech with less word-finding difficulty and more significant sentence structure. He even was able to ask if, given his improvement, the psychiatrist would support having his driver's license reinstated. While this was not practical, the patient reveled in being at home with his family. After about six months at home, he began to decline, and placement in a nursing home was once again a possibility.

The case examples above illustrate some of the positive effects of the use of medications in the treatment of AD. However, the result of treatment is often not so positive. At times, individuals demonstrate intolerability to these medications. Use of acetylcholinesterase inhibitors often leads to problematic gastrointestinal side effects. The magnitude of these side effects has been less with more conservative, slower titration of dose. Despite this, some patients develop severe side effects that at times prohibit the use of the drugs. Sleep disruption, muscle cramps, and fatigue are examples of other side effects that may occur with use of acetylcholinesterase inhibitors (Cummings 2004).

Memantine has had fewer side-effect problems. Clinicians have seen one adverse effect as particularly troubling—the occasional increase in confusion and agitation that may occur early in the course of treatment. Some geriatric psychiatrists in active clinical practice find that in many patients this adverse effect is often time limited, disappearing in a few weeks. Most patients can attain the full recommended dose of 10 mg twice daily.

Many patients taking any of the dementia medications see limited benefits. They continue to demonstrate decline in memory and other cognitive functioning. Family members and other caregivers often report subtle global benefits that are indeed difficult to measure. Perhaps the most important measure of these medications is the burden of providing care. If the medications are helpful with activities of daily living and behaviors, then family and caregivers receive a treatment "benefit."

How might we measure this benefit? With many other chronic diseases there is more quantifiable, objective evidence of improvement. The cardiologist can match specific physical exam findings with EKG, X-ray, and blood tests to demonstrate improvement in patients. The internist can quantify fasting blood glucose and hemoglobin A1C to measure current insulin needs and glucose control over recent weeks. There are numerous other examples of how medical specialists measure treatment benefit in their patients.

For patients who have dementia, no such diagnostic tests exist, at least none that are readily available and easy to administer by the primary care physician. There are examples of neuropsychologic batteries that could be performed at baseline and then at the time of follow-up visits. Such tests might be able to more adequately quantify any improvement or stabilization in global or specific neurocognitive functioning. A number of these are currently being marketed; however, most clinicians are not putting them to use. They have their drawbacks, including the time needed to administer them as well as the variability that often occurs with patients, variability that can affect the outcome significantly. Therefore, getting a static picture of neurocognitive functioning today might not accurately represent how the patient has been doing over time.

Clinicians have more regularly used simple scales that are less time con-suming to administer and that review the patient's recent functioning. These can then be scored and compared to how the patient has done since the time of the last visit. Scales include those that measure ADLs, behavior, and care-giver burden (Burns, Lawler, and Craig 2001). The caregiver burden scales may be the most important. When caregivers can no longer appropriately take care of patients, there is often some negative consequence. This might in-clude the need for long-term-care placement. In long-term-care settings, this burden on caregivers might lead to caregiver burnout or less appropriate care being delivered to that patient.

For many patients and clinicians, a global assessment of "improvement" is often used as the measure of whether to continue or stop a dementia medica-tion. This family-identified improvement includes a robust placebo benefit, be-cause clinicians and caregivers are hopeful that a patient will receive a significant benefit. Many of us ask a question such as "On the whole, how do you think your husband (wife, mother, etc.) is doing?" While it is difficult to appreciate the benefit of "slowing of the progression of the disease," we often try to have caregivers estimate this. Our objective view of the patient and the changes since the last visit is often difficult to quantify. One novel approach would be to videotape patients briefly and then compare videos at follow-up visits. It may be easier to appreciate changes in language function, social in-teraction, and other subtle changes by comparing such prior function to the present.

As clinicians, we have all at times treated patients with these medications and seen essentially no significant improvement. How long should one con-tinue with limited or no evidence of a benefit? Many clinicians will suggest stopping the medication after three to six months of such treatment. Some-times treatment is inappropriately continued. Family members may view con-tinued use of these medications as their only hope for some benefit for their loved one, and they may be reluctant to stop despite the lack of any significant improvement.

Another difficult treatment decision is the decision to stop the medication as the patient enters the final stage of their disease. While family and clinician share a positive view of the prolongation of the mild stage of the disease and in some cases of the moderate stage, few view prolongation of function as a benefit once the patient has entered the final or severe stage of the disease. We question whether at this point we are prolonging the patient's dysfunction rather than allowing the disease to take its toll. There are, however, patients who have taken the medications until entering this final stage, and who still seem to enjoy some activities, some social interaction, and for whom life seems tolerable or even joyful. Does the clinician advocate stopping the medication at that time? Family input into such a decision is vital.

With the addition of memantine, new questions arise. These include whether to start memantine or an acetylcholinesterase inhibitor when a patient is first seen during the moderate stage of his or her disease. Another question is when to add memantine to an acetylcholinesterase inhibitor, and if this leads to little improvement, the next question is when to discontinue it (Tariot et al. 2004). For many patients such dual treatment adds significantly to their medical expenses, which may already be burdened by their being prescribed a number of other medications.

For psychiatrists, neurologists, internists, or family practitioners, the management of dementia care continues to be complex and challenging. Certainly there are realistic limits on the treatments that are available today. Some patients respond minimally or not at all. Others experience side effects that limit use of the medications. For patients who seem to have some beneficial response, the perplexing question of when to stop medication has little scientific rationale to offer guidance to clinicians. Often the decision resonates from family, at times motivated by the cost of medication weighed against the more limited benefit of treatment as the disease progresses. We all would readily welcome a "more curative" treatment for AD and other dementias. Hopefully one will come soon to prevent the ballooning of cases as baby boomers come of age for this disease over the next 10 to 20 years.

Clinicians are aware that these medications have their limits. They may not be exerting much of a clinical benefit as the patient enters the last stage of the disease. Fortunately most do not cause many side effects. There is, however, the cost of maintaining medications for years despite the limited benefit of medication. Perhaps 10 or 20 years from now we will look back on these times and view the situation differently. As more substantive treatments become available, we might muse upon the minimal benefits of the "ancient" dementia treatments. We hope that this time will come soon.

One thing is certain: dementia is a terrible disease. It often robs patients of their identity. It can steal them from their spouse and family. It causes great stress for many. With the current estimate of up to a third of individuals getting the disease by age 85, most of us who live long enough will experience the hardships of this illness either by having dementia or being married to or closely related to someone suffering from the disease. Studies demonstrate nearly a 50 percent incidence of depression in spouses of people with AD (Rabins, Lyketsos, and Steele 2006). Indeed, the current treatments are often limited in the magnitude of benefit they provide. For such a devastating illness, any treatment benefit, no matter how trivial or short acting, is a blessing for the patients and families who continue to suffer.

REFERENCES

AD 2000 Collaborative Group. 2004. Long-term donepezil treatment in 565 patients with Alzheimer's disease: Randomized double-blind trial. *Lancet* 363:2105–15.

Bullock, R., et al. 2004. A long-term comparison of galantamine and donepezil in the treatment of Alzheimer's disease: Effects on attention and cognition. Poster session at the 17th annual meeting of the American Association for Geriatric Psychiatry, Baltimore.

Burns, A., B. Lawler, and S. Craig. 2001. *Assessment scales in old age psychiatry.* London: Martin Dunitz.

Burns, A., B. Spiegel, and P. Quarg. 2004. Efficacy of rivastigmine in subjects with moderately severe Alzheimer's disease. *International Journal of Geriatric Psychiatry* 19:243–49.

Cummings, J. L. 2004. Use of cholinesterase inhibitors in clinical practice: Evidence-based recommendations. *Focus* 2:239–52.

Cummings, J. L., et al. 2004. Donepezil improves behavioral symptoms in patients with Alzheimer's disease. Poster session at the 17th annual meeting of the American Association for Geriatric Psychiatry, Baltimore.

DeJong, R., O. W. Osterlund, and G. W. Roy. 1989. Measurement of quality-of-life changes in patients with Alzheimer's disease. *Clinical Therapeutics* 11:545–54.

Farlow, M. 2002. A clinical overview of cholinesterase inhibitors in Alzheimer's disease. *International Psychogeriatrics* 14:93–126.

Feldman, H., S. Gauthier, J. Hecker, B. Vellas, P. Subbiah, and E. Whalen, Donepezil MSAD Study Investigators Group. 2001. A 24-week, randomized, double-blind study of donepezil in moderate-to-severe Alzheimer's disease. *Neurology* 57:613–20.

Geldmacher, D. S., G. Provenzano, T. McRae, V. Mastey, and J. R. Ieni. 2003. Donepezil is associated with delayed nursing home placement in patients with Alzheimer's disease. *Journal of the American Geriatric Society* 51:937–94.

Hollister, L. E., and J. Yesavage. 1984. Ergoloid mesylates for senile dementias: Unanswered questions. *Annals of Internal Medicine* 100:894–98.

McKeith, I., T. Del Ser, P. Spano, M. Emre, K. Wesnes, R. Anand, A. Cicin-Sain, R. Ferrara, R. Spiegel. 2000. Efficacy of rivastigmine in dementia with Lewy bodies: A randomized double-blind placebo-controlled international study. *Lancet* 356:2031–36.

Mohs, R. C., et al. 2001. A 1-year, placebo-controlled preservation of function survival study of donepezil in AD patients. *Neurology* 57:481–88.

Parnetti, L., U. Senin, and P. Mcocci. 1977. Cognitive enhancement therapy for Alzheimer's disease: The way forward. *Drugs* 53:752–68.

Potkin, S. G., et al. 2002. Impact of Alzheimer's disease and rivastigmine treatment on activities of daily living over the course of mild to moderately severe disease. *Progress in Neuro-Psychopharmacology and Biological Psychiatry* 26:713–20.

Rabins, P. V., C. G. Lyketsos, and C. Steele. 2006. *Practical dementia care,* 2nd ed. New York: Oxford University Press.

Reisberg, B., et al. 2003. Memantine in moderate-to-severe Alzheimer's disease. *New England Journal of Medicine* 348:1333–41.

Small, G., et al. 2004. Rivistigmine demonstrates efficacy over 5 years in Alzheimer's disease. Poster session at the 17th annual meeting of the American Association for Geriatric Psychiatry, Baltimore.

Tariot, P. N., M. R. Farlow, G. T. Grossberg, S. M. Graham, S. McDonald, and I. Gergel, Memantine Study Group. 2004. Memantine treatment in patients with moderate to severe Alzheimer disease already receiving donepezil. *JAMA* 291:317–24.

Watkins P. B., H. J. Zimmerman, M. J. Knapp, S. I. Gracon, K. W. Lewis. 1994. Hepatotoxic effects of tacrine administration in patients with Alzeimer's disease. *JAMA* 271:992–98.

Winblad, B., and N. Portis. 1999. Memantine in severe dementia: Results of the M-Best Study. *International Journal of Geriatric Psychiatry* 14:135–46.

CHAPTER 6

Managing Dad

JUDITH LEVINE

On the Alzheimer's wing in the nursing home where my father lives, everyone is kind.[1] The rooms and halls are clean and cheerfully decorated; as in a kindergarten, paper turkeys go up in November, wreaths in December, pastel-colored eggs in April. There is hardly ever an odor of urine in the air or even a scrap of litter on the linoleum. Except for the woman who screeches night and day, the place feels calm. In this Catholic institution, a saint benignly gazes from every wall.

I fought my mother about sending Dad here. When I wrote a book that was partly about this fight, she stopped speaking to me (Levine 2004). That's how big a fight it was. At the time, a dozen years into his slowly progressing dementia, Dad was living in their apartment with a talented caregiver named Nilda. Mom had moved to her beau's apartment farther uptown. She oversaw Dad's care with the help of a care manager, a former social worker who had known him for a decade. We each visited Dad once a week.

Dad was doing well with Nilda. He devoured her Argentine chicken stews and fruit Jell-Os and let her bathe him, though it could take two hours to get the job done. Nilda called Dad "my friend." Dad called her "darling." Once, when she was picking him up at his day program, a new aide asked who she was. "Is this your sister? You grandma?" the aide teased.

"Him?" Dad said, stalling until a word bubbled up from the marsh of his memory. "Oh, him." He patted Nilda companionably. "That's my sergeant." It was a compliment.

Dad got kicked out of that day program after some contretemps with the music therapist and started traveling uptown to another program, which welcomed him. The whole thing may have been too much, though, and he soon took to sinking imperturbably to the floor or growling at the chauffeur when it was time to get on or off the van. Only Nilda could (eventually) humor him to cooperate. About this time, Dad also ceased to be able to tell the toilet from the chairs in his bedroom, so Nilda spent hours scrubbing the house with disinfectant. He was up a lot more at night, too, which was wearing her out. Turning 70, Nilda began developing a host of health problems herself.

Still, in the fall of 2004, at a meeting with the care manager, my family decided Dad should keep living at home. If Nilda was no longer willing or able, a new caregiver could be hired. Mom agreed, but she was too worn out to stick to the plan. Less than a month later, on a Thursday, she informed me that a bed had become available at the nursing home, and Dad was moving the following Monday.

I had the usual worries. Although the home had a good reputation and a new Alzheimer's unit director whom Mom knew, I feared that Dad would deteriorate quickly there. I imagined him scared outside of familiar surroundings and depressed by institutional life. Worst of all, he would lose his beloved Nilda, who had promised to keep working as long as he lived in the apartment. Mom insisted that he no longer knew where or with whom he was—that the move, in other words, would not upset him.

My misgivings resonated beyond the details of what his days and nights would be like. The medical and therapeutic professionals in his life, along with my mother, described him in the language of stages and symptoms; he was already taking a number of psychotropic medications. Still, I believed that as long as Dad had an apartment in a neighborhood with children, dogs, shopkeepers, beggars, cops, and bus drivers—and Nilda—he was protected from the wholesale medicalization of his self. As long as he had a home, my father had a fighting chance of remaining a person. Once inside the red-brick walls of an institution, I feared, he would become a patient.

On my first few visits to the nursing home, I was relieved. Dad's hair was trim, his cheek freshly shaven. He was starting to get chubby around the middle—a combination of more food and less exercise—but he had not deteriorated, certainly not physically. In fact, noticing his expanding girth, the staff had reduced his portions and stepped up efforts to get him to move around more.

I liked both Loretta and Desiree, the aides Mom had employed to be with him during the day (the place is not staffed sufficiently for individual care). My partner Paul and I met with the unit director, whom we found intelligent, progressive, down to earth, and attuned to Dad's needs. He was being well looked after.

Moreover, he seemed to have adjusted quickly to the new place and the new routines. Arriving on the fifth floor, even in the first weeks, I usually found him in his room. He was doing nothing, but he seemed content, even cheerful. Paul and I felt better because it appeared that Mom had made the right decision. Dad wasn't doing so well at home; he was doing pretty well here. He wasn't traumatized to leave Nilda and his apartment; he was growing attached to his new caregivers and his new room.

Still, I knew my relief to be one of the myriad perversities that stem from the conflicting needs of the person with dementia and his family or caregivers. I didn't want Dad to be unhappy, in part because that would make me unhappy. If he was going to be in an institution, I wanted him to feel like a naturalized institutional citizen. So I was *glad* that Dad apparently could not tell "home" from "the home." Great news: My father doesn't know where he is!

Some months later, Loretta told me that Dad did not immediately adjust to the new place. For weeks, he kept asking to go home. He was, and sometimes still is, disturbed by the routines, especially at the beginning and end of the day. He flails and strikes the orderlies who try to bathe him. In the evening, he resists staying in bed when he's put there. When he's had a fitful night, he dozes during the day and refuses to walk to the dining room for meals.

To smooth out these bumps, the nursing home administers drugs. There's nothing new about this. My father has been drugged since his diagnosis with Alzheimer's almost 15 years ago. Back then, there were no cholinergic AD drugs. The current vogue was megadoses of vitamin E. Twice a day Dad took a giant capsule along with Lipitor for cholesterol and a couple of aspirin for his heart.

His doctor also prescribed the antidepressant Zoloft. There was nothing new about his depression either. The only child of a brittle, narcissistic single mother who never wanted children and paid him little but punitive attention, all evidence is that my father was a depressed boy, a depressed young man. He was depressed when I was a child. Now, a professional and an intellectual losing his ability to think and communicate, what else would he be but depressed?

The psychiatrist at the aging and dementia center who evaluated Dad's first battery of memory and language tests wrote in the records, "I feel he probably is demented and that his high scores reflect his premorbid function." He translated this to Dad and Mom: "The smarter you are, the more you have to lose." I wondered which part of this double message Dad heard loudest—the abundance of his personal resources or the depths of his potential loss. This doctor also diagnosed depression.

In spite of a lifetime of borderline depression, though, that's not the word I would use to name my father's feelings at the onset of dementia. He was afraid. His fear reflected the general cultural terror of the "loss of mind," which we believe means the loss of self. Once, early on, he told me he saw "a tall, black wall" where his future was. Watching his extravagant vocabulary, his analytic acuity, his wit—the pillars of his personality and self-image—crumble, Dad was grieving. No doubt, Zoloft damped these feelings, relieved some of his hopelessness. Ironically, though, it was the advance of his disease that took better care of them. When awareness of his deficits fled, so did his sorrow. Dad became happier than I'd ever known him. The Zoloft was discontinued.

By the time Aricept came on the market, vitamin E was no longer considered effective, and anyhow the pills were too big for Dad to swallow and the oil inside them too nasty-tasting to disguise in his food. His psychiatrist prescribed Aricept, even though Dad was beyond the stage when it is claimed the drug makes any difference. Indeed, at that final meeting when we decided to keep Dad at home, the care manager did not attribute his good physical and emotional health to any medication. One of the reasons she recommended continuing the "current care plan" was the obvious effect of the excellent attention he had received from Nilda and his other caregivers, including Mom. Still, the care manager's attitude toward Aricept, like the psychiatrist's, was the usual one: *it can't hurt*. Dad took the drug for seven or eight years.

At the nursing home, Dad's two caregivers keep his spirits up, his body comfortable and clean, and his mind more or less stimulated. But his equilibrium is maintained with a cocktail of the anticonvulsive Neurontin and the antipsychotic Seroquel, along with nightly doses of the sleeping pill trazadone. I don't know exactly how the docs calibrate Dad's prescriptions. But the general strategy is, if he becomes overly aggressive, the dosages are increased. If he starts nodding off every time his butt hits a horizontal surface, the doses are lowered. The trazadone is given at an hour that will bring him sleep from bedtime until a decent hour in the morning, with minimal wandering in between and minimal sleepiness at other times.

Sleepiness is still a problem. Often when I visit, I find my father with his chin on his chest, drool dripping from the corner of his fleshy lips. He cannot be roused. But aggression, touchiness, and nighttime wandering are problems not just for Dad but for the institution. If nearly full-time napping is the cost of peace, it seems, the naps will be tolerated.

All these people have Dad's interests at heart. But it is easy to conflate his interests with those of the institution and of his caregivers. A July 2004 press release from AstraZeneca, the maker of Seroquel, reveals this conflation. Reporting on findings that the drug reduced agitation in elderly patients who have dementia and are living in long-term care with no evidence of increased cerebrovascular risks, the release concludes with a quote from one of the researchers, Dr. Pierre Tariot, professor of psychiatry, medicine, and neurology at the University of Rochester. "Agitation is a significant issue for patients suffering from this condition and their caregivers," says Dr. Tariot. "It is an aspect of dementia that is both difficult to manage and emotionally troubling for those who care for patients suffering from dementia" (AstraZeneca 2004).

Other than being an "issue," it's hard to know how or whether Seroquel benefits the people who take it. Indeed, Seroquel, approved for control of manic episodes in bipolar disorder, may have paradoxical effects when prescribed off label to elderly patients with dementia. One English study found rates of cognitive decline twice as high in subjects taking the drug as in those taking a placebo (Ballard et al. 2005).

One thing is for sure: the docility these drugs bring benefits people with dementia by putting them in the good graces of the ones who take care of them, and that's no small thing. Loretta and Desiree, who try their best to keep Dad awake, report that he is "good" or (as they tell him) "a good boy." The psychiatrist and social workers express it differently. They say he is "well managed."

Alzheimer's disease has effects on personality. I know this. Perhaps medication is helping Dad feel happier, more in control, less fearful. If this is so, then it is good. It is not true, however, that our trust in Aricept and the other drugs that allegedly retard or control dementia "can't hurt." Whatever the benefits of drugs, they are gotten at a cost.

The United States pours virtually all available resources into biomedicine while neglecting the quotidian needs of people with dementia and their caregivers. The National Institutes of Health granted $633 million for scientific research on Alzheimer's in fiscal year 2004, the lion's share going to inquiries into DNA, neurotransmitters, or proteins.[2] At the Alzheimer's Association's massive, weeklong International Research Conference last July, only one panel was devoted to the so-called psychosocial aspects of dementia.[3]

These fiscal and scientific priorities reflect a conception of aging as an engineering problem, a compendium of destructive processes to be managed and diseases to be cured. With stem cells to regenerate worn-out body parts, bioengineers promise to cure death itself. The medical model of dementia dictates where social-service dollars go too. One reason Dad is in a nursing home is that the government pays for hospital-like nursing home placement but is stingy when it comes to the less expensive option of home care and community-based services. Whenever legislative challenges arise to these priorities, the nursing home industry sends in its lobbyists to keep them in place. Of course, they want to defend their turf. They are hurting too. And because the United States—unlike other industrialized nations—has no coherent policy or ongoing funding for eldercare, the interests with the best-paid lobbyists are likely to continue to shape the ways that elderly people are cared for.

The medicalization of my father's dementia translates all his living expressions into "behaviors" and all these behaviors into symptoms of brain decay, or secondarily, of over- or undermedication. Call me literal minded, though: Dad's "behaviors" (a.k.a. his outbursts of anger or bouts of intransigence) don't look like symptoms. They look like the expression of feelings, and legitimate ones at that.

In the morning, strangers appear. They take him to a cold tiled room and soap and hose him down, an experience that is at best humiliating, at worst terrifying (this procedure is a little more benign now, as the same aide, a woman, toilets him whenever she is on that shift, and Loretta or Desiree help if they have arrived). A lifetime night owl, Dad isn't ready to sleep when the staff dress him in his pajamas at 7:30 p.m. When they keep dragging him back to bed, he gets frustrated. That's not hard to understand.

As for nodding off at all hours, there's not much to keep Dad's eyes open. Here at the nursing home, an already small life is further diminished. He has lost patience with his dentures, and rather than force him to wear them (then constantly searching for them when he pulls them out), he is allowed to go without. The unfortunate side effect of this humane policy is that he has forfeited one of his remaining pleasures, eating. At meal times, he dully ingests the gums-only pap of pre-masticated vegetables, meat, and cereals. Similarly, he has cast off his bothersome eyeglasses, so he sees less. This may exacerbate his waning ability to focus on the paintings in the hallway or the flowers in the gardens outside.

Aside from the occasional recreational program or disjointed conversation with another resident in the hall, Dad has few distractions in his day. When the weather is good, his caregiver takes his hand, leads him to the elevator, presses him into the corner so as to defeat the alarm set off by his ankle bracelet, and walks him outside. There he may stroll around a little circular path under the trees. ("Up the hill!" he says, as the sidewalk rises, almost imperceptibly. Then, "Down the hill now.") After this tiny excursion, he is settled on a bench a dozen yards from the building's front door. If his caregiver—who gets a half-hour lunch break in her 10-hour day—takes the opportunity to chat with another worker, Dad is soon snoring.

When I mentioned my father's reluctance to look at the paintings to one of the nurses passing us in the hall, she replied, "Oh, they don't look at the pictures." "They"—people with dementia—are presumed incapable of interest and thus are not enticed to be interested. If he doesn't see the flowers, it is because "they" do not see flowers. If Dad falls asleep, he must be overmedicated. On the Alzheimer's wing, the idea of boredom is deemed inapplicable.

So, it seems, is ordinary unhappiness. My father's dining room tablemate is almost always in a fury or in tears at meal times. "She's a bad one," an aide tells me. To me, an occasional visitor, her misery seems justified. The poor woman is restrained in a chair with a strap she cannot open.

The aides in the dining room deserve my sympathy too, for they are also in institutional restraints. Three or four of them have to feed 35 residents at once, in about an hour; they can't have people wandering off. Still, watching Lily cry out and try, futilely, to free herself, I feel locked with all of them in the tautological restraints of the medical model of dementia. This woman has Alzheimer's; ergo, she is likely to be agitated. Because she is agitated, she must be restrained. If the restraints make her more agitated, perhaps she needs psychotropic medication. If the medication deprives her of emotions both negative and positive, so be it. At least she does not have agitation, that "aspect of dementia that is both difficult to manage and emotionally troubling for those who care for patients suffering from dementia."

On April 7, 2004, the *New York Times* reported on an Alzheimer's conference at the Johns Hopkins University at which several researchers (including some of the editors of this volume) declared that the benefits of AD medications are modest at best and are far outweighed by their high costs. If promising drugs are on the horizon, they said, it is a distant horizon. The only indisputable beneficiary of medicating people with dementia is the pharmaceutical industry, whose sales of five related drugs have soared into the billions of dollars (Grady 2004).

This news, reprinted from Kansas City to Sydney, Australia, whipped up a predictable storm in the Alzheimer's world. In letters to the editor of the *Times*, some applauded these revelations, pointing to the harmful effects of medication and calling for research stripped of profit-motivated bias. But many condemned the doctors at the conference and chided the newspaper for running the story. The Alzheimer's Association posted its unpublished letter of "concern" on its website. It cited "more than 100 new compounds in the pipeline" and its lobbying efforts for $40 million to accelerate clinical trials. The letter expressed the notion that drug therapy isn't perfect but that "even a slight improvement" benefits a sufferer's whole family (Tangalos 2004). A letter to the *Times* from an Alzheimer's activist and caregiver put it this way: "The approved drugs are the closest to a miracle we have so far" (Walsh 2004).

These letters imply two things: (1) that drugs are the only way of treating dementia, and (2) that ceasing to prescribe them not only would deprive sufferers of this meager help but also would rob them and their families of hope. My reaction to the story was the exact opposite. For the first time in years, I felt hopeful.

My family's experience teaches me that the difference in the life of a person with dementia is not medical, it is social: predictable routines; a connection to home or community (and an institution can be a community); and the generosity, respect, and creativity of those around. The *New York Times* reported on two U.S. studies that found that Alzheimer's patients (just like everyone else) are less depressed and agitated if they get enough exercise, participate in stimulating activities, and live in pleasant environments (O'Conner 2003). Other research has found that that high-quality nonmedical treatment, even in the last stages of global deterioration, can retard cognitive decline and even help people recover intellectual powers that were considered irretrievable. The late British psychologist Tom Kitwood, who observed similar effects at his clinic in Bradford, England, called this process "rementia" (Kitwood 1997). It is not achieved by a pharmaceutical compound.

On Dad's 86th birthday, in March 2005, an interesting thing happened. One of the social workers gave him a ball about the size of a soccer ball, covered with multicolored patches of velvety plush, stuffed and smooshy as a teddy bear. When the ball was tossed to Dad, he caught it firmly. Then he tossed it back, with accuracy and strength. He could do this fast or slow. He could pass it to someone else. He could even, with a sly look in his eye, throw a feint.

A couple of weeks later, out on the bench in the early spring sun, Dad and I played catch. He laughed and joshed in his half-gibberish speech. For the first time in months, I saw the agile tennis player, powerful swimmer, and home handyman I'd known all my life. Here was not a bad boy or a good boy, not an AD "sufferer" with frazzling brain cells, not a well-managed patient. Here was my confident, competent, competitive father. Tossing that ball back and forth, I wondered what else he might be able to do if given the chance.

Giving him the chance requires new thinking, new research, new creativity, and new priorities. It also requires a new kind of hope. That hope will not be found in chemicals but in relationships and communities; it will not come in a tablet or a capsule. For me, for now, hope is shaped like a large, fuzzy, multicolored ball, grasped in my father's still-strong hands.

NOTES

1. Theodore Levine died in January 2006. This chapter was written in 2005.

2. "Estimates of Funding for Various Diseases, Conditions, Research Areas (FY2004)," U.S. National Institutes of Health website. My conclusion about the proportion of funding going to biomedical research derives from searches of NIH-awarded grants lists, as well as testimony of researchers in the field. fairfoundation.org/NIH_funding_2003–2008.pdf.

3. Program, Ninth International Conference on Alzheimer's Disease and Related Disorders, Philadelphia, July 17–22, 2004.

REFERENCES

AstraZeneca. 2004. Study examines Seroquel for the treatment of agitation in elderly patients with dementia. Press release issued July 22. www.prnewswire.com/cgi-bin/stories.pl?ACCT= 104&STORY=/www/story/07-22-2004/0002215779&EDATE=.

Ballard, C., et al. 2005. Quetiapine and rivastigmine and cognitive decline in Alzheimer's disease: Randomised double blind placebo controlled trial. *British Medical Journal* 330:874–78.

Grady, D. 2004. Minimal benefit is seen in drugs for Alzheimer's. *New York Times*, April 27, A1.

Kitwood, T. 1997. *Dementia reconsidered: The person comes first.* Buckingham, UK: Open University Press.

Levine, J. 2004. *Do you remember me? A father, a daughter, and a search for the self.* New York: Free Press.

O'Connor, A. 2003. Exercise and setting ease Alzheimer's effects. *New York Times* (November 4): F5.

Tangalos, E. 2004. Unpublished letter to the editor of the *New York Times,* Alzheimer's Association website (April 7; no longer available).

Walsh, J. B. 2004. Letters, *New York Times,* April 11, A4.

CHAPTER 7

Making Sense of the Language of Benefit for Alzheimer's Disease Treatments

JASON H. T. KARLAWISH, M.D.

> You don't believe in the current Alzheimer's drugs.
> —*A colleague in conversation with the author*

> No measurement, no science.
> —*Anonymous*

Nearly half a century has passed since Alzheimer's disease (AD) began its transformation from what was once a part of nature that we simply accepted as life's course to a disease we must fight, conquer, and even cure. As a physician, I am pleased that this is happening. I have a clinic full of patients and their families who suffer with this disease. A key to the success of this transformation is the development of evidence-based treatments.

No doubt, current treatments for AD have an effect on the disease. Multiple randomized and well-controlled clinical trials show this. Yet despite a decade of these trials, the nature and significance of that effect remain controversial. For example, the American Academy of Neurology's evidence-based guidelines for the treatment of AD recommend only that the most common class of treatments, the acetylcholinesterase inhibitors, be considered in the treatment of mild to moderate AD. They are not labeled "standard of care." Why? An appendix to that guideline explains the problem: there is no standard approach to determining the magnitude of the benefits of treatments for dementia.

The singular problem in the testing and use of AD treatments is the lack of a coherent language to represent the benefits of those drugs. By "coherent language," I mean a language of benefit that makes sense across the communities of researchers, clinicians, patients, and policy makers. Until we develop a coherent language, controversies over whether an AD treatment is "worth it" will continue. Researchers will squabble over the best way to measure whether a drug has an effect on the disease. Clinicians will agree to disagree on whether and how best to use the treatments. Families will wonder if the drug is working. Policy makers will question whether the drug is worth its cost.

In this chapter I will develop the concept of a coherent language of benefit and examine why AD lacks such a language, how the field will likely develop such a language, and how that language will transform the way we understand the disease we currently call "Alzheimer's disease."

A key event in the emergence of AD as a medical problem is the development of diagnostic criteria. The most popular of these is the National Institute of Neurological and Communicative Disorders and Stroke and the Alzheimer's Disease and Related Disorders Association (NINCDS-ADRDA) criteria published in 1984. These criteria gave clinicians and clinical investigators a common language to say what AD is. The criteria, as well as others such as the American Psychiatric Association's *Diagnostic and Statistical Manual of Mental Disorders*, require declines in at least two domains of cognition that interfere in the ability to perform usual and everyday activities.

What is notable in these criteria is not what they say, but what they do not say. The document lists multiple possible cognitive and functional tests that may be used to evaluate a patient, but it concedes that these many tests are simply suggestions because there is continued debate about what tests are best. The criteria are more akin to general guidelines to shape clinical judgment. AD researchers and clinicians continue to struggle with the question, what measures are both valid and valuable measures of the disease?

I assert that history explains why this struggle continues (Karlawish 2002). The fields of AD drug development, diagnostics, and staging began simultaneously. We are trying to do three things at once. This is strikingly different from many other common diseases of aging, such as diabetes, hypertension, and cancer. For those diseases, medicine developed a reasonable expertise at diagnosis and staging before we developed a commensurate expertise at treating the diseases. Frustrating as this was for clinicians and their patients, it meant that when medicine began to use the randomized and controlled trial to develop treatments, a reasonable language was in place that allowed clinical researchers to say to clinicians that the treatment worked.

For example, in the case of hypertension, medicine knew that measures such as blood pressure, kidney or heart failure, and stroke were all valid and clinically meaningful representations of the disease. A study that showed that an intervention could affect them was a study reporting on an intervention worth using in the clinic. Results from such a study were coherent because they made sense to clinical investigators, clinicians, and even patients. Everyone was speaking the same language, more or less.

The features of such a coherent language of benefit include that the same terms work in the contexts of diagnosis, staging, and treatment. Hypertension is diagnosed using blood pressure measured in millimeters of mercury. Its severity is graded using the same measure. And the response to an intervention—whether in a clinical trial or clinical practice—is measured using blood pressure in millimeters of mercury. In sum, this measure is valid because scientists accept that it adequately captures the disease. In addition, the measure is valued because clinicians, policy makers, and patients map their particular ideas of what is "good," "beneficial," etc., onto this measure.

Other common diseases have similar histories. Diabetes is well understood as a disease whose signature is elevations in blood glucose. Clinicians and patients can measure this in the office or at home. Clinical trials of promising new diabetes drugs can show that the drug has properly lowered blood glucose. In the cases of both hypertension and diabetes, there is general consensus not only on what is the proper measure but also on what is a "normal level" of blood glucose and blood pressure.

"Consensus" is the operative term in achieving a coherent language. That is, the measure or measures work well enough for the variety of communities that use them, communities such as clinicians, investigators, and policy makers. Consensus means that controversies only simmer. They do not disrupt the progress of experiment. There are multiple sources of controversy. They include whether the measure reflects sufficient clinical benefit to the patient. In the case of hypertension, for example, the benefit of lowering blood pressure does not consistently translate into achieving the goal of improving a patient's health and well-being. Another controversy is the decision about what is a "normal" blood pressure. Though data describe the normal distribution, the cutoff of what is above and below normal is a judgment informed by these data but not determined by them. Humans make that judgment, and a variety of ethical, political, and even economic considerations inform it. When new data or ethical, political, or economic shifts occur, the consensus may be disrupted, and thus coherence breaks down.

Such coherence of a language of diagnosis, treatment, and progression is essential for the progress of testing new therapeutics. Specifically, a coherent language allows us to confidently narrow down the reasons why a promising drug failed to benefit the subjects of the clinical trial. A so-called negative trial, that is, a trial that fails to show substantial change on the primary endpoints, has multiple explanations for this failure. One explanation, and the one we reach for first, is that the drug did not work. It did not affect the disease.

But there are other possible explanations. The problem may be in the way we measure the disease. Problems with our measures may have led us to enroll people in the study who do not actually have the disease, or our measures of how the disease progresses may not adequately capture it. The fault is not with the drug but with the language that we construct to talk about the disease. We may not be talking about it correctly.

In the case of developing new therapies for which we have a coherent language of benefit, we can be reasonably confident that a negative study reflects the failure of the drug to affect the disease. Our language is good enough. We need to pick a different drug. But in the case of developing new therapeutics for which we do not have a coherent language of benefit, the progress of experiment is intermittent, disputed, and comparatively slow. The problem may be the drug, how we measure whether people have the disease, how we measure the drug's effect, or a combination of these issues.

In AD drug development, we do not have a coherent language of benefit. Instead, we have many different measures of many different perspectives to say what we think is AD. Moreover, many of these measures are not shared among clinicians and clinical researchers. They are instead "private languages," meaning they are largely understood within an exclusive community, such as the community of clinical investigators.

For example, one of the primary endpoints of an AD clinical trial is the cognitive subscale of the Alzheimer's Disease Assessment Scale (the ADAS-cog). As ubiquitous as it is in clinical trials, it is entirely unused in clinical practice. Moreover, at the same clinical research centers where trials commonly occur, the ADAS-cog is gathered only in the context of clinical trials. The federally funded Alzheimer's disease research centers do not include this measure in their "uniform data set." The most common measure of cognition, the Mini-Mental State Exam (MMSE), is used as an inclusion criterion for studies, but it is rarely used as an outcome measure. Moreover, its use is increasingly restricted because the measure is under copyright and the holders of that copyright are more and more determined to collect their fees. This point reiterates how the coherence of a measure of benefit is influenced by extrascientific considerations such as whether one must pay to use the measure, that is, to speak the language.

Similar problems exist with several of the common measures of staging. One of the more popular measures, the Clinical Dementia Rating scale, known commonly as the CDR, involves a detailed and structured interview lasting up to one hour. While this measure is widely used in clinical research settings and is part of the "uniform data set," it is rarely, if at all, used in clinical practice. Although loss of function is a hallmark sign of AD, measures of function, such as the instrumental activities of daily living, are not typically used as primary endpoints and are not commonly performed in clinical practice. Only recently has the U.S. clinical research enterprise settled on a preferred measure, the Alzheimer's Disease Cooperative Study measure of activities of daily living.

In short, the problems with the language of benefit for AD illustrate why even when a clinical trial shows a statistically significant effect of a drug compared to a control, the results are not easily translated into clinical practice and readily supported by institutions that pay for the drugs.

How will we develop a coherent language for the diagnosis, staging, and treatment of AD? The answer to this question requires close attention to one particular feature of a coherent language. The language is typically biological, that is, the words describe things that we measure "in the laboratory" as opposed to asking questions, filling out forms, and then summing up scores to arrive at the truth.

This feature is likely not accidental. Biology gives a measure's truth the veneer of objective truth. It removes the vagaries introduced by the skills and enthusiasm of the person who is making the measurement and the interaction between that person and the patient being measured. In AD, clinicians and especially families are well aware that a patient may have a bad day of testing with a callous tester. Such real-world events can introduce substantial variance into the measure. But blood is blood. Once a vein is found, the interaction between the patient and the phlebotomist has little relevance to the accuracy of what the laboratory measures in that blood. This, of course, assumes that the biological measure does not depend on the skills and equipment used to measure it. Because if it does depend on these factors, then it is just as inadequate as the statistically noisy clinical measures it was intended to replace.

There are likely other reasons why medicine favors biological measures. They seem to get us closer to the disease as opposed to the symptoms of the disease. As well, they are easily reimbursed, and sometimes reimbursed handsomely.

The desire to develop a biological language of AD leads to my final point about the creation of a language of benefit for AD: AD clinical trials are designed not simply to test whether a drug is effective but to test whether the language of benefit is valid.

Current clinical trials now routinely include "biomarkers" of AD. The term refers to measures in blood, urine, or spinal fluid or detailed images of the brain that scientists reason "are" AD. The logic of the biomarker is that it signifies the disease. As levels of the biomarker increase, the disease worsens. A successful intervention is one that reduces the level of the biomarker and in turn reduces the severity of the disease. All of this makes sense, but it is contingent upon the validity of the biomarker. In fact, none of the candidate biomarkers is a validated biomarker. Instead, in what may seem to be circular logic, the clinical trial is testing the validity of the biomarker to measure AD.

To the degree that this effort is successful, it will in turn reveal one final aspect of the construction of a language of benefit: coherent languages of benefit change the disease they measure. This may at first seem paradoxical. A disease is an entity, like the elements of the periodic table. How can the way we talk about treating a disease change the disease?

Properly understood, the biological reality of the disease does not in fact change. But the way clinicians and investigators talk about their idea of what the disease is does change. For example, osteoporosis was once upon a time talked about as a disease of fractured bones. Physicians diagnosed it by looking for fractures, especially in the bodies of the vertebra. And then medical science discovered how to measure bone mineral density and that normalized scores of bone mineral density predicted not simply having a fracture but the probability over time of experiencing a fracture. In time, the disease became the Z-score measurement of bone mineral density that predicted the risk of a fracture.

AD will likely experience this kind of transformation. As one or more biomarkers are sufficiently validated and interventions affect them, AD as we talk about it will become that biomarker. Depending on the ease of the biomarker's measurement, its cost, and the size of the effect of treatment, it is entirely possible that it will change how we diagnose AD. It will transform from being a diagnosis made when a person has dementia to a diagnosis made when the biomarker is "positive." A person will not have to have dementia to have AD.

Alzheimer's disease is as real as the Earth we live on. I have a clinic full of patients who repeat the same question over and over, cannot pay a credit card bill, accuse their partner of infidelity, and ask me if they are losing their mind. AD exists. But the way we talk about this disease is in flux. We are like the survivors walking away from the dust of the fallen Tower of Babel, a bit flummoxed, our ears are still ringing from the noise. Slowly we are discovering the contours of this disease and the language to coherently represent them. I neither believe nor disbelieve in the current treatments for AD. I just want a better way to talk about them.

REFERENCE

Karlawish, J. H. T. 2002. The search for a coherent language: The science and politics of drug testing and approval. *Ethics, Law and Aging Review* 8:39–56.

PART III

OBJECTIVITY, LANGUAGE, AND VALUES AT THE INTERFACE OF SCIENCE, MEDICINE, AND BUSINESS

Perhaps the most consistent point of controversy generated by interdisciplinary projects that focus on a particular scientific enterprise is the "objectivity question": Is the enterprise—in the case of this book, the development of drug treatments for dementia—a more or less neutral, value-free endeavor that ensures that it will produce reliable knowledge and practice than other human activities? Or, despite the good intentions of its practitioners, is the scientific enterprise so suffused with human ambition and fallibility that it is no more or less reliable than anything else that people produce?

The three chapters in this section problematize the objectivity question by scrutinizing in different ways language practices that mediate the relationships among science, medicine, and business in the development of drug treatments for dementia. Each approaches the question of what is possible and desirable from a different perspective, and, perhaps not surprisingly, they reach different conclusions. We present them not to resolve the question but in the hope that together these different perspectives can lead to a more nuanced approach to the question. As previous interdisciplinary work—including earlier work on the concept of Alzheimer's disease by two of this volume's editors (Whitehouse, Maurer, and Ballenger 2000)—has suggested, the answer to the objectivity question is complex. As a result, it is not possible to capture the essence of the scientific enterprise in a simple either/or formulation. This is equally true in the context of drug development for Alzheimer's disease, though the financial stakes are higher and the attractiveness of the polarities may be greater. We recognize that for many of our readers these may be the most controversial chapters in a book that aims to provoke debate.

In the first chapter of this section, John R. Gilstad and Thomas Finucane argue that the peer-reviewed research literature on donepezil, the most widely used of the acetylcholinesterase inhibitors, rhetorically functions as paid advertising for the drug company sponsoring the clinical trials. They do not criticize the scientific validity of the results generated by these trials but rather the way the description of the results presents a coherent promotional message replete with persuasive turns of phrase and enthusiastic "spin" applied to rather unimpressive and sometimes even negative results. Though Gilstad and Finucane are careful to avoid any explicit claims about the motivations of the researchers involved, the strong implication of this chapter is that the manufacturer influenced the content of the articles, leading the authors to use words and formulations consciously chosen to frame the results favorably and to cause peer reviewers, journal editors, and publishers to look the other way. But whatever the motivations of those involved, Gilstad and Finucane's commitment as clinicians to the normative ideal of objectivity leads them to view the situation as a scandal and to conclude that, in the future, professionals and society will be embarrassed to have succumbed to the manipulations of drug companies.

Clearly Gilstad and Finucane have taken a highly controversial position, one that we believe bears examination. Living in a culture that values free speech means that all sides of an issue can be publicly explored, and a major theme of this volume, that the development of treatments for later-life cognitive decline is a lens through which the values, ideals, and methods of society can be viewed and understood, can only benefit from a careful examination of how one major element of cognitive therapeutics is presented. Intriguingly, Gilstad and Finucane use the term "rhetoric," with its current negative connotations, to describe the language used to market donepezil rather than a more neutral word such as "language." If one adopts the ancient Greeks' use of the term as the discipline that studies the techniques of persuasion, then the rhetoric used by the authors to examine the rhetoric used by those marketing the drug tells us a great deal about how a careful analysis of the words chosen to discuss a topic and the placement of these words in particular positions in articles is a subject worth study. The conclusions a reader draws will reflect both the strength of the arguments on both sides of the question and the values the reader brings to the subject.

Rein Vos advances a much more radical claim in his chapter than Gilstad and Finucane, arguing that the scientific process of drug development itself is fraught with value judgments. Like Finucane and Gilstad, Vos highlights the importance of language, examining the use of words such as "disease" and "normal," terms for processes such as "birth" and "dying," and classification schema such a "genetic," "infectious," and "environmental" to demonstrate that the way these words are used inevitably reflects the values of individuals and society. Moreover, Vos suggests that drug discovery is not a linear process in which advances in knowledge about disease lead to discoveries that result in specific developments but an iterative one in which scientific discovery sometimes is driven by a need to apply its findings, influencing how abnormality, disease, and the development and targeting of a therapeutic agent are conceptualized.

But as a philosopher inclined by discipline to critically examine the truth claims of science, Vos represents this situation less as a scandal than as an inherent, albeit generally unacknowledged, aspect of drug development. He argues that it is worthwhile to acknowledge that drug development is value-laden in order to better appreciate the process as well as the harmful effects that can come from making absolute claims about the primacy of any single approach. Values matter, and an explicit understanding of how values are expressed in language can benefit drug development and society. According to Vos, we should not try to exclude values from the process of drug development but instead make sure the process is equally open to the values of all stakeholders, including patients and caregivers, and that value conflicts are acknowledged and negotiated in a fair manner.

Peter Whitehouse's interest in the concept of quality of life (QOL) reflects a similar concern about how to incorporate values into the way we approach the problem of AD and dementia. Whitehouse writes from the perspective of a neuroscientist who participated early in research that led to the development of cholinergic drugs for AD but who has grown increasingly disenchanted with the biomedical model of dementia. His personal chapter tells the story of how he came to change his views so radically, emphasizing his discomfort with the influence pharmaceutical companies were having on the direction of his own career, as well as the influence they continue to have on the AD field as a whole, and his growing interest in what disciplines like history and anthropology can contribute to dealing with dementia.

Whitehouse recognizes that scientific medicine has difficulty validating and measuring a value-laden term such as QOL, but he believes it must remain the primary goal of treatment and prevention in a medicine that is concerned with the broadest human needs—building and maintaining a just and environmentally sustainable world. Rather than ignore or seek a more scientifically viable proxy for QOL, Whitehouse questions the faith society puts in biomedical science, worrying that viewing age-associated cognitive declines as disease and claiming that they can be cured by pharmaceutical agents has distracted society from important steps that can be taken both early and late in life to lessen their occurrence.

The chapters in this section clearly do not agree on a simple answer to the objectivity question or on the best way to resolve the tension between science and business that, in the case of drug development for dementia and many other conditions in contemporary medicine, complicates and intensifies the problem. Nonetheless, together the chapters reinforce the important point that there are no simple answers and that many perspectives are valuable. The critical disciplines like philosophy, history, and anthropology that Vos and Whitehouse engage can usefully question whether the process of drug development could ever be objective and value-free; at the same time, Gilstad and Finucane passionately defend the ideal that scientific literature should report data in an unbiased manner that retains fidelity to the data generated by clinical trials. Similarly, our quest for objectivity and rational pursuit of effective therapeutics should not keep us from asking fundamental questions about what we are doing and why. In the end, we are left with the task of balancing many different values, imperatives, and perspectives. We hope the chapters in this section stand as a useful contribution to this ongoing process.

REFERENCE

Whitehouse, P. J., K. Maurer, and J. F. Ballenger, eds. 2000. *Concepts of Alzheimer disease: Biological, clinical, and cultural perspectives.* Baltimore: Johns Hopkins University Press.

CHAPTER 8

Science and Marketing

The Promotion of Donepezil in the Primary Research Literature

JOHN R. GILSTAD, M.D.
THOMAS E. FINUCANE, M.D.

Far too large a section of the treatment of disease is today
controlled by the big manufacturing pharmacists, who have
enslaved us in a plausible pseudoscience.
—*William Osler, 1909*

Advertising: the science of arresting the human intelligence
long enough to get money from it.
—*Stephen Leacock, 1924*

Consider the contrast between an educated reader's approach to a
research article on a medication and her or his approach to advertising about
that same medication. In the research article, the reader evaluates the *evidence*: what was measured, how it was measured, whether the results are reliable and generalizable. In advertising, the reader evaluates the *rhetoric* to
discern the underlying truth and distinguish it from the predictably persuasive, hyperbolic, or even misleading presentation. The primary research articles on donepezil, however, share several rhetorical features with advertising:
a coherent promotional message, persuasive turns of phrase, and enthusiastic "spin" applied to outcomes data that may be seen, when analyzed objectively, to be distinctly unimpressive. In this chapter we will describe some of
these promotional rhetorical features, categorized into families of canards:

"symptoms," "momentum," "ethics," "effective versus beneficial," "spinning the negative," "standard of care," "stabilization of disease," and "ignoring the nonpromotional," with brief mention of product placement, indication expansion, and graphical trickery. We emphasize that our discussion is limited to an analysis of the rhetoric; we examine not the scientific validity of the clinical trials' results but the way these results are reported.

Before proceeding, we also emphasize one key difference between the donepezil literature and an advertising campaign. The latter is openly purchased by the manufacturer while the former is the product, for the most part, of clinical scientists, peer reviewers, and journal editors who have ethical standards to uphold and reputations to protect. Is it fair or even rational to suggest that industry has somehow managed to buy advertising from these biomedical professionals in the form of peer-reviewed literature? We do not address that question in this chapter; instead, we simply let the rhetoric speak for itself. The relative importance and the specific mechanisms of overt financial or professional reward, pressure, subconscious obligation, and genuine enthusiasm remain to be elucidated.

The following discussion is based largely on the first 12 published randomized controlled trials (RCTs) of donepezil in which clinical endpoints were measured (table 8.1). The first 10 of these were supported by the vendors of donepezil (studies 1–10 in table 8.1). The results of all these randomized trials are fairly consistent: the drug has had a statistically significant effect on psychometric testing, but the effect appears to be small, heterogeneous, and unpredictable; effects on global assessments, function, and behavior are less consistent. Several simple rhetorical devices in the industry-sponsored randomized controlled trials (SRCTs) create a coherent promotional message, affirming efficacy and encouraging clinical use. Because stabilization of disease is such an important claim in donepezil advertising, and there are no industry-sponsored RCTs with institutionalization as an endpoint, we include a single industry-supported nonrandomized study (Geldmacher et al. 2003) and contrast its findings and rhetoric with an RCT not supported by donepezil vendors that was designed to examine the same question.

The Symptoms Canard

Phrases that contain the words "efficacious treating symptoms" appear repeatedly in the SRCTs, describing data that do not actually address symptoms. In the context of physical diagnosis, "symptoms" usually refer to problems de-

TABLE 8.1
First twelve published randomized controlled trials of donepezil
with clinical endpoints measured

1.	1996	Rogers, S. L., and L. T. Friedhoff	*Dementia* 7 (6): 293–303
2.	1998	Rogers, S. L., et al.	*Neurology* 50 (1): 136–45
3.	1998	Rogers, S. L., R. S. Doody, R. C. Mohs, and L. T. Friedhoff	*Archives of Internal Medicine* 158 (9): 1021–31
4.	1999	Burns, A., et al.	*Dementia and Geriatric Cognitive Disorders* 10 (3): 237–44
5.	2000	Homma, A., et al.	*Dementia and Geriatric Cognitive Disorders* 11 (6): 299–313
6.	2001	Mohs, R. C., et al.	*Neurology* 57 (3): 481–88
7.	2001	Winblad, B., et al.	*Neurology* 57 (3): 489–95
8.	2001	Feldman, H., et al.	*Neurology* 57 (4): 613–20
9.	2001	Tariot, P. N., et al.	*Journal of the American Geriatrics Society* 49 (12): 1590–99
10.	2003	Feldman, H., et al.	*Journal of the American Geriatrics Society* 51 (6): 737–44
11.	2000	Greenberg, S. M., et al.	*Archives of Neurology* 57 (1): 94–99
12.	2004	AD2000 Collaborative Group	*Lancet* 363: 2105–15

scribed by a patient, whereas "signs" are abnormalities discovered by the examiner. The distinction is not absolute, as the example of "negative symptoms of schizophrenia" illustrates; if severe enough, negative symptoms would not be reported by the patient, and would need to be discovered by the examiner. But there may properly be said to be a distinction in the realm of mild to moderate Alzheimer's disease. For families who care for these patients, a claim that a drug treats the symptoms of the disease implies that the patient will himself report feeling better.

The measure that most directly attempts to assess how patients feel about their life—a seven-item, 350-point quality-of-life scale—found no meaningful difference between drug and placebo in the four trials in which it was used, however. Differences were not statistically significant in three of the four, and in the fourth trial a difference of 10 points favored placebo. That is, no genuine "symptomatic" benefit, as reported by patient or caregiver, has been measured in these SRCTs despite what the words "efficacious treating symptoms" suggests. Symptomatic improvement may be inferred by the results of some other psychometrics, but the improvement is small and in some cases inconsistent—not the straightforward success story that the motif implies. For example, in the Clinician's Interview-Based Impression of Change, in which the examiner makes a global judgment about response to therapy after interviewing the patient and a caregiver, these same four trials all showed statistically significant mean improvements, but in all the effect was less than half a point on a seven-point scale (that is, not quite halfway from "no change" to "minimal improvement"). Another global assessment scale, the 18-point Clinical Dementia Rating–Sum of Boxes (CDR-SB), was unchanged in two trials and showed treatment differences of 0.4 and 0.6 in the other two. AD2000 (study 12 in table 8.1), the study with the largest number of patient years in randomization, showed no differences in "behavioral and psychological symptoms (or) carer psychopathology." This trial has been criticized, but the outcomes on its psychometric tests were about the same as those of the industry-sponsored studies.

The Momentum Canard

The body of sponsored donepezil literature creates an impression of established truth through repetition of positive phrases from one paper to the next, assertions of "confirmation" of positive results with references to prior papers, and neglect of the nonsponsored paper that presents a different interpretation. "Well tolerated and effective," "effective and well tolerated," and "well tolerated and efficacious" are examples; in none of these recurring formulations of the same claim of efficacy is the extent or character of the efficacy modified in any way. Instead, a simple, positive message is frequently repeated. As early as the second published SRCT (study 2 in table 8.1), the authors report that their trial "confirms that donepezil is efficacious in treating symptoms of memory loss and cognitive loss." None of the sponsored trials that occur after the first nonsponsored trial acknowledges it or addresses the less favorable interpretation of results—the lack of a simple positive message— that it contains. The monolithic, strongly positive rhetoric of the sponsored trials remains perfectly consistent.

The Ethics Canard

One SRCT refers to prior evidence of the drug's effectiveness and then opines that "results such as ours raise ethical and practical concerns regarding randomization of patients with AD to placebo in clinical trials of more than a few months duration" (Mohs et al. 2001). In mid-discussion, the single nonrandomized study we include, done "under the direction of and with funding from Eisai, Inc., and Pfizer, Inc." makes the same claim, stating simply that "conducting such a study [i.e., a proper RCT] would not be ethical" (Geldmacher et al. 2003). The powerful assertion in both publications is that the drug's effectiveness is so certainly demonstrated and so meaningful to patients that to withhold this drug is to harm patients, and an investigator would be unethical if she participated in such a trial.

"Effective" or "Beneficial"?

Early trials on donepezil use the words "effective" and "efficacious" prominently, and the word "benefit" never appears (studies 1–5 in table 8.1). The seventh (Winblad et al. 2001) uses "effective" but then switches to introduce "benefits" and "beneficial" to the SRCT rhetoric. Subsequent SRCTs attribute "benefits" rather than "effects" (studies 8–10 in table 8.1). The nonrandomized, drug-company-sponsored trial contains an explanation of the rhetorical agenda behind this change from "effect" to "benefit." "Doctors and caregivers need to be educated that, in the same way as the actual benefits of treating hypertension or hyperlipidemia are seen only after years of treatment, treatment of AD with donepezil needs to be maintained to see important long-term benefits." That is, it is no longer necessary to see effects from the drug, it is just necessary to keep prescribing it in order to achieve future SRCT-proved "benefits" for the patients.

"Spinning" the Negative Trial

The penultimate SRCT in our series was a well-designed study of the use of donepezil in nursing home residents (Tariot et al. 2001). Its primary outcome measure was the Neuropsychiatric Inventory–Nursing Home Version (NPI-NH). Three secondary measures were also studied: the CDR-SB, the MMSE, and the Physical Self-Maintenance Scale (PSMS). For the primary outcome measure of the study, the NPI-NH, the authors found "no significant differences observed between the groups at any assessment." The same was true for the PSMS. At study's end no significant difference was seen in the MMSE. (The authors did not state this in the two paragraphs of discussion about MMSE results, but it is seen in the figure.) The CDR favored donepezil treatment by less than a point on an 18-point scale (p < .05).

This trial was completely negative for the primary outcome and nearly completely negative for all secondary outcomes. Nonetheless, the top-line conclusion in the article's abstract is: "Patients treated with donepezil maintained or improved in cognition and overall dementia severity in contrast to placebo-treated patients who declined during the 6-month treatment period." The abstract concludes with a simple promotional statement: this study's findings "are consistent with previous findings in outpatients and support the use of donepezil in patients with AD who reside in nursing homes." The upbeat promotional message grafted onto this negative trial continues in the text's discussion, with only a temporary hesitation: "At the very least, the data in this trial demonstrate that cognition and overall dementia severity are maintained for 6 months in these nursing home patients." Remember that at study's end the MMSE was not different between drug- and placebo-treated patients. Several other SRCTs "spin" their results, but none so egregiously as this.

The Standard of Care Canard

Authors of the nonrandomized trial we consider here, as well as several other authors (Geldmacher et al. 2003; Clark et al. 2003; Cummings et al., 2004), claim that cholinesterase inhibitors (ChEI) treatment is the standard of care for patients with Alzheimer's disease and cite the American Academy of Neurology's "Practice Parameter: Management of Dementia" for confirmation (Doody et al. 2001). In doing this, they are misleading. Here is what the "Practice Parameter" says, in its entirety: "Cholinesterase inhibitors should be considered in patients with AD (Standard), although studies suggest a small average degree of benefit" (Doody et al. 2001).

The Stabilization of Disease Canard

Claims of disease stabilization are founded on a few experimental observations. Treated patients often show an improvement on psychometric testing, such as the cognitive subscale of the Alzheimer's Disease Assessment Scale (ADAS-cog), which rises a point or two, and then falls to baseline after about six months. The decline roughly parallels the decline in patients on placebo. In some cases, as described above, authors simply summarize negative results positively. "Patients treated with donepezil maintained or improved in cognition and overall dementia severity in contrast to placebo-treated patients who declined during the 6-month treatment period" (Tariot et al. 2001)—this in a study where the cognitive measure was not different from placebo at six months.

Some trials have looked at whether nursing home placement (NHP) can be delayed as a surrogate measure for disease progression. The results are contradictory; trials sponsored by vendors of the drugs are positive. Because no SRCTs have been done with NHP as an endpoint, we have included in this discussion a nonrandomized industry-sponsored trial in order to compare it to the only true RCT, one that was not industry-sponsored. The sponsored article is titled, predictably, "Donepezil is associated with delayed nursing home placement in patients with Alzheimer Disease." The study looked at patients on donepezil and compared those who took at least 80 percent of prescribed doses with those who did not for specific numbers of weeks. The top-line conclusion in the abstract is, "Use of donepezil by AD patients resulted in significant delays in NHP" (Geldmacher et al. 2003).

The study's design of comparing a drug's efficacy based on patient adherence has been discredited for decades. In 1980, for example, the Coronary Drug Project found that subjects who faithfully took a lactose placebo at least 80 percent of the time had half the mortality of subjects assigned to placebo who were not as adherent. Those authors did not claim, as the drug-company-sponsored authors of the 2003 publication do, that the lactose placebo "resulted in" anything. They noted that adherent patients differ from nonadherent patients in important ways (CDP Research Group 1980). The 2003 study is perhaps even more implausible. Patients with a coherent fabric of caregiving are more likely to remain adherent and enrolled and more likely to avoid NHP. A variety of other serious criticisms have been leveled at this study, including failure to report known baseline differences between the groups and "lack of a detailed analysis plan, resulting, in reality, in data dredging" (Schneider et al. 2004).

AD 2000 reached the opposite conclusion. "No significant benefits were seen with donepezil compared with placebo in institutionalization (42% vs. 44% at 3 years; p = 0.4) or progression of disability (58% vs. 59% at 3 years; p = 0.4) . . . [or] in behavioral and psychological symptoms, carer psycho-pathology, formal care costs, unpaid caregiver time, adverse events or deaths, or between 5 mg and 10 mg donepezil." The findings of this trial are similar to the findings of SRCTs: psychometric differences were highly statistically significant (MMSE was 0.8 points better at two years in the drug-treated group p < 0.0001), but patient and caregiver could not tell the difference between drug and placebo. In contrast to the findings, however, the rhetoric of the SRCTs and AD2000 is different; the rhetoric of the nonrandomized, industry-sponsored trial of NHP is deeply promotional.

Ignoring Nonpromotional Studies

In addition to AD2000, one other RCT was conducted without drug company sponsorship (Greenberg et al. 2000). Neither of these trials is ever referenced by the industry-sponsored trials, which reference each other promiscuously. Results in this second non-industry-sponsored RCT were about the same as those of AD2000 and of the SRCTs; treated patients were about two points better on the 70-point ADAS-cog (p = .04). The rhetoric is quite different. Effect and benefit are characterized as "modest" and "small," words that are never used in any of the industry-sponsored donepezil RCTs. How to characterize results of this magnitude has been argued; the effective range of the ADAS-cog may be smaller, analogous to the subset of the blood pressure scale that is clinically relevant. But "modest" and "small" are not unreasonable, as reflected in the similar characterization found in the American Academy of Neurology practice parameter (Doody et al. 2001), which summarizes results like these as suggesting "a small average degree of benefit." The SRCTs do not reference opposing interpretations and present instead a uniform positive message.

A variety of other rhetorical features with promotional import are apparent in these and other SRCTs. The brand name Aricept appears in the first line of an early SRCT (Rogers, Doody, et al. 1998) and on the first page of a second SRCT (Mohs et al. 2001); studies that do not receive support from vendors do not use brand names in research publications, as a rule. The drug's indications are stretched to encompass both milder (Rogers, Farlow, et al. 1998) and more severe (Tariot et al. 2001) cognitive impairment. Graphs magnify results by presenting only a small portion of a measure's range on the y axis, creating an intellectual *trompe l'oeil* that suggests marked benefits.

Prominently placed rhetoric may mislead readers who expect to find dispassionate science in peer-reviewed RCTs and who expect advertising to be confined to advertisements. The effectiveness of this embedded fabric of promotional rhetoric is magnified precisely because it is woven throughout the primary research publications on donepezil. The mechanisms by which the donepezil papers acquired features of advertising are likely complex, because they involve more than just drug company investment in an overt ad campaign. Authors, editors, and journals are necessary to complete the presentation of this promotional material. We have no data on actual mechanisms. But the outcome is similar to what one might expect from a formal rhetorical campaign. The rhetoric we have outlined here has been influential in the blockbuster success of this marginally effective drug, a process—and a problem—that Osler described a century ago. Further, we believe that in 10 years we will be embarrassed that we were manipulated by drug companies into channeling so many billions of dollars to the drug companies and away from these tragically ill patients and their valiant and sometimes desperate caregivers.

NOTE

The views expressed in this chapter are those of the author and do not necessarily reflect the official policy of the Department of the Navy, Department of Defense, or U.S. government.

REFERENCES

AD2000 Collaborative Group. 2004. Long-term donepezil treatment in 565 patients with Alzheimer's disease (AD2000): Randomized double-blind trial. *Lancet* 363:2105–15.

Burns A., M. Rossor, J. Hecker, S. Gauthier, H. Petit, H. J. Möller, S. L. Rogers, and L. T. Friedhoff. 1999. The effects of donepezil in Alzheimer's disease: Results from a multinational trial. *Dementia and Geriatric Cognitive Disorders* 10 (3): 237–44.

CDP Research Group. 1980. Influence of adherence to treatment and response of cholesterol on mortality in the coronary drug project. *New England Journal of Medicine* 303 (18): 1038–41.

Clark, C. M. and J. H. T. Karlawish, 2003. Alzheimer disease: Current concepts and emerging diagnostic and therapeutic strategies. *Annals of Internal Medicine* 38 (5): 400–410.

Cummings, J. L. 2004. Alzheimer's disease. *New England Journal of Medicine* 351 (1): 56–67.

Doody, R. S., J. C. Stevens, C. Beck, R. M. Dubinsky, J.A. Kaye, L. Gwyther, and R.C. Mohs, et al. 2001. Practice parameter: Management of dementia (an evidence-based review). Report of the Quality Standards Subcommittee of the American Academy of Neurology. *Neurology* 56 (9): 1154–66.

Feldman H., S. Gauthier, J. Hecker, B. Vellas, B. Emir, V. Mastey, and P. Subbiah. 2003. Efficacy of donepezil on maintenance of activities of daily living in patients with moderate to severe Alzheimer's disease and the effect on caregiver burden. *Journal of the American Geriatrics Society* 51 (6): 737–44.

Feldman, H., S. Gauthier, J. Hecker, B. Vellas, P. Subbiah, and E. Whalen. 2001. A 24-week, randomized, double-blind study of donepezil in moderate to severe Alzheimer's disease. *Neurology* 57 (4): 613–20.

Geldmacher, D. S., G. Provenzano, T. McRae, V. Mastey, J. R. Ieni.. 2003. Donepezil is associated with delayed nursing home placement in-patients with Alzheimer's disease. *Journal of the American Geriatrics Society* 51 (7): 937–44.

Greenberg, S. M., M. K. Tennis, L. B. Brown, T. Gomez-Isla, D. L. Hayden, D. A. Schoenfeld, K. L. Walsh, et al. 2000. Donepezil therapy in clinical practice: A randomized crossover study. *Archives of Neurology* 57 (1): 94–99.

Homma, A,, M. Takeda, Y. Imai, F. Udaka, K. Hasegawa, M. Kameyama, and T. Nishimura. 2000. Clinical efficacy and safety of donepezil on cognitive and global function in-patients with Alzheimer's disease: A 24-week, multicenter, double-blind, placebo-controlled study in Japan E2020 Study Group. *Dementia and Geriatric Cognitive Disorders* 11 (6): 299–313.

Mohs, R. C., R. S. Doody, J. C. Morris, J. R. Ieni, S. L. Rogers, C. A. Perdomo, and R. D. Pratt, "312" Study Group. 2001. A 1-year, placebo-controlled preservation of function survival study of donepezil in AD patients. *Neurology* 57 (3): 481–88.

Rogers, S. L., R. S. Doody, R. C. Mohs, and L. T. Friedhoff. 1998. Donepezil improves cognition and global function in Alzheimer disease: A 15-week, double-blind, placebo-controlled study. Donepezil Study Group. *Archives of Internal Medicine* 158 (9): 1021–31.

Rogers, S. L., M. R. Farlow, R. S. Doody, R. Mohs, and L. T. Friedhoff. 1998. A 24-week, double-blind, placebo-controlled trial of donepezil in patients with Alzheimer's disease. Donepezil Study Group. *Neurology* 50 (1): 136–45.

Rogers, S. L., and L. T. Friedhoff. 1996. The efficacy and safety of donepezil in patients with Alzheimer's disease: Results of a US multicentre, randomized, double-blind, placebo-controlled trial, the Donepezil Study Group. *Dementia* 7 (6): 293–303.

Schneider, L. S., N. Qizilbash. 2004. Delay in nursing home placement with donepezil. *Journal of the American Geriatric Society* 52 (6): 1024–22.

Seltzer, B., P. Zolnouni, M. Nunez, R. Goldman, D. Kumar, J. Ieni, and S. Richardson, Donepezil "402" Study Group. 2004. Efficacy of donepezil in early-stage Alzheimer disease: A randomized placebo-controlled trial. *Archives of Neurology* 61:1852–56.

Tariot, P. N., J. L. Cummings, I. R. Katz, J. Mintzer, C. A. Perdomo, E. M. Schwam, and E. Whalen. 2001. A randomized, double-blind, placebo-controlled study of the efficacy and safety of donepezil in patients with Alzheimer's disease in the nursing home setting. *Journal of American Geriatrics Society* 49 (12): 1590–99.

Winblad, B., K. Engedal, H. Soininen, F. Verhey, G. Waldemar, A. Wimo, A. L. Wetterholm, R. Zhang, A. Haglund, and P. Subbiah, Donepezil Nordic Study Group. 2001. A 1-year, randomized, placebo-controlled study of donepezil in-patients with mild to moderate AD. *Neurology* 57 (3): 489–95.

CHAPTER 9

Profiling Drugs and Diseases

The Shaping, Making, and Marketing of Drugs for Alzheimer's Disease

REIN VOS, M.D., PH.D.

The drug-discovery field is tightly connected to the dream of developing magic bullets for the treatment of disease. This applies to biomedical research into Alzheimer's disease (AD). Strong feelings of hope and expectation are expressed with the emergence of new technologies in genomics, molecular biology, and biotechnology. Much hope is therefore invested into science- and technology-driven research toward therapies for AD. This hope is inspired by the view that medicines are developed for diseases and that this is an objective and scientific process devoid of values and norms, which should enter the development process only in later stages when assessing the social, economic, and cultural effects of the drugs on persons, families, and society at large. Science comes first, and ethics follows, because they seem to be separate activities.

In this chapter I will argue the opposite—that in reality diseases are developed for drugs and drug discovery is an intrinsically value-driven process. To support and elaborate this view, I will try to get rid of the science-driven vocabulary of "disease model," "hypothesis," "pathway," "animal model," "disease entity," and other related terms and concepts. Although these terms are relevant for talk in the respective scientific fields of biomedicine, they mask some important features of the drug-discovery and drug-development process, which is a bidirectional, back-and-forth process, a synthesis of laboratory sciences and clinical medicine and an integration of facts and values, of science and ethics. We need a coherent language to elucidate how the two sides of the traditional dualistic conception of the relationship between medicine and society interact. I will use the concept of drug profiles and disease profiles, showing that the drug-discovery process is largely one of profiling drugs and diseases, of attempts to match such profiles, and of communicating back and forth through profiles of drugs and diseases between the various levels of the human organism studied in biomedicine: the molecular, the clinical, and the personal. Stated as simply and provocatively as possible, my thesis is that drugs are looking for diseases, that diseases are developed for drugs, and that this process is value driven throughout.

The Ontological Disease Concept and Its Hidden Moral Talk

To state that diseases are developed for drugs seems odd. AD is widely considered a devastating disease, a biological disorder with a material substrate of tangles and plaques destroying the brain. Therefore, most people view the drug-discovery process as a scientific undertaking that aims at achieving disease models of these plaques and tangles, disentangling the relevant pathogenetic pathways and their crucial components to find targets for drugs. This biomedical model of disease and therapy rests on an ontological concept of disease in which disease is conceived of as a separate and distinct entity (or process) "inside" the patient. If one knows the "truth" of the disease, one is able to develop a therapy or a drug. Thus, the ontological view implies the notion that disease is some kind of fixed entity or process that can be detailed and targeted. Once the intricate details of the target are spelled out, one is able to develop strategies for intervening.

Although AD and other forms of dementia are a biological reality, and a devastating one at that, the ontological concept of disease masks two things. First, saying that there "is" a disease hides the normative aspects of discerning the normal from the pathological. In the philosophy of medicine, there is a long tradition of debating the concepts of normality and disease. Murphy in the 1970s differentiated among various uses of the concept of normal (whence also abnormal) in clinical medicine (for example, "commonly encountered in its class," "most representative in its class," or "most suited to survival and reproduction"). Thus, a broad spectrum of notions of normality can be denoted, ranging from the "distributional" aspect, as in a Gaussian or other kind of measure of "normal" and "abnormal" values regarding height, weight, age, blood pressure, plasma cholesterol, etc., to the "functional" aspect, as in a beating heart that suddenly arrests or a brain slowly losing control over memory. In past decades, the so-called functional failure model emerged as the fundamental model to formulate the basic features of normality and disease.[1] The concept of disease as a functional failure of a programmed biological process is indeed a powerful model, because it makes sense in that many diseases, with enzyme defects as the prime example, expose disruptions or frustrations of normal functioning. Granted that biological processes are real, diseases are real. Thus, diseases such as AD, but also symptoms such as pain, fatigue, and headache and signs such as temperature, color, swelling, and heart murmur, may all be indicators of functional failure, which can be explained as disruptions of biological functional processes. As Albert, Munson, and Resnik (1988) formulate the analogy: "If a machine such as a clock does not work properly, then in order to understand its failure and to repair it in the most efficient and effective way, we must have knowledge of the mechanisms by which the clock operates" (163).[2]

There is a long history in philosophy and biology of talking about biological functions—reproduction, health, survival, and well-being—which attempts to reduce functions to causal processes. Thus, the function of the heart is to pump blood, and the intrinsic features of the causal machinery of the cardiovascular system, including the heart itself, are geared to let the heart perform its function. So construed, no one can object. However, we should not let this obscure the normative character of functions: biological processes can be described as functions only with respect to some set of values, namely, survival, reproduction, health, or well-being.[3] Thus, functions cannot be reduced to causal notions only and have to be set in terms of a furtherance of a set of values that we hold. In other words, they are observer relative. To take the analogy of the clock again: it makes good sense to use clocks for the function of "telling the time" and to analyze the processes in terms of this function, but first we have to set the end of telling the time as a valuable thing in itself. We may have good and preferably (scientific) evidence-based reasons to do so, but the ends themselves have to be merited as valuable.

I realize that to extrapolate this analysis to devastating diseases such as AD is difficult to swallow. Aren't plaques and tangles in the brains of patients with AD disrupting important biological processes with a consequent loss of functions such as cognition, memory, and awareness? Yes, indeed, but the point is that we have to distinguish between agentive or intentional and nonagentive or nonintentional functions: "Thus we say 'The heart functions to pump blood' when we are giving an account of how organisms live and survive. Relative to a teleology that values survival and reproduction, we can discover such functions occurring in nature independently of the practical intentions and activities of human agents; so let us call these functions 'nonagentive functions' " (Searle 1995, p. 20). Hearts and brains continue to function as hearts and brains even when no one is paying any attention. In contrast, when we use artifacts to perform certain functions, such as chairs, screwdrivers, and cars, there is implied a continuous use to which we intentionally put these objects. Thus, the heart's function of pumping blood is a nonagentive, nonintentional function, whereas the "artificial heart" is otherwise.[4] There is no need to end up in postmodernist stories of fiction and social or cultural fantasy here; good science is needed to tease out the complex causal machinery of AD. However, to frame such causal processes in terms of (disruption of) functions implies an observer-relative notion of a set of values. Kitcher puts the same issue in a context-relative sense: to be able to denote any causal, biological process (for example, to identify certain genetic "defects," as in the case of sickle-cell anemia) requires that we refer to context. In the context of technology-driven Western societies (that have eliminated swamps, developed antimalaria drugs, etc.), sickle-cell anemia can be considered "dysfunctional," whereas in swampy areas lacking antimalaria drugs, sickle-cell anemia can be considered "functional," that is, serving values such as life, survival, reproduction, and health (Kitcher 1996).

In the case of AD, there is the additional problem that the difference between disease and ("healthy") aging is highly diffuse and fluid and might even, in the end, implode. Scientists are right to consider Alzheimer's a disease, because so many people at 70 or 80 or 90 years old are well functioning. In the end, however, it will be interesting to see what normal or abnormal aging would look like at the age of 300 years or at some Methuselah's age. Suppose that scientists find out that the function of "aging" is to eliminate old people in order to let new generations survive—therefore, everybody would die from AD if they did not die from some other cause first. Would this be "functional" or "dysfunctional"? Humans get white hair or have skin changes with aging that we do not consider disease—but are they functional or dysfunctional? The counterargument here is that this is not the fundamental issue, because the important task is to sort out the boundaries or the interaction between normal aging and "abnormal" aging just as is the case in the nature-nurture debate on genetics. However, the most apt analogy is the long debate in obstetrics over whether giving birth should be considered a "physiological" or "pathological" process, with the latter relegating to the sidelines those who make pleas for giving birth at home versus in the hospital. The pragmatic stance in obstetrics as developed in modern medicine, namely, providing medical service when things go wrong, leads in gerontology to the paradoxical situation of providing medical service when things go normal. The concept of "good dying" in palliative care provides an analogous case. Here, it is not the distinction between normal and abnormal that helps medical professionals provide good-quality care but a set of values that includes relieving pain and giving social support. Also in question is what sort of values are to be important when we consider different functioning at different levels (for example, biological, psychological, and social).

The second point masked by the ontological concept is that therapy always implicates a normative decision expressing what a therapy or a drug should do. This normative judgment relates to the purpose of disease classification, which serves the aim not only of coherent data collection and the understanding of the mechanisms of pathology but also of therapeutic decision making. Consider, for example, whether one lists tuberculosis as an infectious disease, a genetic disease, an environmental disease, or a disease of defective immunity. We designate tuberculosis an infectious disease because this appears to indicate the most efficient mode of treating and preventing the condition. There is, however, a great deal of information that social determinants like housing and nutrition affect the morbidity and mortality patterns of tuberculosis, pointing at sanitary and social measures. The point here is that classifications of disease can signal how one should think about treatment and prevention. Even so, the purpose of classification affects what kind of medical knowledge is stored in disease classifications. This applies also to therapy for the most serious diseases. Because AD is a devastating disease that affects deeply the life of elderly people and the lives of their families and dear ones, acting to prevent, relieve, or alleviate this condition is a self-evident response and has a natural appeal. These actions are *valued* actions expressing what we value and what we don't.

In opposition to this ontological concept of disease, the history of the disease concept of Alzheimer's shows a vast literature expressing social and cultural views on AD. These views articulate the *nominalist* view that a disease is what physicians *say* a disease is or, closely related, a relativistic view that what *counts* as a disease is relative to a given society or culture at a particular time.

Examples of what were once called diseases are masturbation and hysteria. Some of what we now know to be diseases were once called "sins to God," such as Black Death and AIDS. In this sense, concepts of aging, senility, mental illness, and dementia express more of culture than of biology (for example, the emphasis of AD as a decline of cognitive function against the background of a "hypercognitive" culture and society) (Post 2000).[5]

Although one can read these biological and cultural perspectives on AD as the expression of a deep gap between biology and culture, this need not be the case. In between lies a third concept of disease, a *pragmatist* concept, which holds that what counts as a disease is determined by what *can be done about it* (Vos and Willems 2000). This pragmatist definition acknowledges what biological and cultural perspectives express: it matters that a condition is called a disease because this implies action, a commitment to medical intervention and cure as well as broader societal consequences such as public investment in science and medical care and the shaping of the patient's self-image and the family's expectations and behaviors (Holstein 2000). However, the pragmatist conception emphasizes that disease concepts originate from proposed therapeutic solutions. It reverses the order of finding solutions for problems. Instead, solutions define the problem: the hammer defines the problem as the need for a nail to be driven in and the drug as the need for treating the disease with a pill.[6] The technological tool at hand frames the way the problem is seen and approached. Consequently, difficult issues such as whether the graying or loss of hair or the decline of cognitive function should be considered as normal or as a disease are bypassed. Instead, the problem becomes whether tools are available that can efficiently and effectively repair such (dys)functional processes. The question therefore is not whether disease concepts and models are framed by drugs or whether drug discovery is a value-driven process, but how and in what respects. It is not the aim of this chapter to settle the superiority of the pragmatist concept to the ontological and nominalist concepts. In the remainder of this chapter, I will show how and in what respects drug development for AD is a value-driven process in which concepts and models are framed by drugs rather than vice versa.

Drugs Defining the Disease

The preceding analysis shows that drug discovery is inherently a value-loaded process but still leaves the matter of how exactly drugs can define diseases. Let me elaborate this perspective a bit more in two ways, one empirically, the other conceptually.

Empirically, it is worth noting the dynamic landscape of drugs and AD and other neurodegenerative diseases. The drugs of today are the result of research of 10, 20, or 30 years ago. The development of cholinesterase inhibitors such as tacrine and donepezil, the first drugs approved for AD in the United States, was the result of research in the preceding decades. In fact, these drugs have a long history, starting with the development of physostigmine in 1864 and a host of other compounds derived from the calabar bean, a plant that came into notice in 1846 (Weatherall 1990). During the 1950s and 1960s, more than 50,000 anticholinergic compounds were known and investigated. The cholinergic hypothesis was "hanging in the air" at that time, with the availability of so many chemical tools to manipulate the cholinergic system.

The landscape of current biomedical research into drugs for neurodegenerative diseases is similarly dynamic. The compounds now in the pipeline—Kwon et al. (2004) stated that 270 compounds are in development for the different neurodegenerative disorders—will come out in the next 5 to 10 to 15 years, and many hundreds of compounds will follow. Among these compounds will be substances that have been developed for other disorders, but look out for new application of the following in the area of neurodegenerative disorders: anti-inflammatory drugs such as nonsteroidal anti-inflammatory drugs (NSAIDs), estrogen-replacement therapy, and NMDA antagonists. The notion that drugs are developed for diseases is much too simple. The history of medicine, typically celebratory (Whitehouse 2004), focuses on the development of disease concepts rather than on the development of techniques and compounds. As Whitehouse describes: "It is clear that an important part of the history of AD has been determined by the development of biological technologies. When biologists have a new and creative technique to apply to the disease (e.g., the microscope, microtome, molecular probe), they tend to dominate the discussion and the literature" (Whitehouse 2000, p. 299). This applies also to drugs and other chemical technologies, as the history of the anticholinergic drugs exposed below will show. It is often neglected or concealed that drugs and other chemical compounds and the wide variety of biological technologies have been an impetus for biomedical research and clinical medicine.

It is worth strengthening the point here that modern drug development is conceived of as the construction of target molecules as basic science pharmaceutical companies have the ability with high-throughput screening libraries to quickly find chemical compounds to act on those molecules. The key is the interface between clinical phenomena and molecular targets: "Find me a target and we will find you a chemical that could become a drug." I have shown in other works, however, that this is in fact a two-way process: identified targets do lead to drugs, but drugs ("old" drugs and "new" chemical compounds as reference substances) help to identify and validate new disease targets (or new aspects of known disease targets) (Vos 1991, 1995; Kuipers, Vos, and Sie 1992; Weeber et al. 2001).

Let me elaborate the conceptual point with the help of the historical case of the cholinesterase inhibitors. The research community realized that a therapeutic strategy could be developed on a preliminary view, albeit a dominant, revolutionary, and enthusiastic one. No assumption lay behind this view, as if some "fixed" disease entity had to be developed. After all, it was called the cholinergic *hypothesis*. Every scientist in the field knew that if this hypothesis would come to be true, the concept of AD would fundamentally change. This indeed happened. Along the road, new criteria for assessing AD, and hence for evaluating the success of Alzheimer's drugs, have been developed (for example, the improvement or at least slowing of the loss of memory and cognition and maintaining independent function as assessed by the cognitive subscale of the Alzheimer's Disease Assessment Scale, the Clinical Global Impression of Change Scale, the Clinician Interview-Based Impression of Change Scale, and the Mini-Mental State Examination). With the arrival of new cholinesterase inhibitors, criteria for diagnosis, testing, and evaluation were developed. Hence, the concept of disease comes along with the development of the drug, how perfectly or imperfectly the drug turns out. Only *afterward,* after much testing in numerous clinical trials, have the developed cholinesterase inhibitors come to be labeled as "symptomatic" or "palliative" drugs, that is, drugs that result in small but measurable benefits in terms of cognitive-test results as compared with placebo or no treatment (Mayeux and Sano 2004, p. 1673).

The fact that the developed cholinesterase inhibitors such as tacrine and donepezil appeared not to be the magic bullets hoped for has changed the view of AD once more. For these drugs have created two important distinctions: one that the cholinergic pathway is not *the,* or certainly *not the only,* important pathway; the other that whatever "*disease-modifying*" drugs for AD might be, the (currently available) cholinesterase inhibitors aren't the right ones. The scientific paradigm is now that the cholinergic deficit is the result of the death of neurons, with the ensuing question of why neurons die. The amyloid hypothesis, which proposes that the accumulation of amyloid beta peptide in the brain is the primary pathogenic mechanism in AD, can be considered the next step in this process, a step that has been constructed through the development of the cholinesterase inhibitors. To summarize: the very idea of "palliative" or "symptomatic" drugs in AD has come along with the development of the cholinesterase inhibitors.

Multiple Routes of Drug Discovery

Pharmaceutical discovery is a dazzling, complex process of defining and redefining disease and outcome measures of disease and drugs at the molecular, cellular, organ, and patient level. How could this complexity be described in terms of a simple, linear process of developing a drug for a disease? Drug discovery can be thought of as a "reverse" kind of process; drugs (or newly developed drugs) are used by scientists to characterize disease and relevant aspects thereof (Vos 1991). Let me give two categorical examples. The first concerns the assessment of the validity of disease models in the field of AD and can be found in Studzinski, Araujo, and Milgram 2005. The authors claim to have been able to establish the aged beagle dog as a model for human aging and dementia "*by testing the efficacy of certain compounds such as phenserin*" (emphasis added) in their model. The authors conclude: "These findings collectively support the utilization of the dog model as a preclinical screen for identifying novel CETs [cognitive-enhancing therapeutics] for both age-associated memory disorder and dementia" (Studzinski, Araujo, and Milgram 2005, p. 412). Here drugs help to define the animal model, which in turn will be the reference point for developing new compounds. Whether the findings of these authors are scientifically correct has to be judged by the scientific community. The point is that this example—as do many other examples—illustrates an important pattern of how disease models at the cellular, tissue, organ, or animal level are carved out and validated with the help of drugs and other technologies.

The second example is the distinction of subtypes of disease through the aid of biological technologies, among which are drugs, for example, the discriminating effect of the apolipoprotein E (APOE) genotype in predicting responsiveness to cholinesterase inhibitors. APOE genotyping is being investigated in several multicenter clinical trials; the results, if confirmed, will lead to selecting subpopulations for an effective treatment by cholinesterase inhibitors (Issa and Keyserlingk 2000). The history of medicine shows many examples of drug- or technology-driven distinctions in nosologic entities, such as insulin- and non-insulin-dependent diabetes mellitus or steroid- and non-steroid-sensitive chronic obstructive pulmonary disease (COPD). These distinctions are not just a matter of "representations," as if they are different images or presentations of the disease. On the contrary, they have produced new (subtypes of) diseases, new nosologic entities. Nowadays these distinctions can be considered static models of diabetes and COPD, or even obsolete categories, since medical science has moved on to newer definitions. Once, these definitions were important, dynamic, and novel distinctions providing new questions in basic research, epidemiology, and clinical research in COPD and diabetes. This illustrates how drugs and other biological tools entail a modification in disease ontology.

However, drugs and technologies do not accomplish such changes on their own but in conjunction with other measuring devices, substances, laboratory tools, imaging techniques, epidemiological methods, and clinical observation. Making differences in disease ontology is integral to the practice of medicine, of which biological technologies and drugs are a crucial component (Vos 1991; Willems 1995; Vos and Willems 2000). Many routes in biology and medicine are possible, and it is not claimed here that this is the only route to discovery. What is claimed is that the relationship between theory, experiment, technology, and clinical observation is much more differential and multiple than envisaged in the retrospective, linear kind of history telling in biomedical and pharmaceutical research. This is aptly phrased by the philosopher Ian Hacking: "Theory and experiment have different relationships in different sciences at different stages of development. There is no right answer to the question: Which comes first, experiment, theory, invention, technology . . . ?" (Hacking 1983, p. xii). Thus, there is something fundamentally wrong with our notions of disease and therapy. This I will explicate, before showing why we need the concept of profile and profiling, which actually is not a philosopher's invention; the term is part and parcel of the practice of drug discovery and medicine.

Profiling Drugs and Diseases

Suppose we had the ideal drug in our hands, some kind of drug that attaches to the enzyme β-secretase, which is supposed to reduce the deposition of β-amyloid plaques in the brains of Alzheimer's patients and in this way to relieve memory loss. Let us call this drug an "antisecretase." A simple defini-

TABLE 9.1
Disease characteristics and therapeutic characteristics
of a drug against Alzheimer's disease

Disease	Drug	Therapeutic
Memory loss	Antisecretase	Reduction of β-amyloid plaques

tion of this antisecretase as a remedy to treat AD can be easily identified, as indicated in table 9.1.

Let us accept this for a moment and assess the distinction between therapeutic and disease characteristics. No one would deny the obvious difference between "reduction of β-amyloid plaques" and "memory loss." However, the clinician—and the patient and his or her family—might argue that reducing the number of β-amyloid plaques in the brain is a therapeutic goal, as is the relief of memory loss—the last one the significant denominator of the patient's and family's distress and of the problem the clinician has to face. This is particularly so because, as scientists presumably would argue, both goals are causally related. The difference is not as clear as suggested, and a further distinction has to be made, as shown in table 9.2.

In this hypothetical case, AD is characterized by an increased presence of β-amyloid plaques and memory loss, making the two therapeutic goals specified in table 9.2 desirable. However, therapeutic and disease characteristics are still different things. Therapeutic characteristics determine what a drug *should do;* disease characteristics determine what a disease *is.* Although disease concepts apparently represent objective states of affairs—whereas drugs express purposefully desired goals in human life—they are in reality represented as negative things that are to be prevented and excluded. Although we as humans might have good reasons to represent disease concepts this way, we have to be aware that this is an intrinsic evaluative process because it presupposes the relevant aspects of the bad state of affairs that should be prevented. Disease characteristics express how AD has been carved out from "normal aging." Disease profiles are distinguished from "normal" or "healthy" profiles.[7]

TABLE 9.2
Therapeutic and disease characteristics of Alzheimer's disease

Therapeutic	Disease
Reduction of β-amyloid plaques	β-amyloid plaques
Relief of memory loss	Memory loss

Now suppose our hypothesized drug antisecretase does something else, say dilate the gall bladder or stimulate hair growth. This is an effect in the human organism but certainly not a therapeutic characteristic. So, a drug produces a variety of effects in the organism, but some are *judged* as therapeutically useful and others as useless. When considering the functional characteristics of a drug, two sets have to be distinguished: *operational* functional characteristics and *wished for* functional characteristics. The term "operational" refers to a drug's actually having certain effects in the organism, whereas the term "wished for" denotes the functional characteristics that are considered therapeutically useful, that is, desirable features.

The distinction between wished for and operational is crucial (Vos 1991). What the effects of a drug are is an empirical matter. However, to treat a disease implies that we wish the treatment to act in a certain way. If the drug possesses the characteristics wished for, it is a good drug; if it does not, then it is a bad drug. The profile of wished-for (functional) characteristics expresses what we desire a certain drug to do. The profile of operational (functional) characteristics represents what a drug actually does. The extent to which these two profiles fit determines our judgment of the drug. Suppose we have the ideal drug, the magic bullet for the treatment of AD. The distinction between wished for and operational holds in spite of the perfect match between the two profiles, because the match can always be severed. We all experience in other domains of life what happens when this match breaks down. When our car runs out of gas or our bike has a punctured tire, we suddenly become aware of the insufferable difference between what we want a car or bike to perform and what these objects actually do, and we become angry. In our hypothetical case of the antisecretase drug, we do not have a perfect drug for the treatment of AD. However, the drug might be almost perfect as long as the effects of dilating the gall bladder or stimulating hair growth are not considered too dramatic or as long as other therapeutic goals are not added.

In a similar way, the distinction between wished-for and operational characteristics can be applied at the physical and chemical structural properties of a drug, say, its three-dimensional configurations, its lipophilic character, and the presence of certain chemical groups in its molecular structure (figure 9.1). The set of physical and chemical structural characteristics represented by the drug antisecretase is considered to be responsible for the reduction of β-amyloid plaques, which in turn relieves the memory loss experienced by so many patients with AD. However, the particular molecular structure of this drug, which may be characterized by a variety of physicochemical parameters, does not need to be (or not in all respects) specific for reducing β-amyloid plaques and memory loss, just as the exact physical makeup of a clock might not be essential for determining time (a mechanical and a digital clock both serve the function of "telling time"). There may be many compounds with different structures that reduce β-amyloid plaques and memory loss.[8] The extent to which the profiles of wished-for characteristics and operational characteristics fit determines our judgment of the drug, as indicated in figure 9.1.

The three-compartment model illustrates these concepts and also that drug discovery can be described as a back-and-forth process between the profiling of drugs and diseases. New compounds might enable scientists to disentangle functional patterns of drugs hitherto indistinguishable. New functional insights might enable clinicians to assess relevant aspects of disease differently. However, the backward process is as realistic: new insights into the conditions of disease might lead to new functional demands of clinically relevant drugs, hence to new demands of the structural features of the drugs desired. Another important result of this three-compartment model is that it shows that drug discovery is a goal-and-value-driven process through and through.

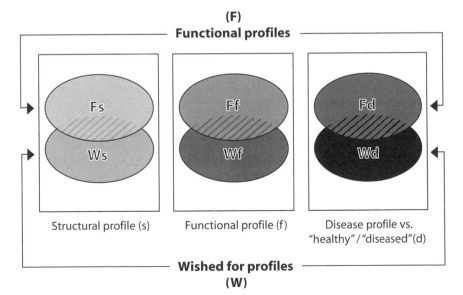

Figure 9.1. The three-compartment profiling model

Drug Discovery as a Two-way Process

Currently, there are no cures and few symptomatic treatments for neuro-degenerative diseases such as AD, Parkinson's disease, multiple sclerosis, amyotrophic lateral sclerosis, Huntington's disease, and a vast array of related neurological and psychiatric disorders. For that reason, it is strongly believed that much work has to be focused on the molecular and cellular level, because basic research is the science behind medicine: its discoveries will lead to the development of tools, techniques, and finally drugs and other treatments that address and prevent these diseases. This view simply states that the road of drug discovery is from laboratory breakthroughs to clinical treatments. I am not claiming that the path from laboratory to the clinic is a wrong one; indeed, that is how many conceive that the antibiotics were developed. In previous work I have shown that this is indeed an important route, but only one among many. If one seriously believed that the lab-to-clinic path were the only one, then, as Oates once cynically wrote, "each molecule should arrive at the bedside for the first clinical investigation with the package insert already written" (Vos 1991, p. 12).

The one-way or linear view of drug discovery is illusory and unrealistic, as the three-compartment model shows and a real-life example of the Alzheimer's field illustrates. Currently, much research is invested in the potential efficacy of NSAIDs in treating AD, and various clinical trials are continuing to explore whether these drugs may help to *prevent* the disease. It is instructive to see how this research developed.

Originally, it was reported in clinical studies in rheumatic disease and arthritic disorders that the onset of dementia is delayed in patients taking NSAIDs. Epidemiological studies further indicated that prolonged usage of NSAIDs may be beneficial in AD. Although some longitudinal clinical studies and double-blind placebo-controlled clinical trials showed positive effects, other studies reported negative findings (Gasparini et al. 2004). Animal studies and cell culture studies showed that the various NSAIDs had differential effects on Aβ metabolism—increasing or decreasing the production of Aβ-peptides, which are the amyloidogenic components of the plaques in AD—leading to the concepts of Aβ42-lowering NSAIDs or NSAIDs with Aβ-lowering properties. The view emerged that some NSAIDS might have positive effects in AD and others not, explaining why some trials produce positive results and other trials do not. This view inspired further preventive trials. Rapidly, the complexity of effects of the different classes of NSAIDs on AD

pathology became apparent, with differential effects on Aβ40 and Aβ42 secretion, Aβ-aggregation into fibrils, microglia, or astrocyte activation. Only
some NSAIDs possess properties that reduce the inflammatory reactions associated with the formation of Aβ plaques.. However, in late 2004, a large government study designed to test whether the anti-inflammatory drugs na-
proxen (an NSAID sold as Aleve) or Celebrex (a pain reliever related to Vioxx
and known as a COX-2 inhibitor) are effective, was halted after researchers
noted that these drugs may cause an increased risk of heart attack and stroke.
The issue here is not whether the question posed by the government study was
answered or whether it was legitimate to ask if these drugs could prevent AD.
The point is that through this research differentiations could be made between compounds once considered a homogeneous group, leading to insights
of how pathological pathways can be differently influenced.

Although the issue of the use of NSAIDs for the treatment of AD is complex
and controversial, the case shows that a continuous transfer of information
from the laboratory to clinical trials and epidemiology and back again takes
place. This conclusion is independent of the outcome of the process. Either it
will be shown that (some) NSAIDs have a profile potentially relevant to their
clinical use in AD or it will not, but in both cases the back-and-forth communication between the various levels of medical information holds. Even in the
age of genomics, proteomics, metabolonomics, or any "-omics," we will see this
bidirectional process of upstream and downstream information.

The common impulse is to separate scientific issues from norms and values. It
is presumed that at the fundamental (ontological) level of the concept of AD,
"technical issues" have to be sorted out first: are the Baptists (proponents of
the *beta*-amyloid protein of neuritic plaques) or are the Tauists (proponents of
the *tau* protein of the neurofibrillary tangles) right? Is there a "plaque-only
AD," a "plaque-and-tangle dementia," a "plaque-and-vascular AD," etc.
(Whitehouse, Maurer, and Ballenger 2000)? After resolving such technical issues, we can identify targets for disease and develop therapy. When therapies
have been designed, developed, and tested in clinical research, then finally social, economic, and cultural effects on patients, families, and society can be assessed. Ethical analysis concerns the *consequences* of drugs and therapies.

However, as we have seen, this neat separation of science and ethics does
not work. The three-compartment model shows that the drug-discovery process is intrinsically a value-driven process in a twofold way. First, an evaluative decision has to be made for the carving out of something as a disease, par-

ticularly so because a disease is inherently connected to the idea that pain, suffering, and discomfort have to be relieved, treated, and prevented. Second, values enter the process of designing the desired profile of a therapy, as some set of functions (and structures) must be specified as desirable targets. All along the road of the discovery process, technical information flows together with normative issues. What are relevant outcome measures? What side effects are acceptable? What are the responsibilities of patients, families, and clinicians?

Therefore, it is understandable to see the discussion of AD treatment goals not only as a scientific, technical, or clinical issue but also as a normative issue. Should cognitive decline, in the sense of progressive loss of memory and cognitive function, be considered the central feature of AD rather than other aspects of behavioral and functional change? And, if so, where should outcome measures in terms of loss of memory and cognition be set? Thus, the FDA set the cognitive subscale of the Alzheimer's Disease Assessment Scale as one important standard to assess as the primary outcome measure for the approval of new-drug applications for AD. This leads to the fundamental discussion of what, actually, a (six-month) 4–5 percent change on this 11-item assessment of memory, orientation, attention, reasoning, language, and motor performance signifies *clinically* (see Mayeux and Sano 2004). I would add also, what it signifies *normatively*. This shows that it is of no use to deny the role of values and norms in pharmaceutical discovery and biomedicine, nor to tease out or separate facts from values. It is much better to understand how and in what respects norms and values play their roles, namely, through the incorporation of values as elements of disease profiles and wished-for characteristics of drug profiles. This is a matter of science, but also of ethics and power struggle. Pharmaceutical companies have understood this for some time, for which reason they promote disease and drug profiles as constructs through social marketing, as illustrated by the examples of mood-enhancing drugs, erectile-dysfunction drugs, or hair-restoring drugs. This is played out in a similar way through images of AD and consequently of certain compounds as fighting or relieving the "mind robber," the "slow death of the mind," or the "neverending funeral."

The above analysis points out two sets of consequences. The first concerns what values to incorporate into biomedical and pharmaceutical research, and the second concerns who is to do the incorporating. Conceptualizing drug discovery as a bidirectional process of matching drug and disease profiles shows not only that drug discovery is a normative process throughout but also in what ways norms and values become incorporated in pharmaceutical research. Ethics is not an *ex post factum*. It is not something that happens after the research proposal has been finished and handed over to the research ethics committee. On the contrary, in many ways norms and values are embedded in pharmaceutical and biomedical research as they are taken up as wished-for characteristics in drug profiles, for example, safety, comfort and ease of drug use, but also in valued aspects of the treatment of diseases, such as the emphasis on wishing to repair memory loss, loss of cognitive function, etc., in AD. So do we wish to include loss of cognitive function in disease and drug profiles, and if so, what should be the rate of loss? And what about other cognitive, physical, emotional, and social abilities? Such matters are of concern to patients and their families and caregivers. Scientists mostly consider these features as a matter of empirics. The crux is that these features are incorporated in drug profiles because we consider them valuable things to strive for (however much scientists have provided sound, evidence-based reasons to do so). Norms and values are part of the texture of biomedical and clinical research. A public deliberation about these norms and values is essential. As Whitehouse (2000, p. 303) notes: "Perhaps the most critical issue is how our concepts of AD can be applied to better understand our therapeutic goals. If AD is a form of aging, albeit often premature, can we try to reverse aging? When is it appropriate to consider AD as a terminal illness and thus palliate symptoms and promote a good death? How can we frame and put into practice attempts to prevent, cure, reverse, or even just slow the progression of disease? How do we balance our goals when we use a medication that might improve behavioral symptoms but make a person's thinking less clear?"

The second set of consequences concerns who has the power to make such judgments. The process of developing new drugs for AD goes together with developing norms, criteria, and guidelines for evaluating models, animal experiments, and other laboratory tests, for deciding to take the step from the laboratory to clinical trials, and for modeling clinical studies. But interesting normative questions are not only which norms become developed, but also which stakeholders (researchers, clinicians, industry, patient organizations) and which disciplines (medicine, engineering, pharmacy, gerontology, social work) play a role in that process, which arguments and perspectives are discussed, which compromises are negotiated between different stakeholders, and how this is publicly accounted for. Patients and their relatives, along with their caregivers and social workers who deal with the daily experiences of affected individuals and their families, have to be given a more important role in the development, testing, and evaluation of emergent therapies for AD. Not only should patients be protected as subjects of research and science through informed consent and an exit option, but also they and their families should be much more fully involved in medical and clinical research.

The history of pharmaceutical discovery in AD shows that it is of no use to see doing science and doing ethics as two entirely different things, as radically different "rationalities," disjunctive discourses, or different modes of communication. Rather it is the conjunction of the different logics, rationalities, and value sets that is at stake. The normative worlds of the researcher, the clinician and the patient with his or her family need to be coordinated, not separated (Vos, Willems, and Houtepen 2004). Drug discovery is a multifaceted process connecting many branches of medicine and many stakeholders, ranging from the scientist, to the clinician, to the patient and his or her family. The integration and coordination of the rationalities and value sets of these parties is crucial. Alois Alzheimer himself is a paradigmatic example, presenting in his papers of 1906 and 1907 the case of Auguste D., a 51-year-old woman from Frankfurt who exhibited arteriosclerotic changes, senile plaques, and the devastating symptoms of "presenile" dementia. The interfaces in his discovery were, so to speak, between his own brain cells that stored information on chemistry, pathology, psychiatry, and careful patient care, and these neural connections enabled him to identify this woman as an example of a new nosologic entity. Through his intervention, novel insight and understanding were gained and new goals, norms, and values for therapy and patient care were set.[9]

NOTES

1. For a good introduction and exposition of this model, see Albert, Munson, and Resnik 1988, particularly chap. 7, pp. 151–80. The authors here defend the "descriptive" or "empirical" concept of disease, whereas I follow the opposite track with John Searle's analysis of the concept of function as the basis. See Searle 1995.

2. In this way, Albert, Munson, and Resnik (1988) are able to reject cultural views of the concept of disease, arguing that disease concepts are always driven by the norms and values of a society; for example, masturbation was denoted a disease by nineteenth-century medicine. "Thus, the functional-failure concept makes sense out of saying (as we do) that physicians in the eighteenth century *failed* to identify SLE [Systemic Lupus Erythematosus] as a disease, although it existed then. Similarly, it makes sense of saying that physicians in the nineteenth century were *wrong* to identify masturbation as a disease: masturbation does not and never did involve any functional failure" (163).

3. Cf. the work of Ruth Garrett Millikan, Larry Wright, Elliott Sober, and others. In the philosophy of medicine there is extensive literature on the disease concept, with claims of disease as a "natural" phenomenon (Boorse) and as the result of an evaluative or normative decision (Sonderfeldt, Engelhardt). See, for an entry into the discussion in the 1970s, Engelhardt and Spicker 1975, and for recent discussion the journals *Theoretical Medicine and Bioethics; American Journal of Medicine;* and *Philosophy and Medicine, Health Care, and Philosophy.* I follow the illuminating analysis of Searle (1995).

4. In fact, the artificial heart shows the gradient between the agentive and nonagentive function. It is agentive because humans have intentionally imposed the function on this artifact, but it is nonagentive in that even when no one is paying attention, a once-construed artificial heart will perform its function. Similarly, most car drivers are unaware that the function of the drive shaft is to transmit power from the transmission to the axles, but all the same that is its agentive function.

5. Behind this lies also the fundamental discussion in neurophilosophy and neuroscience about the distinction between "mind" and "brain"; see the work of Daniel C. Dennett on this topic.

6. The psychologist Abraham Maslow, known for his "pyramid of need" concept, commented: "If the only tool you have is a hammer, you will see every problem as a nail." This phrase is widely known, albeit in different forms.

7. The difference with drugs is that the disease profile includes characteristics *not* wished for!

8. A philosophical and technical way to put the problem faced here is to say that "structure underdetermines function."

9. This is a "free" interpretation of a quotation that describes Withering's 1785 discovery of digitalis for the treatment of heart disease. Withering "needed little help from those in other branches of science because he himself was a botanist, clinician, mineralogist, and chemist. The interfaces in his discovery were between his own brain cells that stored information in botany, chemistry, and medicine, and these neural connections quickly enabled him to identify the foxglove as the only ingredient of a Shropshire potpourri that was likely to have potent biological activity" (Comroe 1977, p. 933).

REFERENCES

Albert, D. A., R. Munson, and M. D. Resnik, eds. 1988. *Reasoning in medicine: An introduction to clinical inference.* Baltimore: Johns Hopkins University Press.

Comroe, J. H. 1977. *Retrospectroscope: Insights into medical discovery.* Menlo Park, Calif.: Von Gehr Press.

Dennett, D. C. 2001. *Kinds of minds: The origins of consciousness.* London: Phoenix.

Fleck, L. 1983. Über einige besondere Merkmale des ärztlichen Denkens. In *Ludwig Fleck: Erfahrung und Tatsache,* ed. L. Schäfer and T. Schnelle, 37–45. Frankfurt am Main: Suhrkamp Taschenbuch Verlag.

Gasparini, L., L. Rusconi, H. Xu, P. del Soldata, and E. Ongini. 2004. Modulaton of β-amyloid metabolism by non-steroidal anti-inflammatory drugs in neuronal cell cultures. *Journal of Neurochemistry* 88:337–48.

Hacking, I. 1983. *Representing and intervening: Introductory topics in the philosophy of natural science*. Cambridge: Cambridge University Press.

Holstein, M. 2000. Aging, culture, and the framing of Alzheimer disease. In *Concepts of Alzheimer disease: Biological, clinical, and cultural perspectives*, ed. P. J. Whitehouse, K. Maurer, and J. F. Ballenger, 158–60. Baltimore: Johns Hopkins University Press.

Issa, A. M., and E. W. Keyserlingk. 2000. Apolipoprotein E genotyping for pharmacogenetic purposes in Alzheimer's disease: Emerging ethical issues. *Canadian Journal of Psychiatry* 45 (10): 917–22.

Kitcher, P. 1996. *The lives to come: The genetic revolution and human possibilities*. London: Simon & Schuster.

Kuipers, T. A. F., R. Vos, and H. Sie. 1992. Design research program and the logic of their development. *Erkenntnis* 37 (1): 37–63.

Kwon, M.-O., F. Fischer, M. Matthisson, and P. Herrling. 2004. List of drugs in development for neurodegenerative disorders. *Neurodegenerative Diseases* 1:113–53.

Mayeux, R., and M. Sano. 2004. Drug therapy: Treatment of Alzheimer's disease. *New England Journal of Medicine* 341 (22): 1670–79.

Post, S. G. 2000. The concept of Alzheimer disease in a hypercognitive society. In *Concepts of Alzheimer disease: Biological, clinical, and cultural perspectives*, ed. P. J. Whitehouse, K. Maurer, and J. F. Ballenger, 245–56. Baltimore: Johns Hopkins University Press.

Searle, J. R. 1995. *The construction of social reality*. London: Penguin Books.

Studzinski, C. M., J. A. Araujo, and N. W. Milgram. 2005. The canine model of human cognitive aging and dementia: Pharmacological validity of the model for assessment of human cognitive-enhancing drugs. *Progress in Neuro-psychopharmacology and Biological Psychiatry* 29 (3): 489–98.

Vos, R. 1991. *Drugs looking for diseases: Innovative drug research and the development of the beta blockers and the calcium antagonists*. Dordrecht: Kluwer Academic.

———. 1995. The logic and epistemology of the concept of drug and disease profile. In *Cognitive patterns in science and common sense*. Groningen studies in philosophy of science, logic, and epistemology. Poznan studies in the philosophy of the sciences and the humanities, vol. 45, ed. T. A. F. Kuipers and A. R. Mackor, 69–86. Amsterdam: Rodopi.

Vos, R., and D. L. Willems. 2000. Technology in medicine: Ontology, epistemology, ethics, and social philosophy at the crossroads. *Theoretical Medicine and Bioethics* 21 (1): 1–6.

Vos, R., D. L. Willems, and R. Houtepen. 2004. Coordinating the norms and values of medical research, medical practice and patient worlds: The ethics of evidence based medicine in "orphaned fields of medicine." *Journal of Medical Ethics* 30:166–70.

Weeber, M., H. Klein, L. T. W. Jong-van den Berg, and R. Vos. 2001. Using concepts in literature-based discovery simulating Swanson's Raynaud–fish oil and migraine-mg discoveries. *Journal of the American Society for Information Sciences* 52 (7): 548–57.

Weatherall, M. 1990. *In search of a cure: A history of pharmaceutical discovery*. Oxford: Oxford University Press.

Whitehouse, P. J. 2000. History and the future of Alzheimer disease. In *Concepts of Alzheimer disease: Biological, clinical, and cultural perspectives*, ed. P. J. Whitehouse, K. Maurer, and J. F. Ballenger, 291–305. Baltimore: Johns Hopkins University Press.

————. 2004. The history of therapeutic trials in dementia. In *Trial designs and outcomes in dementia therapeutic research*, ed. K. Rockwood and S. Gauthier. London: Taylor & Francis.

Whitehouse, P. J., K. Maurer, and J. F. Ballenger, eds. 2000. *Concepts of Alzheimer disease: Biological, clinical, and cultural perspectives*. Baltimore: Johns Hopkins University Press.

Willems, D. L. 1995. Tools of care: Explorations into the semiotics of medical technology. Ph.D. diss., University of Maastricht.

CHAPTER 10

Can We Fix This with a Pill?

Qualities of Life and the Aging Brain

PETER J. WHITEHOUSE, M.D., PH.D.

What is quality of life (QOL)? How can it be measured and improved? Whose QOL is important? For me as a clinician, scientist, and human being, QOL echoes in my mind and heart as a daunting challenge. It is an elusive concept, but it is essential in our daily lives. We all acknowledge intuitively its importance to health, yet it remains mysterious. Although relatively easy to define as a multidimensional concept that incorporates behaviors, values, abilities, expectations, external forces, and inner subjectivity, it is difficult to fathom its complexity and especially to measure it objectively. It pushes science to the limits and stimulates our moral imagination. Like wisdom, good QOL is perhaps something to strive for rather than to expect to fully achieve. Perhaps, like life itself, QOL is better viewed as a process than a state. To achieve a high QOL, we must decide the best strategies for living our lives within socially just, ecologically sound communities populated by other human beings and living creatures.

Addressed in this chapter are perspectives I have gained as a practitioner and researcher during 25 years of assisting persons diagnosed with dementia and their families maintain and even enhance QOL (Whitehouse and Rabins 1992; Whitehouse 1998, 2000). A related issue is how this work over the last quarter-century has affected my own QOL and that of my colleagues. Ultimately, we must also ask how investing in interventions to improve the quality of lives of patients with dementia and their caregivers may compete with other health and social issues that affect the lives of people with other diseases. Does the race to find a cure, or at least better drugs, for AD limit our abilities to improve public education or environmental health, for example?

Because of the focus of this book, the emphasis will be on the role of medications to treat Alzheimer's disease (AD) and related disorders and their potential effect on QOL. Issues surrounding drug development and marketing are critically important to personal and public health. Social concern about the pharmaceutical industry will continue and likely grow in the future as the costs and value of drug treatments in dementia and other chronic diseases are increasingly debated in the United States and around the world. In fact, the United Kingdom's National Institute for Clinical Excellence, after review of the evidence for current therapies, is recommending that the National Health Service significantly limit payment for AD drugs. This recommendation is due, in part, to the drugs' lack of clearly demonstrable benefit to QOL and to health care costs (Whitehouse et al. 1998; Jonsson et al. 2000).

Drugs and Quality of Life

As a scientist who contributed to the discovery of the mechanisms of brain failure—particularly those that involve cholinergic systems in AD and related conditions—I expected that drugs acting on this neurotransmitter system might improve cognition (Whitehouse et al. 1981). My hopes were that if we could enhance thinking for patients, better QOL would emerge. As it became clear that AD is a multisystem disorder and that the actions of a single drug on a single neurotransmitter system might be limited, my goal of improving QOL with drugs of this class seemed overly optimistic. We explored and tested the so-called cholinergic hypothesis, that is, that reductions in acetylcholine and other related markers contribute to the cognitive impairment in AD and related dementias. Evidence to support the cholinergic hypothesis came mostly from animal and autopsy studies. However, the true test of the cholinergic hypothesis was whether drugs developed to enhance that neural system could improve function in daily life and lift people out of their dementia to enjoy a higher QOL. Ideally, such a cholinergic drug would work not just in carefully controlled studies involving highly selected research "subjects" but also for more typical patients in nonacademic practice settings.

As a contributor to the guidelines for antidementia drugs that were developed by the FDA and other regulatory bodies, I saw standards set low for the first drugs. As a result, tacrine (Cognex) was approved as the first cholinesterase inhibitor to treat AD, despite modest positive effects on cognition and clinical global ratings. The initial positive (but ultimately misleading) report of tacrine's effects (Summers et al. 1986) described people returning to work and playing golf (Davis and Mohs 1986; Whitehouse 2006; see also Ballenger, chapter 11 in this volume). However, this study was flawed, both scientifically and ethically. Patient selection, follow up, and assessment were unclear. The first author had an undisclosed financial interest in the drug. Having organized four international conferences on the pharmacoeconomics of drugs for dementia and having led the movement to elevate interest in QOL in the field as the key outcome of interventions, I began to see the limitations of these drugs in individual people as well as from a societal perspective. As drugs moved from the laboratory to the clinic and to the market, I witnessed the pervasive effects of the pharmaceutical industry's marketing efforts (particularly direct-to-consumer marketing and influencing so-called opinion leaders) on raising people's hopes and fears and in shaping our very conceptions of health and disease.

I also became aware of the challenges of using the concept of QOL to guide care in my clinical practice. As I aged in place in Cleveland, I became a senior expert on the diagnosis of dementia. I believed that my relationships with patients and caregivers were keys to whatever healing I offered people with cognitive challenges and their families. I not only referred people to our research studies but also obtained memantine and other medicines from Europe before they were approved in the United States. Patients sought me out as an expert on the latest drugs to treat dementia, and that knowledge was an important part of their hope. I also scoured Asia for complementary and alternative medical approaches. My patients came to know that I was informed about the potential benefits, as well as risks, of medications in the United States and from around the world.

With varying degrees of enthusiasm, I prescribed the four cholinesterase inhibitors that were eventually approved in the United States, hoping that some of my patients would see meaningful benefits. Some did, but relatively few, and I was always uncertain how much of the benefit was due to a placebo effect. When an effect was present that could be linked to cholinesterase inhibition, it seemed to enhance attention rather than improve memory. Although families reported that the patients appeared brighter and better able to sustain conversations, there were few glimpses of improved function and, rarely, improved QOL with these drugs.

Caregivers encouraged patients to stay on cholinesterase inhibitors not because they saw improvements but because they were afraid that if they stopped the drugs, their loved ones' conditions would worsen. Postmarketing studies conducted by industry were used to convince physicians and families to start these medicines early in the disease and never stop. Such studies were mostly not prospective and often involved unmatched control groups. Differential dropout was perhaps the most fundamental flaw in these studies; participants who got worse on the drug or who could not tolerate it did not stay in the study, so by the end of the study those who remained on the drug looked better than those who did not remain on the drug. In personal communication with Paul Leber, a dominant figure at the FDA during the development of the draft antidementia drug guidelines and the approval of tacrine, he warned that postapproval studies of these drugs might well be scientifically flawed and subject to exaggerated positive interpretations. Moreover, underreporting of negative trials in medicine has become a major practical and ethical problem. How can you avoid believing that drugs are effective if only positive studies are published and/or disseminated by drug company representatives and become part of scientific and public knowledge?

Expectations about the Future of Drug Treatment

Many thought leaders and drug company employees seem sincerely to believe that cholinesterase inhibitors are more helpful to patients than I do. Ironically, those who prescribe the drugs may obtain better effects in their patients than I do because of the power of their own beliefs in the medications. However, I came to observe two important correlates in physicians with strong beliefs that current drugs worked well and that future drugs were just around the corner in the drug-development pipeline: high expectations for the power of science and high expectations for being paid by industry as consultants. First, some physicians, particularly psychiatrists and neurologists, believe strongly in the message of the public education campaign called "the decade of the brain," that is, that we now understand enough about the basic mechanisms of neural plasticity that we will soon be able to restore brain function. Proposition 71, California's Stem Cells and Cures Act, illustrates high (and false) expectations that gene modification and stem cells will be used to treat (and perhaps cure) AD in any kind of short, intermediate, or long term. This constitution-modifying action allowed three billion dollars from California taxpayers to be invested in companies and universities in stem cells. Lawsuits and concerns from both the right and left sides of the political spectrum delayed distribution of the funds.

AD was constantly mentioned as a target of this stem-cell effort, yet most experts believe that stem therapies are a remote possibility for treating dementia. Part of this political message is that drugs are the way to improve human cognition and that science is a powerful force for improving QOL. These same therapeutically aggressive and enthusiastic clinicians have no qualms about ordering costly and invasive spinal fluid tests and neuroimaging studies. The contentious, but successful, effort to get the Centers for Medicare and Medical Services to allow reimbursement, fortunately in a limited way, for diagnosis of dementia using PET scan to measure the distribution of glucose metabolism is an illustration of the inappropriate drive to employ expensive technology without knowing its full import. This is the second correlation with strong belief in the power of drugs among physicians—consulting, grant, and speaking fees from industry.

The Influence of the Pharmaceutical Industry

As both a scientist and clinician, I became increasingly concerned about the power of industry to influence the attitudes and behaviors of physicians and patients. As a thought leader, was I leading the corporation or being led in my own thinking? Earlier in my career, it was considered not only bad form for academics to collaborate too closely with industry but also a sign of failure to leave the university and work for pharmaceutical companies. I, on the other hand, never had such a negative view of industry; instead, I developed collaborative relationships with those whom I perceived would likely become leaders in industry. Now, thought leaders compete as to how many company advisory boards they can attend, and for many the ultimate ambition is to form their own biotechnology company. Undoubtedly, the cholinesterase inhibitors have improved the QOL of opinion leaders like me. I have traveled around the world, organized and participated in wonderful conferences, eaten delicious meals, and supplemented my organization's and my own personal income considerably through industry funding.

As a clinician-scientist, my life has been improved by the availability of current drugs, but what about persons affected with memory problems, their families, and society at large? The conclusions are less clear. I have significant concerns about the high cost of the drugs and the missed opportunities to improve QOL through other means. Why did tacrine cost four dollars a day when it was introduced, and why do all the other cholinesterase inhibitors cost about the same? Given that the pharmaceutical industry is supposedly a prime example of the success of global capitalism, driven by a competitive market for drugs, why do we not see more price competition? Undoubtedly some aggressive competition occurs in the closed-door negotiations between industry and large purchasers of drugs such as health maintenance and other organizations. At the level of my individual patients, though, there appears to be relatively little variation in price among the drugs. To be frank, I doubt that these drugs are worth the amount of money we pay. I would like to see lower prices through a combination of genuine competition and more balanced information about the effects (for good and ill) of drugs available to consumers and the market.

Yet, more comprehensive and novel kinds of nonpharmacological interventions to improve cognitive vitality and QOL do not receive enough emphasis. The pharmaceutical companies push the message that every ill has a pill. In fact, once a pill is marketed for one use, companies look to find other conditions that could be treated by their already profitable drugs. The prelaunch activities surrounding the treatment of pseudobulbar affect (PBA) are an illustration of this market creep. PBA is a sudden outburst of crying or laughing that happens involuntarily and without strong underlying subjective emotion. It occurs in conditions like multiple sclerosis and amyotrophic lateral sclerosis. PBA often has a sudden onset and ending and can be precipitated in stereotyped ways. Currently available drugs are not usually very effective. Avanir was developing a marketing campaign focusing on expanding conceptions of PBA in expectation of the approval by the FDA of their drug combination for treating PBA in ALS and MS. In my view, PBA is best managed by informing the patient and family that the symptoms, although concerning, do not imply that the patient is necessarily depressed or that their emotional state is necessarily intensely unpleasant. The company might like us to presume that the emotional incontinence or lability that is common in AD is the same as PBA in MS and ALS. If this were the case, then the indication for drug treatment with any new agents approved to treat PBA might be extended in physician's minds to other common conditions like dementia. I believe that we should not extend the market to broader indications without better evidence for the effect of new treatments in conditions that have not been adequately studied in the early phases of drug development. Yet Avanir was supporting efforts to develop a new term, "involuntary emotional expression disorder" (IEED), to include PBA and other more general categories such as emotional incontinence and emotional lability.

In general, physicians are too quick to try new medications, even though older ones are available whose safety profiles are better known. Physicians should be more cautious about off-label use of new medications, particularly in older persons. Geriatricians understand the danger that this optimistic attitude represents, especially the hype surrounding newly approved medications. After all, they invented the concept of "polypharmacy," which highlights the dangers of drug interactions and medication errors.

Arguing that the high cost of current drugs is the price that consumers pay for future breakthroughs, big pharma has been explicit about creating hope for future pills. It is true that we live in the exciting time when the human genome has been mapped. Admittedly, the promises of molecular and genetic approaches, such as stem-cell and gene therapy, may come true for certain diseases. However, it is also true that there is often more hype than hope associated with claims for future progress, especially when it comes to complex, multisystem diseases like AD.

The Vaccine for Alzheimer's Disease

Consider the AD vaccine (Rosenberg 2005). Scientists discovered that in genetically modified mice that overproduce amyloid, active immunization against amyloid protein prevented and actually cleared this allegedly toxic substance from the brain. Clinical studies claimed to show encouraging results. Yet significant scientific, clinical, and ethical issues persist. The vaccine caused an immunological response in some patients that resulted in harmful encephalitis. Some have argued this autoimmune response should have been predicted and monitored more carefully. The company involved has already been investigated by the Securities and Exchange Commission for accounting problems and has had problems with undisclosed or partially disclosed conflicts of interest with thought leaders associated with the company. The same company has also sold diagnostic tests for AD based on cerebrospinal fluid measurements and genetic tests. These measurements are judged to have little usefulness by many experts, including me. The positive hype associated with profit- and fame-seeking (Nobel Prize–seeking) behaviors may have supported, at least temporarily, some companies' images on Wall Street and hence stock prices. However, the short-term creation of shallow and ultimately false hope may undermine the long-term credibility of the industry investors and potential consumers of their products.

Thus, as a clinician and scientist I came to believe that the principal way to improve QOL for patients with dementia is not through current medicines and promises of future therapies. I began to argue for the importance of measuring QOL and using those measurements to determine the value and price that should be associated with therapies. After all, if we can measure QOL, we can compare drugs with each other and with nondrug interventions.

Measuring Quality of Life: The Power of Stories and Numbers

Through funding from the National Institute on Aging (NIA) and others, we embarked on a project to assess QOL using a variety of approaches, both qualitative and quantitative (Whitehouse and Rabins 1992; Whitehouse 1998; Brod, Stewart, and Sands 1999; Selai, Rossor, and Harvey 2000; Whitehouse 2000). We felt it important to ask those affected by AD about their attitudes toward QOL and current therapies. We started with focus groups that revealed high expectations for current and future drugs and supported (in my view) the importance of QOL as a concept to guide treatment. Conversations with groups using too many structural questions proved limiting, however. We pursued individual interviews with affected persons and their caregivers. Other federally funded research examined factors that affect life decisions in those genetically at risk for AD and provided genetic counseling using quantitative and qualitative research methods. Because these individual interview and focus-group methods allowed limited numbers of people to participate, we also developed surveys to explore attitudes in larger groups of patients, families, and physicians about current therapies and their impact on QOL.

A major part of our effort involved psychological rating scales. Work through our own grants and the NIA Alzheimer's Disease Cooperative Study compared different scales for evaluating both patient and caregiver QOL. Rebecca Logsdon's QOL-AD is the most widely used QOL instrument and includes such domains as physical health, memory, and relationships with others. Based on our focus groups, we have expanded the domains of assessment to include religion/spirituality and enjoyment of nature. We compared the QOL-AD to other longer batteries. We also assessed patients' neuropsychological health to explore the cognitive difficulties that limit patient's abilities to provide reliable QOL data. As part of these studies, we also compared patient and caregiver ratings of the patient's QOL. Initial results of these studies have been published elsewhere (Lindstrom et al. 2006). Linda Teri, Rebecca Logsdon, and colleagues recently demonstrated that offering families information about managing dementia symptoms, through training of professional community counselors, can improve the QOL of patients on these scales (Logsdon et al. 1999, 2000, 2002; Logsdon personal communication). Ironically, no drug has yet to demonstrate a similar effect.

Our final method, the use of utility weights, was the most quantitative. Patients and caregivers watched clinical scenarios presented on a computer monitor and were asked to evaluate the desirability of life in different stages of dementia as revealed in these narratives. Patients and caregivers watched mildly, moderately, and severely affected patients in care situations. Using approaches like "standard gamble" (how much risk would you take?) and "time tradeoff" (how much time would you give up?), we obtained utility weights between 0 and 1 that measured the observer's assessment of QOL associated with each stage.

The overall purpose of this NIH-funded research was to compare different methods for assessing QOL and to determine the characteristics of participants who were able to provide reliable data. Ultimately, we wish to use QOL measures in clinical trials to compare drug and nondrug interventions. We also want to use the knowledge gained in our research program to inform people about making decisions at different stages of disease to maintain QOL. As this project evolved, I was personally impressed by the power of individual stories to both help assess and affect QOL. Stories are part of how clinicians assess what QOL means to individuals and families. They are also a part of the therapy to improve well-being. Stories provide a sense of cohesion and integration as an individual faces the stress of age-related cognitive changes. Clinician authors like Oliver Sacks, Rita Charon, and Rachel Remen argue convincingly that narrative approaches offer much in patient care in general. In my own practice, I am extending these principles to the care of older people facing cognitive challenges. With my colleague Danny George, I have developed a story-rich, life-planning multimedia product, called LifeBook, to guide clinical decision making. Yet in scientific studies, it is difficult to use stories as outcome measures. Stories are often denigrated as mere anecdotes because of their subjective nature. Yet, it is in this subjectivity that the essence of QOL can best be captured.

As I've reflected on these stories of dementia, I've come to learn the importance of the diagnostic label on the QOL of people with memory problems.

People live in fear of being diagnosed with AD and often begin dying prematurely after the diagnosis is made. The label AD is a two-edged sword in the battle against loss of QOL associated with age-related cognitive impairment. Certainly, a diagnosis can give some sense of certainty and open the door to medical interventions, especially drugs. However, a diagnostic label can also create fear and limit the pathways on life's journey that remain for the person with age-associated cognitive challenges.

Is Alzheimer's Even a Disease?

At this stage of my career as a clinician scientist and of my life as a human being, my attitude about QOL is much different from two decades ago. In the beginning, I had greater hope and less skepticism that AD was a biological disease that could best be addressed through drugs and molecular approaches. Now, I see limits to the view that genetics can lead to a more personalized medicine and that academic-industry partnerships are a means to create better effective interventions. Personalized medicine is said to depend on the selection of individualized drugs for patients based on an analysis of their DNA. Yet genes do not determine all or even much of health. Moreover, you cannot do much about them except select your parents carefully. A true personalized medicine should be based on an individual's story, and therapy should be based on this narrative rather than on their genes.

The very ethical fabric of the practice of medicine and the scientific enterprise is being threatened. Bioethics promised to address some of these value issues in medicine. Yet, bioethicists are doing little repair and may in fact be causing additional damage. Bioethicists tend to focus their attention on the needs of medicine, to the exclusion of the larger social and health issues. Has bioethics become too co-opted by medicine in its efforts to make way for medical progress in imaging, genetics, and research and too uncritical of the goals of medicine?

Now the world of dementia appears differently to me. A quarter of a century of claimed scientific breakthroughs have only broken through my confidence in current approaches. I would argue that we are now more confused about the diagnosis and treatment of AD than in the 1980s. The overlaps between vascular dementia and AD and between Parkinson's dementias and AD are more puzzling.

My concerns about the current state of Alzheimer's as a disease concept are considered in greater detail in the chapter in this volume on "mild cogni-

Would a cure for AD mean finding a neurological fountain of youth? Is AD really one disease or even one entity? Is it actually a heterogeneous collection of different age-related biological processes? Should we bring back the nicely ambiguous, formerly commonly used term "senility"? We must be realistic about life's opportunities and death's realities. How many resources can we put into finding a technological cure for the chronic disease of the elderly when the ravages of acute diseases and even seemingly simple shortages of clean water threaten our very species?

As I look to the next decade as a healer and scholar, stories will become even more important to me than drugs. I intend to be more of a constructive critic of industry rather than a passive collaborator, and I expect that the humanities rather than the sciences will dominate my thinking about how to improve QOL. These changes represent shifts in balance, not absolute rejections of any position. Yet I see these subtle shifts as essential to improving the quality of life of not only my patients but also of my community and myself. With Danny George, I have written a book exploring these issues (Whitehouse and George 2008).

The Keys to Quality of Life in Dementia

Missed opportunities to improve QOL occur because we focus too strongly on the power of drugs. Staying mentally and physically active and eating healthy are keys to maintaining cognitive vitality. Having a sense of purpose in life and belonging to a family and community are also critical to individual well-being. Yet if physicians spend all their time talking about drugs, there is little time to discuss these other life options that may contribute to preserving and even enhancing QOL.

Let me illustrate an integrated way to enhance the QOL of elders with memory problems. My wife and I developed the world's first public intergenerational school in Cleveland, Ohio (Whitehouse et al. 2000). It celebrates real-life learning in community for all students, from ages 5 to 95. In TIS, we include older individuals with memory challenges who learn alongside elementary school children, even those with cognitive disabilities such as attention deficit disorder. Together we celebrate life-long learning and the power of shared stories to create collective wisdom. We are beginning to gather the evidence that elders who participate in the education of children improve the QOL of both the children and themselves.

As the health consequences of environmental deterioration and social injustices (toxins, epidemics, and warfare) increase, we will likely see more children and adults suffering from diffuse brain damage and ultimately dementia. How we address the topic of quality of life in dementia will affect the quality of life of our species. Preventing brain damage and dementia is much more a social than a medical task. Shall we continue to pretend that we can realistically hope to develop high-tech fixes for human health and social problems, when such fixes often end up being expensive, only marginally effective, and actually cause unintended, unpredictable, and harmful secondary effects? Or do we recognize that science has limits and find in the depths of our souls the values necessary to educate our children and protect their health as we face our own finitude?

ACKNOWLEDGMENTS

I am grateful for the lessons I have learned from colleagues in Cleveland (Neal Dawson, Danny George, Sidney Katz, Marian Patterson, Mendel Singer, Kathleen Smyth, Cathy Whitehouse) and elsewhere (John Bond, Barry Gurland, Richard Harvey, Heather Lindstrom, Rebecca Logsdon, Linda Teri). Preparation of this article was supported by grant AG/HS17511-01A1, Medical Goals in Dementia: Ethics and Quality of Life from the National Institutes of Health / NIA; a grant from the Shigeo and Megumi Takayama Foundation, Tokyo, Japan; and grant AG10483-13 from the National Institutes of Health / National Institute on Aging and Alzheimer's Disease Cooperative Study—Quality of Lives. I am grateful to my colleagues Iahn Gonsenhauser and Susie Sami for useful editorial comments.

REFERENCES

Ali, K., R. Weinfurtner, C. Gilbert, T. Wolpaw, and P. Whitehouse. 2006. Making lead history: Interprofessional environmental learning and scholarship at the Intergenerational School. Paper presented at the Abstract Association for Medical Education in Europe conference, Genoa, Italy, September 14–18.

Basha, M. R., W. Wei, S. A. Bakheet, N. Benitez, H. K. Siddiqi, Y.-W. Ge, D. K. Lahiri, and N. H. Zawia. 2005. The fetal basis of amyloidogenesis: Exposure to lead and latent overexpression of amyloid precursor protein and beta-amyloid in the aging brain. *Journal of Neuroscience* 25 (4): 823–29.

Brod, M., A. Stewart, and L. Sands. 1999. Conceptualization and measurement of quality of life in dementia. *Journal of Mental Science* 38:25–35.

Davis, K. L., and R. C. Mohs. 1986. Cholinergic drugs in Alzheimer's disease. *New England Journal of Medicine* 315:1286–87.

Jonsson, L., B. Jonsson, A. Wimo, P. J. Whitehouse, and B. Winblad. 2000. Second International

Pharmacoeconomic Conference on Alzheimer's Disease. *Alzheimer Disease and Associated Disorders* 14 (3): 137–40.

Lindstrom, H. A., P. J. Whitehouse, K. A. Smyth, S. A. Sami, N. V. Dawson, M. B. Patterson, J. H. Bohinc, et al. 2006. Medication use to treat memory loss in dementia: Perspectives of persons with dementia and their caregivers. *Dementia* 5 (1): 27–50.

Logsdon, R., L. E. Gibbons, S. M. McCurry, and L. Teri. 1999. Quality of life in Alzheimer's disease: Patient and caregiver reports. *Journal of Mental Health and Aging* 5 (1): 21–32.

———. 2000. *Quality of life in Alzheimer's disease: Patient and caregiver reports.* New York: Springer.

———. 2002. Assessing quality of life in older adults with cognitive impairment. *Psychosomatic Medicine* 64:510–19.

Rosenberg, R. N. 2005. Translational research on the way to effective therapy for Alzheimer disease. *Archives of General Psychiatry* 62:1186–92.

Selai, C. E., M. R. Trimble, M. N. Rossor, and R. J. Harvey. 2000. The Quality of Life Assessment Schedule (QOLAS): A new method for assessing quality of life (QOL) in dementia. In *Assessing quality of life in Alzheimer's disease,* ed. S. M. Albert and R. G. Logsdon. New York: Springer.

Summers, W. K., L. V. Majovski, G. M. Marsh, K. Tachiki, and A. Kling. 1986. Oral tetrahydro-aminoacridine in long-term treatment of senile dementia, Alzheimer type. *New England Journal of Medicine* 315 (20): 1241–45.

Whitehouse, P. J. 1998. Measurements of quality of life in dementia. In *Health economics of dementia,* ed. A. Wimo, B. Jonsson, G. Karlsson, and B. Windblad. London: John Wiley & Sons.

———. 2000. Conclusion: Quality of life: Future directions. In *Assessing quality of life in Alzheimer's disease,* ed. S. M. Albert and R. G. Logsdon. New York: Springer.

———. 2006. The history of therapeutic trials in dementia. *Trial designs and outcomes in dementia therapeutic research.* Oxford: Taylor & Francis.

Whitehouse, P. J., E. Bendezu, S. FallCreek, and C. Whitehouse. 2000. Intergenerational community schools: A new practice for a new time. *Educational Gerontology* 26:761–70.

Whitehouse, P. J., and D. R. George. 2008. *The myth of Alzheimer's: What you aren't being told about today's most dreaded diagnosis.* New York: St. Martin's Press.

Whitehouse, P. J., D. L. Price, A. W. Clark, J. T. Coyle, and M. R. DeLong. 1981. Alzheimer disease: Evidence for selective loss of cholinergic neurons in the nucleus basalis. *Annals of Neurology* 10:122–26.

Whitehouse, P. J., and P. V. Rabins. 1992. Quality of life and dementia. *Alzheimer Disease and Associated Disorders* 6 (3): 135–38.

Whitehouse, P. J., B. Winblad, D. Shostak, A. Bhattacharjya, M. Brod, H. Brodaty, A. Dor, et al. 1998. First International Pharmacoeconomic Conference on Alzheimer's Disease: Report and Summary. *Alzheimer Disease and Associated Disorders* 12 (4): 266–80.

PART IV

THE PROBLEM OF HOPE

Confidence and hope do more good than physic.
—Galen

Ignorance and credulous hope make the market for most
proprietary remedies.
—Samuel Hopkins Adams

And as far as false hope, there is no such thing. There is only
hope or the absence of hope—nothing else.
—Patti Davis

Hope has always rested uneasily at the heart of medicine. From
antiquity to the present, physicians have recognized the power of the patient's hope in overcoming disease and in maintaining quality of life. Hope,
it seems, is essential to humanity. To deprive a patient of all hope seems
cruel, and countless medical aphorisms admonish the physician to do nothing to destroy hope. But an equally long tradition warns of the dangers of
false hope, which can be unscrupulously encouraged to maintain the power,
prestige, and profitability of medicine or paternalistically nurtured to protect
patients and their families from realities that the physician believes they
could not handle.

Paradoxically, the success of medicine in the twentieth century has only
exacerbated the problem of hope. Medical science has developed powerful
treatments for some diseases, and so fostered the hope that such treatments
will be found for all diseases. And this hope has in turn encouraged our society to regard more and more problems as diseases awaiting a cure. But medical science has not given us a reliable calculus for determining when hope is
well founded and when it is not. Suffice it to say that there is no realistic
prospect that the dilemma of hope will be resolved by medical technology.

For better and for worse, our hopes seem always to hinge on the cutting edge.

The chapters in this final section of our book examine how the dilemma of hope is embedded in the development of ideas about cognitive decline in old age and the development of therapeutic agents that target Alzheimer's disease (AD). Together, they identify some of the important social and ethical issues that arise when models of illness and normality, human suffering, treatment development, advocacy for the ill, public health prioritization, and the human ego intersect.

Jesse Ballenger begins by describing the social context in which drug development for Alzheimer's disease took place in the United States in the second half of the twentieth century, arguing that the development of antidementia drugs has embodied our society's dominant hopes and anxieties about aging and cognition. These drugs, whether the psychostimulants and brain metabolism enhancers of an earlier era or the cholinergic enhancers currently licensed for AD, have been dogged by controversy about efficacy. But Ballenger argues that their efficacy has been almost secondary to their social role in making dementia a medical problem for which drug treatments are available rather than an inevitable concomitant of aging for which there is no hope. He concludes that while the medicalization of aging and dementia has had both positive and negative aspects, the social forces driving this reconceptualization are difficult to resist, though they can and should be better recognized and understood.

The overarching theme of the next chapter, by Tiago Moreira, is that contrasting paradigms of "truth" and "hope" have characterized how drug development for Alzheimer's disease has been framed by clinicians, scientists, consumers (patients and their caregivers), and those public authorities responsible for health policy and the approval of therapies to treat the disease. He suggests that the language that underlies the constructs of truth and hope has shaped how scientists study the pathobiology of Alzheimer's disease, how the public perceives the disease and what it demands of treatment for it, how public authorities have developed policies directed toward it, and what therapies are approved to treat the disease.

Moreira gives considerable attention to the distinction between disease-preventing and disease-modifying treatments and suggests that a shift occurred in the target of treatment as the inability of cholinesterase inhibitor drugs to change the underlying biology of the disease became clear. Moreira suggests that this may be an error and traces how therapies developed from

a theory of disease modification are now being used to study disease pathogenesis and to identify biological markers of treatment outcomes. He asserts
that consumers will increasingly be used to resolves "stalemates" that arise
between treatment developers and regulators. Whether treatment developers will use the public to influence the outcomes of such debates in their
favor (one meaning of Moreira's phrase "the fabrication of expectations"),
and to what extent regulators will respond to public pressures when the scientific data are equivocal, are questions that Moreira implicitly raises and
that bear further examination.

Margaret Lock and Adam Hedgecoe explore issues related to one of the
central hopes of the emerging age of genetic medicine—that increasing
knowledge of the genetic basis of disease will lead to scientific tests that
clearly convey important information about risk to individuals, allowing
them to take steps aimed to manage that risk and allowing clinicians to identify individuals who will most benefit from particular drugs. In the case of
AD, this hope is currently focused on testing for a specific allele of the
apolipoprotein E (APOE) gene that has been shown to significantly increase
the risk for late-onset AD. The authors conclude that routine APOE testing
should not be done at present because the complexity of the information the
test provides undermines its usefulness for clinicians and patients. First, the
predictive power of the test remains relatively weak because of apparent differences in how APOE alleles may be expressed in different genetic populations. Second, although there has been some research demonstrating that
carriers of the APOE4 allele for increased AD risk respond at different rates
to existing AD drugs than those without an E4 allele, most clinicians do not
believe that the APOE test is specific enough to be useful for pharmacogenetics. Finally, since the test is merely probabilistic (it cannot tell an individual
whether they will or will not get the disease, only that they do or do not have
an elevated chance of getting it), its potential usefulness to individuals is
limited, while the complexity of the information makes the danger of misin-
terpretation or confusion high. Lock and Hedgecoe present preliminary
qualitative data showing that the meaning of such information is frequently
misunderstood and poorly retained at follow up, even after subjects were educated about the meanings and implications of the data.

Lock and Hedgecoe raise a number of troubling questions that will persist
in the era of molecular medicine: who should ultimately decide whether
such information is made available to consumers and patients, and what are
the bases on which this decision should be made? Should, for example, stan-

dards be based on comprehension by a "typical" person, a demonstration that the harm/benefit ratio favors benefit, or, as the authors note in the last paragraph, the "behavior of the market" (the willingness of people to pay for the test results)? The ultimate question of who "owns" the information remains challenging.

In the concluding chapter, Peter Rabins discusses the major themes of this section and the entire book. Rabins recounts the positive and negative aspects of the reconceptualization of dementia, the difficulties in establishing the outcomes to measure in testing drug treatments for dementia, and the problem of managing the legitimate but differing interests of clinicians, pharmaceutical companies, and patients and their families. These issues, he points out, are not unique to the dementia field but are characteristic challenges medicine faces in treating all chronic illness, where therapeutic benefits must be evaluated in a context of only modest overall gains. Our society must undertake a wider discussion of these challenges.

Drawing on several decades of experience in clinical care and research in the dementia field, Rabins identifies some clear dangers that researchers and clinicians must work to avoid in meeting these challenges. Although he believes the reconceptualization of senility as disease has clearly been beneficial to patients and those caring for them, the danger of objectification of the individual must be continually guarded against. Similarly, Rabins argues that there has been a disturbing tendency in dementia advocacy to exaggerate the prevalence of AD, the burden imposed on families, and the failure of families and institutions to provide good care. While no one would dispute that the dementias are devastating, exaggerating the negatives can diminish the opportunities for joy and fulfillment that caregiving can provide and marginalize the contributions of family and professional caregivers to bettering the life of the person with dementia. Rabins also chastises scientists who have since the 1970s continually predicted "cures" or "major break-throughs"; he sees such pronouncements as self-serving and harmful to those struggling with the disease. But Rabins also warns clinicians about the tendency to overreact to the lack of dramatic therapies, adopting an inappropriate therapeutic nihilism. The stance that "nothing can be done" about dementia can lead clinicians to ignore the many nonpharmacological treatments such as education, caregiver support, environmental management, and activity-based treatments that can benefit patients and their caregivers. As always, clinicians must help patients and families steer a course between hype and hopelessness. Thus, he concludes, a balanced presentation of the

likely disease course and the available pharmacological and nonpharmacological treatments available remains the cornerstone of ethically sound
treatment for dementia and other chronic diseases.

The chapters in this section do not provide an easy solution to the dilemma of hope in medicine. But we conclude this book with the modest
hope that together they provide a useful introduction to the challenges facing all those involved in the development, use, and evaluation of drug treatments for dementia, and at the least a warning about some real dangers to
avoid.

There is no ready calculus for delineating false hope from true; indeed in
medicine it may be, as President Reagan's daughter Patti Davis suggests,
that there is no meaningful distinction between the two. But wisdom surely
lies knowing *what* to hope for. While dramatically effective drug treatments
for dementia may remain on the far distant horizon, the experiences of
people with dementia and those who care for them nonetheless constitute
good grounds for hope.

CHAPTER 11

Necessary Inventions

Antidementia Drugs and Heightened Expectations for Aging in Modern American Culture and Society

JESSE F. BALLENGER, PH.D.

Basic and clinical researchers in biomedicine seek to describe drugs in terms of biological specificity and clinical efficacy. Drugs are biochemical agents that reliably produce concrete, measurable effects on bodies. By rationalizing these effects to scientific understandings of the etiology and course of disease, researchers try to develop drugs as tools to prevent, cure, or at least ameliorate diseases. But the social worlds in which drugs are used are complex and powerful, and the specific effects of a given drug on the body can be distorted by the fears, expectations, and motivations of all involved. Researchers, of course, are well aware of this danger and have developed methods and procedures for clinical trials designed to isolate the specific effects of drugs they want to measure in the laboratory or clinic from the social worlds that surround them.

Scholars of society and culture, by contrast, are most interested in precisely what biomedical researchers seek to suppress—how drugs mediate the complex relationships between patients, practitioners, pharmaceutical companies, and regulatory agencies, each driven by a different set of values and desires. Whether the methods and procedures of clinical trials are adequate to draw a bright line between the biological effects of drugs and the highly charged contexts in which they are developed, tested, marketed, and consumed is an open question, and asking this question about drugs for dementia is one of the central objectives of this book. But whatever the answer to this question, it is clear that drugs are much more than simple biochemical agents that can be judged by their usefulness in treating disordered bodies.

In this chapter, I will argue that, whatever their efficacy as biochemical agents and whatever the difficulty clinical researchers have had in measuring meaningful effects in the bodies of patients diagnosed with Alzheimer's disease and related disorders, drugs for dementia have since the 1950s been powerful sociocultural agents. Although they have not thus far and may never amount to a cure and, as several chapters in this volume attest, even their ability to meaningfully ameliorate symptoms is controversial, they played a crucial role in the transformation of old age in twentieth-century American society and culture. The development of antidementia drugs not only signifies this dramatic change but also is one of the most important methods by which this change has been produced.

Aging and Therapeutic Nihilism in Modern America

In the United States at least, the drive to develop drug treatments for dementia has occurred in the context of steadily increasing anxiety since the late nineteenth century about the problems of an aging society. Historians of aging have identified the period between the 1870s and 1920s as a time in which public anxiety about aging intensified in the United States, particularly in discourse around issues of work, retirement, and productivity. The burgeoning U.S. middle class in this period increasingly worried that old age was becoming obsolete in modern society, that the aging body and brain could not possibly keep up with the frenetic pace of change and the stress of working and living in an industrial society (Achenbaum 1978; Haber 1983; Cole 1992; Haber and Gratton 1994). The intensification of this anxiety was connected to the erosion of traditional hierarchical social relations and ideals in the wake of advancing industrialization, mass-market consumerism, and a liberal social order—a transformation that made selfhood increasingly problematic (Wiebe 1967; Lears 1981; Trachtenberg 1982; Lears 1983). In modern America, selfhood was no longer an ascribed status, something established and maintained by the world a person was born into, but was instead something that had to be carefully and willfully constructed by every individual. In this context, the loss in dementia of the ability to independently sustain a coherent self-narrative came to seem perhaps the most frightful of all losses. Senility became possibly the gravest calamity in a land that idolized the "self-made man" (Ballenger 2006b).

American medical writing on aging and dementia during this period re-flected and reinforced these social anxieties. Through the late nineteenth cen-tury, most American physicians approached the subject from a highly specu-lative framework that used basic concepts of inertia and entropy from the physical sciences as metaphors to understand the deterioration they observed in the aging body and mind. Every person began life with a finite quantity of vital energy that could be spent over a lifetime. When this vital energy was de-pleted in old age, the body and mental powers began to deteriorate. Modifica-tions of individual behavior and social environment could ameliorate this to some degree; the way a person lived and the stresses he or she experienced could accelerate or retard the rate at which the body's vital energy was de-pleted. But given a finite fund of vitality, deterioration in old age was un-derstood to be inevitable (Haber 1983). Typical was a description by British psychiatrist Charles Mercier in a textbook that went through several U.S. edi-tions. Mercier compared a person's endowment of vital energy at birth to the inertia of a rolling ball: the greater the force initially given, the further it will go. "So with the living organism; all lives receive at conception an impetus which is to carry them forward to the end, but the impulse is not equally strong in all." Moreover, dementia was often hastened by disease, social fac-tors, or personal habits. As Mercier put it: "Owing to the exceptionally rough nature of the ground, the velocity of the ball is materially diminished at an early stage in its career, and . . . comes prematurely to rest" (Mercier 1908, p. 371).

This medical representation of old age as a state of exhaustion clearly le-gitimated the broader anxiety about aging in the modern world; the pace of industrial work, the complexity of bureaucratic organizations, the seductions of mass consumer culture—all these modern pressures seemed to demand more energy from the individual. Given what medicine was saying about old age, it made sense to think either that elderly people, exhausted by the deple-tion of vital energy, simply could not keep up in the modern world or that that the modern world itself was particularly hard on elderly people, subjecting them to pressures that exacerbated the natural decline of abilities that accom-panied old age. Both of these became standard tropes about aging in Ameri-can society in the twentieth century. In either case, physical and mental dete-rioration in old age appeared to be an inevitable problem in the modern world.

That the highly speculative and metaphorical medicine of the nineteenth century should be so enmeshed in these cultural anxieties is perhaps not sur-prising. But medical progress did not change underlying assumptions, and

the rising prestige of medicine as it claimed the mantle of science only solidi-
fied the idea, both within medicine and beyond, that physical and mental deterioration was an inevitable part of the aging process. As American physicians acquired a more sophisticated knowledge of pathology around the turn
of the twentieth century, the vitalistic model of depleted energy was replaced
by more mechanistic theories of tissue decay and evolutionary cell degeneration. Explicitly metaphoric language was replaced by the more concrete ter-
minology of postmortem dissection and microscopic description. But the
basic medical approach to old age continued to reflect and reinforce the same
modern concern that aging brought inevitable deterioration of physical and
mental abilities (Ballenger 2006b).

The creation of Alzheimer's disease (AD) as a diagnostic category is an excellent example of the way the most advanced medicine remained enmeshed
in cultural anxieties about aging (Ballenger 2006b). As is well known, Alois
Alzheimer's work in neuropathology at the brain anatomy lab in the Munich
clinic directed by Emil Kraepelin was remarkably advanced, and his description of the case of the 51-year-old Auguste Deter in 1906 brought together
the clinical and pathological elements of the modern concept of Alzheimer's
disease, a term that Kraepelin coined in the eighth edition of his influential
textbook on psychiatry (Maurer, Volk, and Garabaldo 2000; Maurer and
Maurer 2003). What has been puzzling is why Kraepelin, whose fame rests on
his replacing the welter of overlapping categories of mental illness with a rigorous and logical nosological system, made a distinction between AD as a presenile dementia affecting people under the age of 65 and senile dementia
affecting the much larger number of patients over the age of 65—a distinction that confounded nosology for decades. Kraepelin was well aware that Alzheimer's work and that of several other psychiatrists demonstrated that the
clinical and pathological features of both categories were essentially identical.
So why, then, did Kraepelin assert the existence of this new entity Alzheimer's
disease? A number of speculations have been offered related to Kraepelin's ri-
valries with Sigmund Freud and Arnold Pick (Torack 1979; Amaducci, Rocca,
and Schoenberg 1986; Myfanwy and Isaac 1987; Ballenger 2006a). All of
these speculations seem plausible, but there appears no reason to believe that
he was being intellectually dishonest. To Kraepelin, it simply made no sense to
call senile dementia a disease, for the pathological processes of old age were
understood to be "normal." But when dementia occurred at earlier ages, even
though associated with the same brain pathology, it seemed to suggest a disease (Beach 1987). This assumption remained powerful within medicine be-

cause it resonated so strongly with broader cultural attitudes toward aging; and it seems to be the reason that the psychiatric literature maintained the distinction between AD as a rare disorder distinct from senile dementia through the 1970s, despite the fact that researchers were well aware of and puzzled by their similarity (Holstein 1997, 2000).

Within medicine, there was little serious thought given to therapeutic interventions to treat or even ameliorate senile physical and mental deterioration during this period—though while physicians worked in a vitalistic model, they did offer some hope for prevention. Although mental and physical deterioration might be inevitable, the point at which it became apparent and speed with which it progressed could be highly variable. Some physicians even thought that senile dementia was not inevitable, if only the individual would take care to avoid dissipating behaviors such as over- or underwork, drinking, and sexual excess that squandered the fund of vitality—following Mercier's metaphor, if they would only take care to avoid particularly rough ground. But as the medical literature became more rigorously focused on the brain and neuropathology, the sense that personal behavior or social factors could modify the onset or course of dementia dropped away. The creation of Alzheimer's disease was perhaps the culmination of this, placing plaque-and-tangle dementia in a sort of therapeutic catch-22: when it occurred among the relatively young, it was a legitimate disease that could be investigated and perhaps prevented or treated, but then it was a rare one unlikely to attract a significant effort; when it occurred among elderly people, it was common enough but was understood as part of the inevitable deterioration of aging that we could not rationally hope to stop or reverse.

The Imperative for Treatment of Dementia in Post–World War II America

Thus it was that as Americans were becoming more frightened of the specter of aging in general and senile dementia in particular, medicine was becoming less and less sanguine about its ability to do anything about it—a situation that would grow increasingly intolerable during the twentieth century. The pressure to develop a meaningful way of treating senile dementia was first felt by American psychiatrists during the 1930s, because the state mental hospital system had become the default institutional setting for patients with senile dementia who could not be cared for in the community, and through the 1950s at least, the legitimacy of psychiatry rested on the state hospitals.

Policy changes in the late nineteenth century making care of mentally ill people the financial responsibility of the state had created a strong financial incentive for families and local welfare authorities to regard senile dementia as a mental illness rather than a part of aging. Psychiatrists running the state hospitals complained bitterly about this but could do little to stem the tide (Grob 1983). Because elderly patients with senile dementia were by definition incurable, their increasing numbers threatened to overwhelm the state hospital system. "Our institutions promise to become in time vast infirmaries with relatively small departments for younger patients with curable disorders," said Richard Hutchings in his 1939 address as president of the American Psychiatric Association (Hutchings 1939, p. 4). Beginning in the 1930s, there was a dramatic upsurge in publications on dementia in the American psychiatric literature, and these articles were frequently framed in terms of apocalyptic demography—that because of the aging of the population these patients constituted a demographic avalanche that threatened to overwhelm psychiatry (Ballenger 2000).

Psychiatrists reacted to the crisis they perceived in the increasing prevalence of senile dementia in the mental hospital in two ways. Many psychiatrists made the argument that alternatives to the hospital for care of elderly people with dementia were necessary, and an alternative was created in the 1960s, when, through provisions in Medicare and Medicaid, the federal government assumed responsibility for funding nursing home care for elderly patients. The result was the transfer of many thousands of elderly patients with dementia out of the mental hospitals and into nursing homes and various community care arrangements as rapidly and dramatically as had been the earlier shift into the mental hospitals (Grob 1983, 1986).

But another group of psychiatrists, led by David Rothschild, who was clinical director of the Worcester State Hospital in Massachusetts, redefined dementia (Ballenger 2000). Seizing on the finding that there was often a discrepancy between the degree of dementia found in life and the degree of pathology found in the brain at autopsy, Rothschild theorized that psychosocial factors might also play an important role in dementia. Rothschild proclaimed in 1941 that "too exclusive preoccupation with the cerebral pathology has led to a tendency to forget that the changes are occurring in living, mentally functioning persons who may react to a given situation, including an organic one, in various ways. When this is taken into consideration, the problem no longer seems puzzling, and at the same time a broader view of senile psychosis emerges, one in which the qualities of the living patient now appear as an important factor in the origins of the disorder" (Rothschild and Sharp 1941, p. 49). Rothschild's psychodynamic model was clearly the dominant approach to senile dementia among U.S. psychiatrists through the 1950s, though it did not have the same currency in the United Kingdom (Ballenger 2000).

Within the sphere of medicine, or at least psychiatry, Rothschild's model seemed to cut through the therapeutic nihilism that had characterized the medical approach to dementia. In the 1940s and 1950s a surge of articles appeared discussing the interest in therapies that had previously been considered inappropriate for aging patients—reflecting both the optimistic avenues that Rothschild's work opened and the desperate empiricism to which psychiatrists were driven by the crisis of the mental hospitals. Virtually every major form of therapy was reported to have been attempted on older patients who had symptoms of dementia—ranging from group and individual psychotherapies to somatic therapies such as electroconvulsive therapy, vitamin and other nutritional therapies, and the drug therapies that will be described in more detail below (Ballenger 2000).

But perhaps more important, the psychodynamic model resonated well with the emerging field of social gerontology. Following World War II, the psychodynamic model of dementia increasingly became a psychosocial model, and ultimately it came to seem like an explanation for aging as a whole. Gerontologists made the case for postretirement educational or recreational programs by evoking the specter of people with dementia piling up in the mental hospitals: "With the number of people who are over 65 increasing significantly each year, our society is today finding itself faced with the problem of keeping a large share of its population from joining the living dead—those whose minds are allowed to die before their bodies do" (Kaplan 1953, p. 3). At the same time, psychiatrists often wrote about dementia as though it were essentially an extension of social issues such as retirement, as when Rothschild described a 75-year-old man whose dementia he attributed not to whatever might be going on in his brain, but to enforced idleness and isolation that followed retirement (Rothschild 1947). Both within psychiatry and beyond among social gerontologists and other aging advocates in various policy fields, researchers increasingly thought of modern social relations as the pathology of senility. The pathology of senile mental deterioration was no longer restricted to the aging brain but now included a society that stripped elderly people of the roles that had sustained meaning in their lives through mandatory retirement, social isolation, and the disintegration of traditional family ties. It seemed that all of the problems of old age, including dementia, could be subsumed into the broad and flexible category of "senility" that psychiatry and gerontology had created.

In this context, the first drugs to treat dementia began to appear. The drugs that came to market in the mid-1950s as treatments for senility followed three broad approaches. The psychostimulants (for example, pentylenetetrazol) were developed and used with the idea that because elderly patients with dementia typically lack energy, alertness, and motivation, drugs that could safely increase their energy would be beneficial. Cerebral vasodilators (such as nicotinic acid) were deployed on the long-held belief that impaired circulation was a cause of senile mental impairment. Cerebral metabolic enhancers (for example, dihydroergotoxine) were thought to improve cell metabolism within the brain. In practice, however, these approaches overlapped (Reisberg 1981). For example, dihydroergotoxine, marketed by a variety of companies but most successfully by Sandoz as Hydergine, began its career as a cerebrovasodilator but was reclassified as a metabolic enhancer (Hollister 1981). But what all of these approaches had in common was that, in keeping with the broad concept of senility that set the context for dementia drug research in this period, they were not aimed at specific pathological mechanisms but at improving the overall mental functioning of elderly patients who had deteriorated in various ways and to various degrees.

A look at the marketing campaign for one of these drugs suggests the way in which they fit into the broader transformation of aging that psychiatry's concern with dementia entailed. Perhaps the most heavily marketed drug for the treatment of senility from the early 1950s through the mid-1960s was pentylenetetrazol, a nervous system stimulant that had been used to produce convulsions in drug-induced shock therapy. Numerous companies sold the drug in a variety of formulas that combined it with vasodilators, vitamins, and hormones, claiming improvement for a wide range of senile symptoms including mental confusion, memory loss, lack of motivation, and emotional and behavioral problems. Advertising for these drugs, which appeared steadily both in geriatric journals like *Geriatrics* as well as broader journals like the *American Journal of Psychiatry*, skillfully positioned them as significant interventions into the broad problem of senility that psychiatrists and gerontologists were grappling with.

An advertisement for Knoll Pharmaceuticals' line of Metrazol products, which included pentylenetetrazol in both a vitamin and a nicotinic acid formula, appeared in *Geriatrics* in 1963, contrasting a small photo of an unkempt elderly woman, frail and disturbed, with a large, striking photo of the same woman, carefully dressed, smiling as she is about to play a card in a four-handed intergenerational card game. The headline: "Before Early Confusion Disturbs the Environment: Help the Geriatric Patient Help Herself." The text explained that the personal habits of older patients often show striking improvement with medication. "The patient becomes neater, more concerned with appearance, more conscious of social relationships. Metrazol helps dispel the mental haze surrounding many aging persons."

An advertisement appearing in the May 1965 issue of the *American Journal of Psychiatry* for Nicozol, a pentylenetetrazol / nicotinic acid mixture, played on similar themes. The headline boasted that Nicozol provided a more cheerful outlook "for the occupationally deprived," and it was illustrated by a six-panel photo montage of an elderly couple seated on a park bench engaged in a light-hearted, spontaneous display of affection for each other. "Normally active men and women tend to stagnate when they reach retirement age or are otherwise deprived of their occupation and responsibilities. Apathetic, irritable, uncooperative, even disoriented, they often become a burden to those around them," the accompanying text explained. Nicozol provided "safe, gentle cerebral stimulation" that would improve their outlook, sociability, personal habits, and appearance, so that the "the occupationally deprived patient becomes more cooperative, cheerful, easier to manage . . . at home, rather than in a home."

Advertisements for these drugs clearly aimed to suggest that they were an effective way of dealing not with a particular set of symptoms but with a much broader set of problems around aging—problems that fell under the rubric of senility as constructed by psychiatrists and gerontologists and that were at the core of society's broader concerns about aging. More fundamentally, the advertisements were both evidence and instantiation of the transformation of aging in American society and culture. Mental deterioration was no longer a problem that could be blandly accepted as an inevitable part of aging that medicine could do nothing about. Rather, it was an intolerable affront to the American dream, which now included the ideal of retirement to a life of active leisure. It had to be taken seriously, and nothing indicated this more than the development of drugs to treat or prevent it.

Perhaps the importance of having drugs to treat dementia explains the persistence on the market of these early drugs despite scant objective evidence that they were effective. Virtually all of the drugs that were marketed as treatments for dementia in the 1950s and 1960s share a similar trajectory.

Initial uncontrolled studies in the literature were wildly enthusiastic, reporting significant and sometimes dramatic improvement in the behavior and
mental functioning of patients with dementia. More rigorous, carefully designed studies using blinded control methods produced results that were ambiguous at best and more often clearly negative. Nonetheless, most of these
drugs remained on the market until the 1980s, generating a medical literature that continued to cycle between positive reports in uncontrolled studies
and negative results in more methodologically rigorous ones.

In the case of pentylenetetrazol, as early as 1955 a controlled study of the
drug found no significant benefits (Hollister and Fitzpatrick 1955). Nonetheless, favorable reports from uncontrolled studies continued to proliferate, and
the 1963 ads described above claimed that "the growing literature on Metrazol
now includes more than 4,000 references attesting to its safety and efficacy."
But a 1965 review in *The Medical Letter on Drugs and Therapeutics* noted that virtually all favorable studies of the drug had been methodologically weak, while
controlled studies consistently reported negative or equivocal results, and concluded that the improvement reported with Metrazol in uncontrolled trials was
likely due to placebo effects (Anon., "Metrazol and other drugs" 1965). Nonetheless, the drug remained in use through the 1970s. In 1979 another major
review noted that none of the 16 published controlled studies had shown that
the drug had a clearly beneficial effect on cognitive function in the aged and reported that the FDA had initiated action to withdraw the drug because it lacked
substantial evidence of effectiveness (Crook 1979).

Despite significant and widespread doubts about their efficacy, the first
generation of drugs for dementia remained a going proposition until the
early 1980s, when—perhaps not coincidentally—the cholinergic hypothesis
seemed to promise that far more effective treatments were on the horizon.
(Several of the early antidementia drugs, including piracetam, cyclandelate,
and dihydroergotoxine are still widely sold directly to patients via the online
"gray market" for "antiaging" or "brain-boosting" drugs.) The early drugs
continued to have a place, albeit an uneasy one, as indicated by a 1981 edited
volume on treatment strategies for dementia that featured some of the most
important researchers in the field (Crook and Gershon 1981). In his introductory chapter, Gene Cohen acknowledged the dismal outlook with regard to
the available treatments for dementia: not only were there no treatments
available to cure, reverse, or stop the progression of senile dementia of the
Alzheimer type (SDAT), but reports that the drugs currently in use produced
positive effects on cognitive impairment were equivocal and controversial.

Still, Cohen credited studies of these early drugs with providing "jumping off points for a number of creative research ideas and studies" (Cohen 1981, p. 4).

Other authors defended the early drugs more directly than Cohen. Steven Ferris made the case that even though psychostimulants and metabolic enhancers had produced discouraging results thus far, it was worth investigating how they might work in combination, and particularly in combination with cholinergic precursors, which on their own had also failed to provide meaningful results (Ferris 1981). Perhaps most interestingly, Barry Reisberg argued that the problem was not so much the drugs but unrealistic expectations among the physicians and researchers who studied them:

> A major source of dissatisfaction with metabolic enhancers relates to the relatively small improvements that have been noted in most studies. While understandable on a human level, the scientific reasoning behind the latter attitude should be questioned. With respect to cancer, physicians learned to accept heroic measures including major surgery, whole body irradiation and chemotoxic therapies in return for increases in survival rates of 10% or less. Precisely the opposite attitude prevails with respect to treatments for SDAT. If an agent exerts no dramatic clinical effect, it may be regarded as virtually useless by the research community. This attitude should be reexamined. (Reisberg 1981, p. 200)

Given the willingness of clinicians to continue using the early drugs for decades despite equivocal findings and marginal gains, Resiberg's argument seems misplaced. If clinicians and researchers in the 1980s were growing increasingly dissatisfied with the first generation of drugs, their belief that better drugs were possible and would soon be available is probably the more likely explanation. Overall, it seems that the majority of clinicians and researchers from the late 1940s on were committed to having some kind of drugs available for the treatment of mental deterioration in elderly people, though they did not seem to have terribly high expectations about efficacy. In the 1980s, many found new hope that medical science was ready to deliver a treatment that would make a real difference.

The Reformation of Alzheimer's as a Disease Category and the Cholinergic Era

By the early 1980s, the social and cultural transformation of aging had worked seismic changes in the landscape of dementia. The rise of AD as a medical concept and a public issue is usually characterized as a sharp break with the previous generation's approach to aging and dementia (Fox 1989; Katzman and Bick 2000a). But there were in fact important elements of continuity. However limited and confusing we might find their ideas about the social pathogenisis of dementia and the broad category of senility, psychiatrists and social gerontologists from the 1940s through the 1960s were committed to improving the lives of elderly people, and their work helped usher in a series of policy changes that transformed the experience of aging in the United States after the 1960s and set the stage in important ways for the emergence of AD. By the 1980s, the economic circumstances of aging were markedly improved, with people over age 65 moving from the poorest age group to one of the best off. Significant legal protections had been won against age discrimination in the labor market, negative stereotypes were challenged, and elderly people organized for political action on their own behalf in large and influential advocacy groups like AARP (Calhoun 1978). With these developments, the expansiveness of the broad concept of senility that had provided a rubric for the efforts of psychiatrists and gerontologists in the 1950s began to seem unacceptable.

For a new generation of gerontologists, the word "senility" seemed to evoke "ageist" stereotypes in much the same way that the word "Negro" became an unacceptable term to those committed to improving the lives of African Americans. Robert N. Butler, who coined the word "ageism," led the attack in his Pulitzer Prize–winning book *Why Survive? Being Old in America.* Senility was not a meaningful medical concept, he argued, but a "wastebasket term" for a variety of discrete disease entities, many of them treatable. The continued currency of the term among professionals was a product of their conscious and unconscious fears and hostilities toward old age (Butler 1975).

In this context, clinicians who worked extensively with older patients were increasingly inclined to view the health problems of elderly people as the product of discrete diseases that might be amenable to treatment rather than normal and inevitable deterioration associated with aging, and biomedical researchers searched for insights into the basic biological mechanisms of dementia with renewed vigor. In the 1970s, the Newcastle team of Blessed, Tomlinson, and Roth established more rigorous clinical pathologic correlations for dementia, and a consensus began to emerge around the concept of SDAT as the most prevalent form of dementia, clearly distinguished from other forms as well as the normal process of aging (Katzman and Bick 2000b). This conception retained the original distinction between AD as a presenile dementia occurring before age 65 and SDAT, occurring after age 65, but suggested at the very least that common pathophysiological mechanisms were at work in both.

Although controversy continues about the relationship of Alzheimer-type dementia to both normal aging and other forms of dementia (Huppert, Brayne, and O'Connor 1994; Morris 2000), the concept of AD as a discrete entity distinct from aging retains great currency. Not least of the reasons for this is that the conceptualization was and continues to be politically effective. Researchers and family members of dementia victims have been able to forge a tremendously successful lobbying effort for increased federal funds for research into what they argued was one of the most devastating diseases of the twentieth century, a disease that threatened to overwhelm the health care system and our capacity to care for the millions who are afflicted. Seen this way, finding treatments that can delay the onset of if not cure AD appeared to be an unquestionable economic and social if not moral priority. In 1976, federal funding for AD research was less than $1 million; by 1983 it had risen to $11 million (Fox 1989); by 2005 it had reached nearly $650 million (Alzheimer's Association 2006).

By the early 1980s, the investment in finding a treatment for dementia appeared ready to bear therapeutic fruit. In the mid-1970s several labs established that the brains of Alzheimer patients have a pronounced deficit in the neurotransmitter acetylcholine, which was known to play an important role in memory (Katzman and Bick 2000a). In the early 1980s, research had identified a cholinergic center of the brain that appeared to be a focal point for cell loss in the disease (Whitehouse et al. 1982; Coyle, Price, and DeLong 1983). These studies allowed researchers to construct a persuasive model of the proximal cause of dementia—the cholinergic hypothesis. Narrowly stated, the cholinergic hypothesis argued that a single aspect of the global cognitive deterioration of AD, the impairment of recent memory, was caused by a pronounced depletion of acetylcholine in the brain, which in turn was caused by the death of a specific group of neurons. Articulated this way, it said nothing about the other cognitive deficits of AD or disturbances of personality and affect. Nor did it say anything about what *caused* the deterioration of this specific population of neurons. But more expansive versions quickly appeared as well, in which the depletion of acetylcholine looked to be the key to unraveling the disease, reducing the complex totality of AD to something that could be managed by scientific research (Dillman 2000).

Most important, the cholinergic hypothesis had therapeutic implications that were clear from the outset, and this was perhaps the major reason for the

excitement it generated. If cognitive deterioration in Alzheimer-type dementia could be linked to the pathological deficit of a specific neurotransmitter,
one could rationally pursue drug treatments designed to either restore levels
of the neurotransmitter or prevent its depletion. This approach had worked in
Parkinson's disease, where a deficit of the neurotransmitter dopamine had
been found. Patients with Parkinson's disease who were treated with L-dopa,
a dopamine precursor, showed dramatic improvement. It was understood
that this would not be a cure; the effectiveness of maintaining the supply of a
neurotransmitter would diminish as the disease continued to destroy neurons
directly. Thus, in the case of Parkinson's disease, the "Lazarus effect" many
patients experienced with L-dopa treatment diminished as the disease progressed. But as long as a sufficient number of neurons remained intact,
cholinergic therapy held out hope for meaningful treatment of the cognitive
symptoms of AD. But it did not prove easy to duplicate the success of
dopaminergic treatment for Parkinson's disease. Loading patients who had
AD with cholinergic precursors like choline and lecithin proved ineffective
and was abandoned in the early 1980s (Bartus et al. 1985). The emphasis in
therapeutic research then turned to developing drugs that would inhibit the
action of cholinesterase, the enzyme that metabolizes acetylcholine after
synaptic transmission, thus keeping the overall level of acetylcholine in the
brain higher.

In 1986, the publication of an article by William Summers and colleagues
in the *New England Journal of Medicine* that reported encouraging results in a
controlled, long-term trial of 17 patients with the cholinesterase inhibitor
tacrine appeared to be a significant breakthrough in this strategy. The authors claimed dramatic improvement for 16 of the patients on the drug: "One
subject was able to resume most of her homemaking tasks, one was able to resume employment on a part-time basis, and one retired subject was able to resume playing golf daily. In other cases, there were improvements in activities
of daily living, such as self-feeding at the family table, where total care has
been previously required." The authors concluded by advising "prudence in
judging these results," going on to explain that tacrine was "no more a cure
for AD than L-dopa is a cure for Parkinson's disease. Just as L-dopa ceases to
have effect in patients in the final stages of Parkinson's disease, we anticipate
THA [tacrine] will cease to have effects as Alzheimer's progresses" (Summers
et al. 1986, pp. 12343–44). Of course, this ostensible call for prudence was
likely to heighten enthusiasm for the drug, because developing a treatment
analogous to L-dopa in Parkinson's was the grail to which the cholinergic hy-

pothesis was supposed to lead. A palliative treatment this effective in providing symptomatic relief in Alzheimer's would be of enormous benefit in the struggle of patients, families, and society to deal with dementia. An editorial that accompanied the Summers article amplified the enthusiasm, noting that for the first time results with cholinesterase inhibitors appeared to have an "efficacy equivalent to L-dopa in Parkinson's disease." The body of the editorial did sound some important cautionary notes, pointing out that the current study would need to be reconciled with an earlier controlled study that had shown much less dramatic improvements. Nonetheless, the editorial concluded by noting that "the findings of Summers et al. represent a triumph of the scientific method" because it was one of the rare instances when drug development followed a rational path, thus providing a "positive reflection of our nation's investment in science" (Davis and Mohs 1986, pp. 1286–87).

But far from standing as a triumph of modern medicine, the Summers study quickly became enveloped in controversy. Six months after publication, five letters appeared in the *New England Journal of Medicine* raising serious questions about the methodology in gathering and reporting the data. Soon after this, the FDA opened an investigation that culminated in accusations that Summers violated regulations pertaining to the proper conduct of clinical research, citing 14 findings that cast serious doubt on his conclusions (Kolata 1988). Additional concerns were raised about Summers's involvement in a for-profit corporation that charged patients $12,000 per year for the tacrine treatment they received in the study, and application for a use patent for the drug—neither of which he disclosed in the 1986 publication. He disclosed both of these at the behest of the *Journal's* editors in a letter published along with the five critical letters (Summers 1987). Summers reached an agreement with the FDA that restricted his research activities on the drug, though he continued to stand by the validity of his conclusions (Scott 1989). In the coming years the drug's fortunes continued to fall. Liver damage emerged as a potentially dangerous side effect, and a major subsequent controlled trial, also published in the *New England Journal of Medicine,* reported far more modest results with the drug: although the study did find statistically significant reduction in the decline of cognitive function, this reduction was not large enough to be detected by physicians' global assessments of the patients (Davis et al. 1992). An editorial accompanying this study argued that the results were in fact so disappointing that the cholinergic strategy ought to be abandoned to focus research and resources on strategies aimed at directly intervening in the degenerative process (Growdon 1992).

Despite ongoing scientific controversy about the drug, tacrine was approved by the FDA as a symptomatic treatment in mild or moderate AD in 1993. The initial publication by Summers et al. ignited public clamor for the drug, and the FDA came under fierce public criticism in 1991 when its advisory board refused to recommend tacrine for approval without stronger evidence of its efficacy. Family members and Alzheimer's advocates followed the lead of AIDS activists in demanding that the FDA quickly approve new drugs to treat deadly diseases when other treatments did not exist (Lockheed 1992). Feverish editorials and op-ed columns appeared around the country that excoriated the agency for letting millions of victims suffer and die while a potentially effective treatment was available. For example, the *Wall Street Journal* consistently attacked the FDA for its "pattern of foot-dragging that in this one case leaves four million patients without any therapy" ("The Alzheimer's morass," March 26, 1991), and in another editorial accused Paul Leber, the FDA official in charge of the division responsible neurological and psychiatric drugs, of "demanding proofs of Euclidean precision" and suggested that the "ironic distance between Dr. Leber's austere and disinterested logic and the ruined landscape of an Alzheimer's life deserves a stage play" ("Marching for Alzheimer's," Sept 24, 1992). Syndicated columnist James Kilpatrick was more blunt: the four million people with the disease "are victims not only of Alzheimer's but also of Dr. David Kessler, commissioner of the Food and Drug Administration. He is the all-powerful czar whose decrees finally govern the availability of new drugs" (Kilpatrick 1992). Without more thorough historical research, it is difficult to assess precisely the impact of public opinion on the FDA's eventual decision to license the drug, however, it seems logical that it played an important role. Leber himself acknowledged that the decision to issue guidelines for drug companies seeking licensure of antidementia drugs was a response to public demand. Leber would have preferred to let FDA guidelines emerge as a codification of best practices based on the experience of bringing several drugs to market, but in the midst of a rising tide of public demand for tacrine, that position was "politically untenable" (Leber 1996).

In any case, the tacrine controversy makes clear how the position of aging in general and dementia in particular has changed in American society and culture across the twentieth century. Although disagreement over the value of the drug itself was sharp, virtually all published commentary in the tacrine debate reinforced a central belief: age-associated dementia was the product of a dread disease that demanded meaningful treatment and eventually prevention or cure. Expectations for aging had significantly risen in the twentieth century, and a drug treatment for a condition that so deeply threatened those expectations was simply a necessity. Given the centrality of having a drug treatment available for dementia to widely held beliefs about aging in modern America, it was perhaps inevitable that, in the absence of any rival treatments, tacrine would win approval. Subsequently, three other cholinesterase inhibitors were approved by the FDA with much less difficulty, each promising to be safer and more convenient than tacrine. Donepezil, approved in 1996, quickly replaced tacrine as the drug of choice because of the convenience of its once-a-day dosing. However, as several other chapters in this volume will attest, debate about the efficacy of these drugs remains as heated as it was over tacrine.

Throughout this chapter I have emphasized continuity rather than change, and there are certainly parallels between the era of psychostimulants and metabolic enhancers and the cholinergic era. In pointing out these parallels, I am not suggesting that no progress has been made in the understanding of the dementias and the pursuit of drug treatment over the past 40 years. The cholinergic hypothesis itself was a significant development in identifying specific mechanisms of the disease, and research has gone much further since then. Similarly, drug evaluation and regulation have become far more robust, and the debate about the cholinergic drugs is grounded much more firmly in data—though for all that I think it also follows some of the same well-worn grooves as debate over the earlier generation of drugs. Perhaps most importantly, 40 years ago patients with dementia and their families played no role in the public discussion about antidementia drugs, but they have been directly and powerfully involved in ongoing controversy about the cholinesterase inhibitors. This last point is actually the essential feature of social and cultural continuity: steadily rising expectations for a healthy, independent, and fulfilling old age. Drug development for dementia has been both a reflection and an instantiation of these rising expectations and the empowerment of older people.

Some of the parallels with the past are obvious: now as then, there are sharp debates over the efficacy of antidementia drugs and even how to measure that efficacy. Now as then, there is nonetheless widespread acceptance of the idea that AD and related disorders must have treatments. One could read the assessment of the state of drug therapy in 1981 as essentially accurate today: there are currently no treatments available to cure, reverse, or stop the progression of AD, and reports that the drugs presently in use produce positive effects on cognitive impairment are equivocal and controversial—though many continue to defend the cholinergic drugs as the best available, providing measurable if not dramatic benefits to patients, and as facilitating further progress in our understanding the disease and developing potential therapeutic strategies. Moreover, now as then, growing dissatisfaction with the cholinesterase inhibitors may be connected to the belief that much more effective treatments are on the horizon. The chapter by Price et al. in this volume (chapter 3) describes the potential for a new generation of drugs that promise to go beyond symptomatic relief to directly slow the progression of the disease.

A less obvious parallel with the past is the way in which antidementia drugs remain intimately connected to rising expectations for old age. An advertisement for Aricept that appeared in *Geriatrics* and many other medical journals in 2003 plays on strikingly similar themes as the ads for Metrazol and Nicozol from the 1960s described above. The Aricept ad is dominated by a close-up of the chiseled, lantern-jawed face of an elderly man with a determined look and a gleam of self-confidence in his eye. The text identifies the man as a 71-year-old patient who has been taking the drug for four years and quotes him as saying, "I haven't retired from the human race . . . and I don't intend to for a long time." Beneath this, the headline proclaims "The Strength to Meet Dementia Head On," which seems meant to describe both the resolute man pictured and the drug he is taking. As a whole, the ad suggests that Aricept is helping this elder to maintain a meaningful and productive position in society, thus addressing not the modest effect the drug has on some measures of dementia but perhaps the broadest and most intense anxiety we have about aging—retaining our status as a human being. Advertising in both eras suggests that antidementia drugs are intimately bound to our most important beliefs about aging.

In trying to summarize the history of modern drug treatment for dementia, I am inclined to paraphrase Voltaire's famous dictum about God: If effective drug treatments for dementia did not exist, it would be necessary to invent them. This dictum should annoy both skeptics and believers. To skeptics for whom the "medicalization" of aging is anathema, it should suggest the inescapable and inevitable importance of drug treatments. Given how deeply therapeutic longing is embedded in widely held ideas about aging, it is not clear how we could or even if we should "demedicalize" dementia. To believers who assume the inevitability of therapeutic progress, this dictum should suggest that their rituals of control and verification are hollow, that their goal of demonstrably effective drugs for dementia may even be a false god. The effect of drugs will never be truly separable from our intense desire for treatment, and the goal itself may be motivated by the desire for domination and control. In the end, the history of drug treatment for dementia provides no simple lessons. Rather, it illustrates that development of these drugs poses a dilemma. It is this dilemma that the remaining chapters in this volume, in different ways, explore.

REFERENCES

Achenbaum, W. A. 1978. *Old age in the New Land: The American experience since 1790.* Baltimore: Johns Hopkins University Press.

Alzheimer's Association. 2006. Statistics about Alzheimer's disease. www.alz.org/AboutAD/ statistics.asp.

Amaducci, L. A., W. A. Rocca, and B. S. Schoenberg. 1986. Origin of the distinction between Alzheimer's disease and senile dementia: How history can clarify nosology. *Neurology* 36 (11): 1497–99.

Anon. 1965. Metrazol and other drugs in emotional disorders of old age. *Medical Letter on Drugs and Therapeutics* 7 (5): 19–20.

Ballenger, J. F. 2000. Beyond the characteristic plaques and tangles: Mid-twentieth century U.S. psychiatry and the fight against senility. In *Concepts of Alzheimer disease: Biological, clinical, and cultural perspectives,* ed. P. J. Whitehouse, K. Maurer, and J. F. Ballenger, 83–103. Baltimore: Johns Hopkins University Press.

———. 2006a. Progress in the history of Alzheimer's disease: The importance of context. *Journal of Alzheimer's Disease* 9:1–9.

———. 2006b. *Self, senility, and Alzheimer's disease in modern America.* Baltimore: Johns Hopkins University Press.

Bartus, R. T., R. L. Dean, M. J. Pontecorvo, and C. Flicker. 1985. The cholinergic hypothesis: A historical overview, current perspective, and future directions. *Annals of the New York Academy of Sciences* 444:332–58.

Beach, T. G. 1987. The history of Alzheimer's disease: Three debates. *Journal of the History of Medicine and Allied Sciences* 42:327–49.

Butler, R. N. 1975. *Why survive? Being old in America.* New York: Harper & Row.

Calhoun, R. B. 1978. *In search of the new old: Redefining old age in America, 1945–1970.* New York: Elsevier.

Cohen, G. 1981. Senile dementia of the Alzheimer type (SDAT): Nature of the disorder. In *Strategies for the Development of an Effective Treatment for Senile Dementia,* ed. T. Crook and S. Gershon, 1–5. New Canaan, Conn.: Mark Powley Associates.

Cole, T. R. 1992. *The Journey of life: A cultural history of aging in America.* Cambridge: Cambridge University Press.

Coyle, J. T, D. L. Price, and M. R. DeLong. 1983. Alzheimer's disease: A disorder of cortical cholinergic innervation. *Science* 219 (4589): 1184–90.

Crook, T. 1979. Central-nervous-system stimulants: Appraisal of use in geropsychiatric patients. *Journal of the American Geriatrics Society* 27 (10): 476–77.

Crook, T., and S. Gershon 1981. *Strategies for the development of an effective treatment for senile dementia.* New Canaan, Conn.: Mark Powley Associates.

Davis, K. L., and R. C. Mohs. 1986. Cholinergic drugs in Alzheimer's disease. *New England Journal of Medicine* 315 (20): 1286–87.

Davis, K. L., L. J. Thal, E. R. Gamzu, C. S. Davis, R. F. Woolson, S. I. Gracon, D. A. Drachman, et al., the Tacrine Collaborative Study Group. 1992. A double-blind, placebo-controlled multicenter study of tacrine for Alzheimer's disease. *New England Journal of Medicine* 327 (18): 1253–59.

Dillman, R. 2000. Alzheimer disease: Epistemological lessons from history? *Concepts of Alzheimer disease: Biological, clinical, and cultural perspectives,* ed. P. J. Whitehouse, K. Maurer, and J. F. Ballenger. Baltimore: Johns Hopkins University Press.

Ferris, S. H. 1981. Empirical studies in senile dementia with central nervous system stimulants and metabolic enhancers. In *Strategies for the development of an effective treatment for senile dementia,* ed. T. Crook and S. Gershon, 173–87. New Canaan, Conn.: Mark Powley Associates.

Fox, P. 1989. From senility to Alzheimer's disease: The rise of the Alzheimer's disease movement. *Milbank Quarterly* 67 (1): 58–102.

Grob, G. N. 1983. *Mental illness and American society, 1875–1940.* Princeton, N.J.: Princeton University Press.

———. 1986. Explaining old age history: The need for empiricism. In *Old age in a bureaucratic society,* ed. D. D. Van Tassel and P. N. Stearns. New York: Greenwood Press.

Growdon, J. H. 1992. Treatment for Alzheimer's disease? *New England Journal of Medicine* 327 (18): 1306–8.

Haber, C. 1983. *Beyond sixty-five: The dilemma of old age in America's past.* Cambridge: Cambridge University Press.

Haber, C., and B. Gratton. 1994. *Old age and the search for security: An American social history.* Bloomington: Indiana University Press.

Hollister, L. 1981. An overview of strategies for the development of effective treatment for senile dementia. In *Strategies for the development of an effective treatment for senile dementia,* ed. T. Crook and S. Gershon, 7–16. New Canaan, Conn.: Mark Powley Associates.

Hollister, L., and W. Fitzpatrick Jr. 1955. Oral metrazol in the psychoses associated with old age. *Journal of the American Geriatrics Society* 3 (3): 197–200.

Holstein, M. 1997. Alzheimer's disease and senile dementia, 1885–1920: An interpretive history of disease negotiation. *Journal of Aging Studies* 11 (1): 1–13.

———. 2000. Aging, culture, and the framing of Alzheimer disease. In *Concepts of Alzheimer disease: Biological, clinical, and cultural perspectives,* ed. P. J. Whitehouse, K. Maurer, and J. F. Ballenger. Baltimore: Johns Hopkins University Press.

Huppert, F. A., C. Brayne, and D. W. O'Connor. 1994. *Dementia and normal aging.* Cambridge: Cambridge University Press.

Hutchings, R. W. 1939. The president's address. *American Journal of Psychiatry* 96:1–14.

Kaplan, J. 1953. *A social program for older people.* Minneapolis: University of Minnesota Press.

Katzman, R., and K. L. Bick. 2000a. *Alzheimer disease: The changing view.* San Diego: Academic Press.

———. 2000b. The rediscovery of Alzheimer disease during the 1960s and 1970s. In *Concepts of*

Alzheimer disease: Biological, clinical, and cultural perspectives, ed. P. J. Whitehouse, K. Maurer, and J. F. Ballenger. Baltimore: Johns Hopkins University Press.

Kilpatrick, J. 1992. Food and drug czar has 4 million victims. *Saint Louis Post-Dispatch*, November 25, 3C.

Kolata, G. 1988. U.S. is considering disciplinary action in Alzheimer's study. *New York Times*, February 12.

Lears, T. J. J. 1981. *No place of grace: Antimodernism and the transformation of American culture, 1880–1920*. New York: Pantheon Books.

———. 1983. From salvation to self-realization: Advertising and the therapeutic roots of consumer culture, 1880–1930. In *The culture of consumption: Critical essays in American history, 1880–1930*, ed. R. A. L. Wightman and T. J. Jackson. New York: Pantheon.

Leber, P. 1996. The role of the regulator in the evaluation of the acceptability of new drug products. In *Psychotropic drug development: Social, economic, and pharmacological aspects*, ed. D. Healy and D. P. Doogan, 69–77. London: Chapman & Hall Medical.

Lockheed, C. 1992. "Deadly over-caution": FDA assailed for slow testing of new drugs. *San Francisco Chronicle*, October 26, A1.

Maurer, K., and U. Maurer. 2003. *Alzheimer: The life of a physician and the career of a disease*. New York: Columbia University Press.

Maurer, K., S. Volk, and H. Garabaldo. 2000. Auguste D.: The history of Alois Alzheimer's first case. In *Concepts of Alzheimer disease: Biological, clinical, and cultural perspectives*, ed. P. J. Whitehouse, K. Maurer and J. F. Ballenger. Baltimore: Johns Hopkins University Press.

Mercier, C. 1908. *Sanity and insanity*, 2nd ed. New York: Macmillan.

Morris, J. C. 2000. The nosology of dementia. *Neurologic Clinics* 18 (4): 773–88.

Myfanwy, T., and M. Isaac. 1987. Alois Alzheimer: A memoir. *Trends in Neuroscience* 10:306–7.

Reisberg, B. 1981. Empirical studies in senile dementia with metabolic enhancers and agents that alter blood flow and oxygen utilization. In *Strategies for the development of an effective treatment for senile dementia*, ed. T. Crook and S. Gershon, 189–206. New Canaan, Conn.: Mark Powley Associates.

Rothschild, D. 1947. The practical value of research in the psychoses of later life. *Diseases of the Nervous System* 8:123–28.

Rothschild, D., and M. L. Sharp. 1941. The origin of senile psychoses: Neuropathologic factors and factors of a more personal nature. *Diseases of the Nervous System* 2:49–54.

Scott, J. 1989. FDA allows doctor to continue testing Alzheimer's drug. *Los Angeles Times*, May 19, 3.

Summers, W. K. 1987. Fee-for-service research on THA: An explanation. *New England Journal of Medicine* 316 (25): 1605–6.

Summers, W. K., L. V. Majovski, G. M. Marsh, K. Tachiki, and A. Kling. 1986. Oral tetrahydroaminoacridine in long-term treatment of senile dementia, Alzheimer type. *New England Journal of Medicine* 315 (20): 1241–45.

Torack, R. M. 1979. Adult dementia: history, biopsy, pathology. *Neurosurgery* 4 (5): 434–42.

Trachtenberg, A. 1982. *The incorporation of America: Culture and society in the gilded age*. New York: Hill & Wang.

Whitehouse, P. J., et al. 1982. Alzheimer's disease and senile dementia: Loss of neurons in the basal forebrain. *Science* 215 (4537): 1237–39.

Wiebe, R. H. 1967. *The search for order, 1877–1920*. New York: Hill & Wang.

derstanding such debates is key to comprehending the dynamics of biomedical knowledge and practice but also that these controversies have consistently been organized through a dichotomy between the "regime of truth" and the "regime of hope." Our argument is that researchers, clinicians, patients, regulators, and policy makers draw on the vocabularies of "truth" or "hope" to make sense of the purpose and process of knowledge creation, evaluation, and use. In this same juncture, these actors also imbue their research findings, models, clinical practice, guidelines, and policy documents with these "paradigmatic" versions of biomedicine. This process is generative, in that by drawing on the vocabularies of truth and hope, actors are able to engender knowledge change and to instigate, through debate, new lines of demarcation between groups and new forms of identity and viewpoints around the issue at stake. While this tension between truth and hope cannot be seen as entirely novel (Marks 1997), the generative dimension of this model enables us to understand two key features of the dynamics of biomedical science and technology. On one hand, it sheds light on the process underpinning the emergence of new groups and constituencies who, in contemporary society, engage in the production, evaluation, and distribution of biomedical knowledge—from new biotechnology firms to patient organizations (Epstein 1997; Rabeharisoa and Callon 2002), to Internet lists (Nettleton and Burrows 2003), to pharmaceutical companies' marketing departments (Angell 2004; Sismondo 2004). On the other, it might help explain how this heterogeneity has introduced a hitherto unknown level of unpredictability to the possible outcomes of technical controversies (Callon, Lascoumes, and Barthe 2001).

The regimes of truth and hope can be broadly characterized as follows. The regime of truth draws on a vocabulary mainly concerned with the fabrication of "proofs." Medical research appears, in this regime, to be grounded in the strength of the knowledge it endorses (Latour 1999). Practice is thus oriented toward achieving *knowledge robustness*. Such robustness is constructed by organizing experiments to evaluate the strength of the links, both within and between the knowledge and its socioeconomic context. These experiments can take various forms: in apparatuses used in laboratories, through protocols used in therapeutic evaluation, or in patients' own evaluation of therapeutic agents (Rabeharisoa and Callon 2002). The regime of hope, on the other hand, is concerned with the *fabrication of expectations* and future possibilities (Brown and Michael 2003). Action is typically oriented toward the potential that knowledge embodies rather than toward its current strength. To enact such knowledge, the regime of hope deploys experimental practices in which tentative, promising links come to existence. Again, these experiments can take a variety of forms, from laboratory work to public assessments of health technology.

The different meanings that each of the regimes allocates to the practice of experimentation encapsulates the main distinction between them. While the regime of truth emphasizes the power experiments can have in ascertaining the quality of propositions, settling disputes, and substantiating claims (Shapin and Schaffer 1985), the regime of hope sees experiments as occasions in which new entities and possible therapeutic solutions are explored. The regime of truth associates testing with the "will to know" (Foucault 1979), whereas the regime of hope links it with the "will to experiment" (Rabinow 1999; Moreira and Palladino 2005). At any one time, in any actual experiment in biomedicine, these two organizing logics are likely to confront each other as actors try to make sense of the situation.

This chapter argues that through this interrelation between hope and truth, researchers, clinicians, patients, regulators, and policy makers were able to interactively transform the practices of therapeutic innovation and evaluation in AD. This process has underpinned the shift from cholino-mimetic pharmaceutical agents to "disease-modifying" drugs.

Negotiating the Effects of Cholinesterase Inhibitors

Researchers in the field of AD usually tell the history of the development of cholinesterase inhibitors in one of two differing versions. One emphasizes the rational development of the agents arising from the formulation of the cholinergic hypothesis and progressively extending laboratory results to experimentation with animals and with humans (Thal 2002). The other links the development of cholinomimetic drugs with expectations brought about by the success of L-dopa in ameliorating the symptoms of Parkinson's disease and by the associated neurochemical understanding of neurodegenerative disease in general (Francis et al. 1999). The first version of the story is closely aligned with a sequential, "rational" model of drug development, in which discoveries of basic biological mechanisms made in the laboratory are translated into therapeutic strategies experimented at in various stages until they reach the clinic. The success of therapies is, in this perspective, associated with robustness of the knowledge originally created in the laboratory. The second version of this story links interest in the basic mechanisms underlying AD with the success of therapies achieved in other fields. It thus emphasizes the nonlinear, iterative dynamics between the clinic and the laboratory in drug development (Vos, chapter 9 in this volume). The success of therapies is, in this alternative story, an achievement created by the possibilities and horizons opened in clinical areas and knowledge sites in interaction with the laboratory.

An understanding of the epistemic and political changes that preceded the growth in research in AD and the emergence of the cholinergic hypothesis does not, however, authorize us to favor any of the above versions (Karlawish 2002). One important factor in this was the partial reconceptualization of senile dementia as AD during the 1960s and its definition as a disorder of the nervous system (Katzman and Bick 2000). Through this process, dementia clinical research was opened to an epistemic field shared with other "diseases of the brain" characterized by degeneration such as Parkinson's. This facilitated knowledge transportability between these domains. Another crucial element was the emergence of what Robert Butler, the founding director of the National Institute on Aging, called the "health politics of anguish" (Fox 1989, p. 82), and the associated establishment of dementia as a research priority of the National Institute of Aging from 1974 onward. This prioritization of dementia in political life itself embodied an understanding of innovation and of therapeutic development that drew on examples in which the application of science was seen to be the key to success. From the onset, it seems that in the epistemic and sociopolitical framing of AD, the two versions of drug development emerged in parallel and in association with each other.

In the mid-1970s, reports started emerging of a possible link between the cholinergic system in the brain and the cognitive deficits observed in patients suspected to have AD (Davies 1976; Perry et al. 1977). These studies and an emerging understanding of the role of acetylcholine in learning and memory led to what has become known as the cholinergic hypothesis of AD. This hypothesis proposed that degeneration of cholinergic neurons in the basal forebrain and the associated reduction of cholinergic neurotransmission in the cerebral cortex and other areas contributed significantly to the deterioration of cognitive function seen in patients with AD (Bartus et al. 1982; Whitehouse et al. 1982). Such speculations gave ground to the hopes put in sequential models of biomedical innovation and were pivotal in interesting the pharmaceutical industry in the activities of AD researchers a few years before the 1980 Bayh-Dole Act[1] (Mowery et al. 2001).

These hopes were not easily fulfilled, and most of the 1980s were characterized by a search for the cholinergic enhancer that would do such a job.

While the rationale for the use of cholinergic drugs for AD lay in enhancing the secretion of or prolonging the half-life of acetylcholine in the brain, it became difficult to find a compound that combined a long half-life with low incidence of unwelcome effects. For the most part the agents chosen in the initial stages of the search (acetylcholine precursors, selective muscarinic agonists, etc.) failed to fulfill either or both of the expectations. Only by the end of the 1980s did a relatively positive picture for cholinesterase inhibitors (ChEIs) start being formed.

In this context, the scientific strength and clinical hopes of the cholinergic hypothesis were crystallized in the National Institute of Neurological and Communicative Disorders and Stroke and the Alzheimer's Disease and Related Disorders Association (NINCDS-ADRDA) diagnostic criteria for AD (McKhann et al. 1984), which can be seen to reinforce the centrality of the "cognitive" dimension of AD by emphasizing that clinical examination should be aided by scores on standardized clinical and neurocognitive tests. It is also in this context of relative optimism that economic agents and scientific and clinical constituencies mobilize regulatory institutions for formulating the methodologic framework for the labeling of possibly forthcoming dementia drugs. Such negotiations rearticulate the alignments between political, clinical, and biomedical interests that arose from the National Institute on Aging's (NIA) prioritization of dementia research. This regulatory framework was configured not only within the context of the new Bayh-Dole Act and the Reaganite neoliberal policy of association between free enterprise and scientific innovation in medicine but also within a reorganized health care system that was now dominated by private insurers in a competitive market and characterized by a loss of monopoly by the medical profession (Schmidt 1999; Light 2000).

The FDA guidelines for the evaluation of antidementia drugs authored by Paul Leber (1990) can be seen as shaped by—but also fundamentally shaping—this configuration of economic and political changes in that they set up standards against which the hope of the cholinergic hypothesis was to be tested. It is interesting to note though that by the time these guidelines were formulated, the strength of the cholinergic hypothesis had been already modulated. This process occurred on three interrelated fronts: first, the picture of the biochemical basis of cognition of dementia was widened (Francis et al. 1999); at the same time, what later became know as the amyloid hypothesis (Hardy and Higgins 1992) was taking root in the dementia research field; and finally, there was a parallel curbing of expectations about the therapeutic power of ChEIs. As a result, Leber, while restricting the definition of antidementia drugs to those that can show that they "beneficially affect the ability to learn new and retrieve old previously learned information" or "those that cause an improvement in, or slow the rate of deterioration of, the various functions (memory, reason, etc) that fail increasingly as the dementia process progresses," acknowledged that these drugs were unlikely to become a "definitive treatment for Alzheimer's" (Leber 1990, p. 2).

That is to say that, by requiring randomized clinical trials (RCTs) to include a design of sufficient length to appreciate a meaningful effect of a drug in improving performance in a cognitive test and changing the clinical impression of the dementia, Leber's guidelines recognized the shortcomings of the cholinergic hypothesis while still upholding a model of therapeutic innovation in which success stems from the full understanding of the "etiology and or pathogenesis of the dementing process" (Leber 1990, p. 2). The Leber guidelines thus represent a pivotal turning point by supporting a model of social organization of biomedical knowledge and health care while modulating the expectations arising from one of the more hopeful products of that model—the cholinergic hypothesis.

Against this backdrop, results of the clinical trials of ChEIs started being disseminated. These results were aligned with the low expectations that had emerged in the clinical research constituency: clinical insignificant results of physostigmine (Davis et al. 1976; Thal 1991) were followed by the disappointing performance of tacrine (Davis et al. 1992), which nonetheless became the first approved cholinomimetic antidementia drug in the United States. By the time donepezil was approved in the United States for the treatment of dementia, a more or less consensual view had emerged among clinical researchers that ChEIs could produce only modest results if held against the cognitive and clinical improvement benchmarks set by the Leber guidelines.

As the drugs entered clinical use, there was also a growing sense of the disparity between these benchmarks and the more subtle behavioral and functional effects claimed to be observed in clinical practice (Farlow 2002). This view was reinforced by the decision of European regulators to consider maintenance of activities of daily living (ADLs) as an outcome for the evaluation of antidementia drugs (Committee for Proprietary Medicinal Products 1997). If, on the one hand, it is possible to connect this to the committee's acceptance of the views of European experts, expressed on behalf of health and social care systems in which the economic burden of disability had become a central political issue, this decision represents, on the other hand, a further turning point in the extension and reconfiguration of the effects of ChEIs. The process, which lasted for most of the 1990s, effectively opened methodological considerations and regulatory debates both to international comparison and to adaptation.

When the International Working Group for Harmonization of Dementia Drug Guidelines formed in 1994, researchers, economic agents, and regulators had become aware of the tension between a global, increasingly competitive and concentrated pharmaceutical market and differing national parameters of drug evaluation (Whitehouse 1997). This tension was seen to be hindering the innovative capacity and efficiency of universities and pharmaceutical companies in developing therapies for AD. The differences between the European, American, and Japanese regulatory frameworks presented themselves as an opportunity for opening the spectrum of effects that could be attached to antidementia drugs.

During the later part of the 1990s, however, it proved difficult to mobilize the U.S. regulatory authorities in the expected direction of including behavioral and functional outcomes as antidementia drug efficacy indicators, which it continued to view as related to "pseudospecific claims" (Leber 1990, p. 2). This attachment to the original expectations created by cholinesterase inhibitor developers and marketers in the late 1980s aligned—in opposition—the interests of clinical researchers, bioscientists, the pharmaceutical industry, and patient organizations/charities. Motivated by the therapeutic potential of a variety of approaches both within the cholinergic model (nicotinic agonists, etc.) and outside it (glutamate, cardiovascular agents, antiamyloid agents, etc.), these constituencies were interested in making visible the effects of antidementia drugs that remained unaccounted for in RCTs designed either for regulatory approval or for taking the "Leber guidelines" as the closest to the ideals of evidence-based medicine (Stewart 2001).

In this rearticulation of the effects of ChEIs, the role of the patient organization was pivotal. Through the support networks that define them, patient organizations were able to echo and reconfigure some of the academic and clinical criticism of outcomes used in antidementia drug trials. The UK Alzheimer's Society's evaluation of dementia drugs is a case in point. Designing and conducting its own "research in the wild" (Callon 1999), the Alzheimer's Society presented an appraisal of antidementia drugs that focused on user-defined outcomes in its submission to the then newly formed National Institute for Clinical Excellence (NICE) (Alzheimer's Society 2000). In the results of the questionnaire, the ability to maintain functional abilities of daily life and improvement in attitude and mood were considered more important than the cognitive scores achieved by patients. The emphasis on maintenance of abilities and quality of life (Bond 1999) rather than cognitive enhancement was, in this way, attached to patients' and caregivers' experience of the process of dementia and correlative evaluation of pharmacotherapy. Such emphasis, helped, in turn, the clinical researcher constituency to make the argument that "the maintenance of baseline levels in a progressive condition such as Alzheimer's disease may be a more relevant goal to . . . individual patients than transient cognitive improvement" (Winblad et al. 2001, p. 656).

This reformulation of the evaluative framework for antidementia drugs not only facilitated a revision of the effectiveness of ChEIs—based primarily on open-label extended observation studies (Winblad et al. 2001, p. 661–62)—but also contributed in important ways to the stabilization of the redefinition of "response" to antidementia therapy from an improvement in outcome measures to a clinical stabilization or maintenance of baseline scores. This is relevant to our purposes from two perspectives. In this process, ChEIs' effects have become partially detached from the hopes of the cholinergic hypothesis and the "rational" model of drug development that it embodied. At the same time, they have been partly associated with a variety of effects that can be said to be embedded in the hopes brought by a variety of competing sequential models of AD formulated during the 1990s. The definition of AD as a progressive but potentially reversible disorder with a long prodromal, preclinical period seems thus to be the epistemic framework against which ChEIs are progressively being judged, with research on the cholinergic mediation of amyloid deposition and tau hyperphosphorylation reinforcing this picture (Giacobini 2001). However, to understand this last configuration of the expected effects of ChEIs, one must understand the epistemic, economic, and political changes in the field of AD that led to such an understanding of the disease and to the *rearrangement* of associated expectations from antidementia drug development.

Effects Looking for an Agent

When AD reemerged in the middle of the twentieth century, its definition relied on a combination of clinical diagnosis of dementia with postmortem verification of pathological lesion in the brain—the plaques and tangles. The NINCDS criteria for the diagnosis of probable AD (McKhann et al. 1984), negotiated during the strengthening of research efforts in AD in the 1980s, detailed this definition by advising the use of auxiliary diagnostic items such as computerized tomography to exclude other abnormalities and document Alzheimer's-related brain atrophy. While in the NINCDS criteria brain imaging appeared as secondary, in the next decade, brain imaging played a major role in changing the clinical and biomedical understanding of AD. This was, of course, not specific to AD and dementia, and it was part of the wider transformation of structural and functional imaging's role in the clinical neurosciences (Beaulieu 2002).

In the field of AD, brain imaging acted as intermediary between established knowledge constituencies, and through this role, it was possible to make volumetric atrophies in the medial temporal lobe important areas to mark the onset of AD (Scheltens et al. 2002). While the use of imaging in the clinical setting is still dependent on the economic circumstances of the clinic, in the research field, it provided the resources to compose an in-vivo description of progressive reduction in cortical volume and blood uptake that would effectively mediate between the other two widely used staging models of the natural history of AD: the pathological staging of dementia—the Braak tangle staging system (Braak and Braak 1991) and the Consortium to Establish a Registry of Alzheimer's Disease (CERAD) plaque-based system (Mirra et al. 1991); and the clinical staging of dementia—the Clinical Dementia Rating (Hughes et al. 1982; Morris 1993) and the Global Deterioration Scale (Reisberg et al. 1982). This relationship between clinical and pathological expertises has significantly stabilized professional relations around AD and, with this, the scientific definition of the disease itself. As in previous processes of introduction of imaging in neurological and psychiatric work (Moreira 2000), structural and functional imaging in AD made visible "silent," preclinical disease developments, reallocating therein scientific and clinical interest.

The clinical neuroscientific understanding of AD as a phased deterioration was also reinforced by transformations in the understanding of the molecular processes underpinning AD. Drawing on animal models of the disease and in vitro biomolecular techniques, bioscientists were able to formulate a series of alternative hypotheses on processes that instigate the formation of plaques and tangles and of neuronal death. The first of these hypotheses became known as the amyloid cascade hypothesis (Hardy and Higgins 1992). This hypothesis emphasizes the critical role of Aß42 deposition in the flow of events that initiate plaque formation and lead to synaptic loss, neuronal dysfunction, and eventually clinical dementia. Despite being the most successful of the causal theories of AD both in enrolling researchers and in attracting industrial sponsors, controversy about the validity of the theory has increased over the years, not least because it suggests a temporal sequence and spatial contiguity between plaque and tangle formation that does not coalesce with pathological data (Joachim et al. 1989). A competing theory about pathogenesis of AD emphasizes the hyperphosphorylation of the tau protein, which is thus prevented from stabilizing the microtubules of the neuronal axon (Lovestone and Reynolds 1997).

The controversy between these two hypotheses has been a distinctive feature of the field of AD research, with the beta-amyloid protein advocates being dubbed "the Baptists," in contrast to "the *Tau*ists." The shared assumptions about the molecular basis of the disease process that both parties in the controversy hold are, however, more revealing than the conflict itself. This agreement has enabled a partial shift of the resources and practices that generate knowledge in AD from neuropathology. Aß42 and tau proteins detected in the cerebrospinal fluid have thus tentatively become signifiers for the presence of AD pathology in the (research) clinic and possible surrogate markers in trials. They have also contributed, along with brain imaging, to a devaluation of neuropathological expertise (Blennow and Hampel 2003)—albeit not pacifically (Braak, Tredici, and Braak 2003). Another shared assumption is the confidence put on sequential models of disease. Furthermore, once the hope for a single genetic key to late-onset AD was repudiated, the epidemiology of dementia, and in particular the growing importance of longitudinal designs, contributed to this epistemic framework that linked life events—diabetes, depression, congestive heart disease—to the processes that mediate neuronal dysfunction in AD.

The enhanced traceability of the process of dementia—by cognitive testing, brain imaging, and cerebrospinal fluid (CSF) analysis—and the shift toward a preventive paradigm in the search for therapeutic solutions were contemporaneous with increased public awareness of the disease and its symptoms (Yankner 2000). This was the result of a series of medical and public education initiatives led by government, university researchers, patient organizations, and the pharmaceutical industry that started with the "politics of anguish" in the 1970s, gained momentum with the advent of ChEIs, and achieved symbolic notoriety when Ronald Reagan became the public face of AD. This information policy reinforced the link between biomedical models of research and the hopes of finding a cure. As a result, a coherent set of expectations has arisen in the age groups that, through continuous engagement with dementia-awareness initiatives, have experienced the process of dementia of their parents as an unnecessary, preventable tragedy. They are also experiencing increased anxiety in relation to their own cognitive status and fear the loss of self that is associated with dementia (Corner and Bond 2004). This generation of "baby boomers" is expected to demand, individually and collectively, a fulfillment of the promises that the public-information policy embodied (Freedman 1999). The agents most responsible for the fulfilment of the policy—pharmaceutical companies—will have their practices of innovation increasingly subject to criticism (Angell 2004) and public scrutiny (Abraham and Lewis 2002).

Within this social context, "disease-modifying" therapies started being tested in animals and humans. Most of these pharmacological agents target the molecular mechanisms that precede neuronal death. From this perspective, they should be used by individuals as early as possible, ideally presymptomatically. This presents methodological, regulatory, and economic problems that rearticulate the experimental framework that was prefigured by later trials of ChEIs discussed in the previous section. Because these drugs hold no enhancement claims, they present a complex problem: how can a drug be seen to be acting when its effect is defined by the absence of change in clinically relevant outcomes? The accepted approach, derived mainly from the design of trials in cardiovascular medicine, is to test the therapy in populations that are at calculable risk of developing the disease within a measurable period of time. The creation and the regulatory recognition of risk categories such as mild cognitive impairment (MCI) and of surrogate outcomes such as brain imaging can be understood to partially address this experimental requirement (Food and Drug Administration 2001).

Such conceptual changes, however, only partially solve the main regulatory problem posed by disease-modifying therapies, namely, that only a small risk is acceptable for presymptomatic individuals, whereas a greater ratio of risk to possible benefit is accepted in patients with clinical symptoms of dementia. Companies and researchers are also still required to test their therapies in populations diagnosed with probable AD. In addition, trials in presymptomatic populations entail longer, larger, and costlier studies, making trials in mild AD more likely to be funded (Citron 2004).

A useful example of the tension between these three problems is the AN1792 immunization trial. Following documented achievements of Aß-based immunotherapeutic approaches in animal AD models (Schenk et al. 1999), a clinical trial for safety testing in humans, co-sponsored by Elan Pharmaceuticals and Wyeth-Ayerst Laboratories, was initiated. Disseminated results from this phase I trial suggested that the vaccine was adequately tolerated in human subjects and was able to stimulate the formation of anti-Aß42 antibodies. These promising results led to the initiation of a phase IIA study in 2001 to assess efficacy, optimal dosage, and safety. This trial enrolled 372 subjects with mild to moderate AD. However, by mid-January 2002, the sponsors announced the suspension of the phase IIA study due to the development of central nervous system inflammation in participants of the study (Orgogozo et al. 2003).

The choice of trial populations denotes the investigators' and sponsors' intention to abide with the experimental requirements set by regulators and methodologists that antidementia drugs demonstrate efficacy in patients with clinical diagnosis of AD before therapy is tried in other, presymptomatic populations. This was possible due to the conviction that amyloid clearance after immunization would have the same direct effects in the cognitive performance of human subjects that were demonstrated in "cognitive tests" performed by transgenic laboratory mice (Schenk, Hagen, and Seubert 2004). The timing of immunization therapy in the AN1792 trial was thus able to conform more closely to what could be seen as the old paradigm in antidementia drug testing: improvement in cognitive scales rather than maintenance of baseline scores. The cognitive effects were also considered to be immediate enough to support this trial design.

The specific way in which the AN1792 trial resolved the tension described above was crucial in keeping the trial (and the immunization approach) open for reinterpretation after risk considerations dictated its termination. This was achieved in three different strategies that worked to further interlock the regimes of hope and truth in the parallel reinvention of therapeutic possibilities and experimental frameworks. The first has to do with the reassessment of the results of the trial. In this, disease-modifying outcomes were emphasized in relation to cognitive outcomes. In contrast to the modest cognitive benefit shown in a small number of patients (Hock et al. 2003), neuropathological analysis of the deceased subjects' brains (Nicoll et al. 2003) suggested clearance of neuritic plaques in some cortical areas. Magnetic resonance imaging (MRI) analysis of subjects in the treatment arm of the trial has also unexpectedly shown considerable reduction in brain volume in the areas associated with AD, which was interpreted as a consequence of amyloid clearance (Fox et al. 2005). The disease-modifying outcomes partially redefined the value of the trial from a therapeutic experiment—aligned with the regime of truth—to an experiment in the possibilities of the immunization approach and the use of surrogate markers in evaluating disease modification.

Second, for this reevaluation to succeed it was necessary also to question the timing of the trial. While it is accepted that the AN1792 trial conformed to risk assessment requirements in testing pharmacotherapy initially in patients that would possible benefit the most from it, it fell partially outside the new, emerging understandings of the disease processes in AD. By relying only on the amyloid hypothesis for its potential success, the trial ignored both the possible independence of neurofibrillary pathology and the role of mediating factors between amyloid deposition and clinical dementia. Thus, in an editorial in *Neurology*, Bennett and Holtzman suggest that the use of an amyloid-based approach in a population where "measures of neurofibrilary tangles may correlate better with the presence and severity of dementia than . . . measures of neuritic plaques" may have been a miscalculation. In addition, they argue that "it may be important to initiate immunization therapy prior to the onset of overt dementia" (Bennett and Holtzman 2005, p. 64). The AN1792 trial served paradoxically to reiterate and reinforce the importance of prevention in AD therapies, which had not been addressed in the original trial conception.

The third aspect of the reinterpretation of the trial is of particular importance, as it concerns what risk-benefit ratio is acceptable within antidementia drug trials. It is an increasingly accepted opinion in the field of dementia research that disease-modifying therapies will have significant side effects. However, rather than drawing on the changes in the understanding of AD, this argument is positioned at the boundary between expert and lay constituencies of AD that resulted from the public information policies discussed above. Recognizing that at present in Western societies, AD is probably one of the most feared diseases of old age, clinical researchers and sponsors have argued that the risk-benefit ratio required by regulatory authorities might be at odds with the evaluations that patients and carers make of that same ratio. In an interview by the author of a neurologist, such rearticulation of the role of patients in evaluating therapies was clearly put:

> *Interviewee:* I think there's been a change in terms of how much carers and patients will direct the course of research . . . but I think there will also be aspects of patients and carers having a role in evaluating . . . treatments.
>
> *TM:* Right. Evaluating from the patient's point of view. Do you mean past the kind of health technology assessment, randomized controlled trials kind of technology, a different kind of evaluation that is more patient-centered and qualitative . . .

I: That's absolutely right [TM: yes]. And putting in context what people feel about the choices and the ethics, for example, a decision may be made that the medication that carries a two, three, five, I don't know what percent risk of some serious side effect . . . maybe it's a level of risk that the regulators or the doctors find unacceptable [TM: yes] but actually patient and carers might say, *actually,* that is acceptable for a particular gain, and so they may change that risk-benefit threshold . . . The HIV lobby even changed the regulatory framework in the U.S.

It is interesting to note that, in the exchange, I associated the interviewee's mention of the role of patients in evaluating treatments with the kind of "research in the wild" initiatives described in the previous section: qualitative and/or patient-derived outcomes to evaluate drug performance. The interviewee's answer, however, presents another possibility of lay involvement in research that is more than an extension of the participation achieved in ChEI evaluation. In this, his use of the case of the interaction between researchers, regulators, and patients in HIV trial design is revealing. In his study of the lay-expert knowledge dynamics in HIV research, Epstein has shown that this interactive relationship between lay, expert, and regulatory constituencies generated unpredictable results both in terms of research and of the lay-expert boundary (Epstein 1996). The blurring of this boundary was effectively what enabled a negotiated reevaluation of the risk-benefit thresholds that became acceptable in HIV trials. By drawing on such history of lay participation in research, AD experts seem to hope that patients and carers might follow a similar path and lower their expectations in relation to risk-benefit threshold in AD therapy trials.

The expected consonance between expert and lay constituencies seems to be supported by studies of the role of patient organizations in AD research in the United States (Beard 2004). Contrary to HIV research, in which a strong, independent movement of identity politics interlocked with biomedical knowledge practices, lay participation in AD research has been traditionally framed within the parameters of mainstream politics. However, as described in the last section, other patient organizations involved in AD research and policy have been more proactive in questioning models of research and the expectations that experts deploy in antidementia drug therapy experiments (Blume and Catshoek 2002). There are also significant changes in the way biomedical research and its relation with pharmaceutical companies is evaluated by the lay public. A fuller engagement with AD therapy research might mean that patients and their carers are more aware of the complex processes that mediate the dementia and of the social and economic forces that shape the therapeutic hopes that are made available to them. They might thus be less prepared to stake so much in only one of the competing approaches that claim to be able to cure AD. This possibility is, however, part of a story yet to unfold.

Considerable advancements have been made in the understanding of AD and the therapeutic and clinical management of dementia in the past 30 years. In those years, the knowledge instigated by biomedical research was extended, adapted, and evaluated by various actors in a variety of settings, producing new, tentative technoscientific, clinical, and social outcomes that then became the context for further experimentation. In this, the hopes and expectations produced by a succession of innovations interacted with an heterogeneous group of "tests"—in the laboratory, in clinical trials, in the clinic, but also in patients' homes. These "tests" themselves were constructed and adapted through an understanding of the character of the hopes embodied in therapeutic innovations.

Through this interaction between truth and hope, the forms of evaluation applied to cholinomimetic pharmaceutical agents have progressively given way to more "patient-centered measures" and to a concern with maintenance of cognitive and functional abilities rather than their enhancement. This adjustment unfolded in parallel with the consolidation of an understanding of AD as an insidious condition with a long prodromal phase and with the shift toward preventative therapeutic strategies. The redefinition of "response" to ChEIs has progressively aligned the practices of drug evaluation with the therapeutic hopes brought by a variety of competing sequential models of AD formulated during the 1990s. On the other hand, finding the forms of evaluation that best match the new generation of therapies is proving to be more difficult than expected. Drug evaluators and regulators have not yet been able to reset the balance between methodological, economic, and ethical requirements that fit "disease-modifying" agents, and they seem to draw on trial designs best suited for an older generation of drugs. These designs also make these drugs more likely to be consumed by people who have dementia than by those "at risk" of developing it.

In examining this process as a whole, one can see how the hopes to find a cure for AD have been modulated by modest outcomes in the various tests to which possible therapies have been submitted. It is important, however, to emphasize how the present context of methodological and commercial uncertainty is also the outcome of a partial disalignment between the expectations created by disease-modifying drugs and the forms of evaluation used to assess them. In other words, while the effectiveness of cholinergic drugs has been extended through the use of bioclinical frameworks associated with preventive disease-modifying drugs, the drugs themselves have paradoxically been tested in experimental formats and in market contexts constructed for first-generation antidementia drugs. While the new preventive therapeutic paradigm was fundamental to finding which effects to expect from cholinesterase inhibitors and how to evaluate them, it has yet to discover its own truth-finding methods and "proofs." It is particularly significant that patients and their views have been recognized as central to solving the stalemate in which drug developers and therapeutic evaluators have found themselves. The exact character of this new space of intervention for patients is still undecided, but there are signs that patients' expectations concern not only the products of biomedical research but also, and increasingly, the transformation of the economic and political processes that frame therapeutic innovation in AD.

ACKNOWLEDGMENTS

This research was supported by an Economic and Social Research Council grant—"Boundary Work, Normal Aging and Brain Pathology"—inserted in the "Science in Society" program. I thank the following for their helpful suggestions: Jesse Ballenger, John Bond, Michaela Fay, Ben Heaven, Jason Karlawish, Carl May, Tim Rapley, and Peter Whitehouse.

NOTE

1. The Bayh-Dole Act was passed in 1980 and allows for the transfer of exclusive control over many government-funded inventions to universities and businesses operating with federal contracts for the purpose of further development and commercialization.

REFERENCES

Abraham, J., and G. Lewis. 2002. Citizenship, medical expertise and the capitalist regulatory state in Europe. *Sociology—The Journal of the British Sociological Association* 36 (1): 67–88.

Alzheimer's Society. 2000. *Appraisal of the drugs for Alzheimer's disease: Submission to the National Institute for Clinical Excellence*. London: Alzheimer's Society.

Angell, M. 2004. *The truth about the drug companies: How they deceive us and what to do about it*. New York: Random House.

Ballenger, J. F. 2006. *Self, senility, and Alzheimer's disease in modern America: A history*. Baltimore: Johns Hopkins University Press.

Bartus, R. T., R. L. Dean III, B. Beer, and A. S. Lippa. 1982. The cholinergic hypothesis of geriatric memory dysfunction. *Science* 217 (4558): 408–14.

Beard, R. L. 2004. Advocating voice: Organisational, historical and social milieux of the Alzheimer's disease movement. *Sociology of Health and Illness* 26 (6): 797–819.

Beaulieu, A. 2002. Images are not the (only) truth: Iconoclasm, visual knowledge and experimentation in brain mapping. *Science, Technology and Human Values* 21 (1): 53–86.

Bennett, D. A., and D. L. Holtzman. 2005. Immunization therapy for Alzheimer disease? *Neurology* 64 (1): 10–12.

Blennow, K., and H. Hampel. 2003. CSF markers for incipient Alzheimer's disease. *Lancet Neurology* 2 (10): 605–13.

Blume, S., and G. Catshoek. 2002. *Articulating the patient perspective: Strategic options for research*. Amsterdam: PatientenPraktijk.

Bond, J. 1999. Quality of life for people with dementia: Approaches to the challenge of measurement. *Ageing and Society* 19:561–79.

Braak, H., and Braak, E. 1991. Neuropathological staging of Alzheimer-related changes. *Acta Neuropath* 82:239–59.

Braak, H., K. D. Tredici, and E. Braak. 2003. Spectrum of pathology. In *Mild cognitive impairment*, ed. R. Peterson, 149–90. New York: Oxford University Press.

Brown, N., and M. Michael. 2003. A sociology of expectations: Retrospecting prospects and prospecting retrospects. *Technology Analysis and Strategic Management* 15 (1): 3–18.

Callon, M. 1999. The role of lay people in the production and dissemination of scientific knowledge. *Science, Technology, and Society* 4 (1): 81–94.

Callon, M., P. Lascoumes, and Y. Barthe. 2001. *Agir dans un monde uncertain: Essai sur la democratie technique*. Paris: Seuil.

Citron, M. 2004. Strategies for disease modification in Alzheimer's disease. *Nature Reviews Neuroscience* 5:677–85.

Clarke, A. E., L. Mamo, J. R. Fishman, J. K. Shim, and J. R. Fosket. 2003. Biomedicalization: Technoscientific transformations of health, illness, and U.S. biomedicine. *American Sociological Review* 68 (2): 161–93.

Committee for Proprietary Medicinal Products. 1997. *Note for guidance on medicinal products in the treatment of Alzheimer's disease*. London: European Agency for the Evaluation of Medicinal Products: Human Medicines Evaluation Unit.

Corner, L., and J. Bond 2004. Being at risk of dementia: Fears and anxieties of older adults. *Journal of Aging Studies* 18 (2): 143–55.

Davies, P., and A. J. Maloney. 1976. Selective loss of central cholinergic neurons in Alzheimer's disease. *Lancet* 2 (8000): 1403.

Davis, K. L., L. E. Hollister, J. Overall, A. Johnson, and K. Train. 1976. Physostigmine: Effects on cognition and affect in normal subjects. *Psychopharmacology* 51 (1): 23–27.

Davis, K. L., L. J. Thal, E. R. Gamzu, C. S. Davis, R. F. Woolson, S. I. Gracon, D. A. Drachman, et al. 1992. A double-blind, placebo-controlled multicenter study of tacrine for Alzheimer's disease: The Tacrine Collaborative Study Group. *New England Journal of Medicine* 327 (18): 1253–59.

Epstein, S. 1996. *Impure Science: AIDS, Activism, and the Politics of Knowledge.* Berkeley: University of California Press.

———. 1997. Activism, drug regulation, and the politics of therapeutic evaluation in the AIDS era: A case study of ddC and the "surrogate markers" debate. *Social Studies of Science* 27 (5): 691–726.

Farlow, M. 2002. A clinical overview of cholinesterase inhibitors in Alzheimer's disease. *International Psychogeriatrics* 14 (suppl. 1): 93–126.

Food and Drug Administration. 2001. Peripheral and Central Nervous System Drugs Advisory Committee meeting (transcript: vol. 1). March 13, 2001.

Foucault, M. 1979. *The History of Sexuality,* vol. 1. Trans. R. Hurley. London: Allen Lane.

Fox, N. C., R. S. Black, S. Gilman, M. N., Rossor, S. G. Griffith, L. Jenkins, and M. Koller. 2005. Effects of A{beta} immunization (AN1792) on MRI measures of cerebral volume in Alzheimer disease. *Neurology* 64 (9): 1563–72.

Fox, P. 1989. From senility to Alzheimer's disease: The rise of the Alzheimer's disease movement. *Milbank Quarterly* 67 (1): 58–102.

Francis, P. T., A. M. Palmer, M. Snape, and G. K. Wilcock. 1999. The cholinergic hypothesis of Alzheimer's disease: A review of progress. *Journal of Neurology, Neurosurgery, and Psychiatry* 66: 137–47.

Freedman, M. 1999. *Prime time: How baby boomers will revolutionise retirement and transform America.* New York: Public Affairs.

Giacobini, E. 2001. Do cholinesterase inhibitors have disease-modifying effects in Alzheimer's disease? *CNS Drugs* 15 (2): 85–91.

Hardy, J. A., and G. A. Higgins. 1992. Alzheimer's disease: The amyloid cascade hypothesis. *Science* 256 (5054): 184–85.

Hock, C., U. Konietzko, J. R. Streffer, J. Tracy, A. Signorell, B. Muller-Tillmanns, U. Lemke, K. Henke, E., Moritz, and E. Garcia. 2003. Antibodies against beta-amyloid slow cognitive decline in Alzheimer's disease. *Neuron* 38 (4): 547–54.

Holstein, M. 2000. Aging, culture, and the framing of Alzheimer disease. In *Concepts of Alzheimer disease: Biological, clinical, and cultural perspectives,* ed. P. J. Whitehouse, K. Maurer, and J. F. Ballenger, 158–80. Baltimore: Johns Hopkins University Press.

Hughes, C. P., L. Berg, W. L. Danziger, L. A. Coben, and R. L. Martin. 1982. A new clinical scale for the staging of dementia. *British Journal of Psychiatry* 240 (56572).

Joachim, C. L., J. H. Morris, and D. J. Selkoe. 1989. Diffuse senile plaques occur commonly in the cerebellum in Alzheimer's disease. *American Journal of Pathology* 135 (2): 309–19.

Karlawish, J. H. T. 2002. The search for a coherent language: The science and politics of drug testing and approval. In *Ethics, Law, and Aging review* 8: *Issues in conducting research with and about older persons,* ed. M. B. Kapp, 39–56. New York: Springer.

Katzman, R., and K. L. Bick. 2000. The rediscovery of Alzheimer disease during the 1960s and 1970s. In *Concepts of Alzheimer disease: Biological, clinical, and cultural perspectives,* ed. P. J. Whitehouse, K. Maurer, and J. F. Ballenger, 104–14. Baltimore: Johns Hopkins University Press.

Keating, P., and A. Cambrosio. 2004. Does biomedicine entail the successful reduction of pathology to biology? *Biology and Medicine* 47 (3): 357–71.

Khachaturian, Z. S. 2000. Neurobiology of aging: Alzheimer's clinical review series: Bridging bench to bedside: Clinical problems in search of basic solution. *Neurobiology of Aging* 21 (6): 843.

Latour, B. 1999. *Pandora's hope: Essays on the reality of science studies.* Cambridge, Mass.: Harvard University Press.

Leber, P. 1990. *Guidelines for the clinical evaluation of antidementia drugs.* Rockville, Md.: U.S. Food and Drug Administration.

Light, D. 2000. The origins and rise of managed care. In *Perspectives in medical sociology,* ed. B. Phil. Prospect Heights, Ill., 484–503: Waveland Press.

Lovestone, S., and C. H. Reynolds. 1997. The phosphorylation of tau: A critical stage in neurodevelopment and neurodegenerative processes. *Neuroscience* 78 (2): 309–24.

Lyman, K. A. 1989. Bringing the social back in: A critique of the biomedicalization of dementia. *Gerontologist* 29 (5): 597–605.

Marks, H. M. 1997. *The Progress of experiment.* New York: Cambridge University Press.

McKhann, G., D. Drachman, M., Folstein, R. Katzman, D. Price, and E. M. Stadlan. 1984. Clinical diagnosis of Alzheimer's disease: Report of the NINCDS-ADRDA Work Group under the auspices of the Department of Health and Human Services Task Force on Alzheimer's Disease. *Neurology* 34:939–44.

Mirra, S. S., A. Heyman, D. McKeel, S. M. Sumi, B. J. Crain, L. M. Brownlee, F. S. Vogel, J. P. Hughes, G. van Belle, and L. Berg. 1991. The consortium to establish a registry for Alzheimer's disease (CERAD). Part II. Standardization of the neuropathologic assessment of Alzheimer's disease. *Neurology* 41:479–86.

Moreira, T. 2000. Translation, difference and ontological fluidity: Cerebral angiography and neurosurgical practice (1926–45). *Social Studies of Science* 30 (3): 421–46.

———. 2005. Diversity in clinical guidelines: The role of repertoires of evaluation. *Social Science and Medicine* 60:1975–85.

Moreira, T., and P. Palladino. 2005. Between hope and truth: Parkinson's disease, neural transplants and the self. *History of the Human Sciences* 18 (1): 55–82.

Morris, J. C. 1993. The clinical dementia rating (CDR): Current version and scoring rules. *Neurology* 43:2412–14.

Mowery, D. C., R. R. Nelson, B. N., Sampat, and A. A. Ziedonis. 2001. The growth of patenting and licensing by U.S. universities: An assessment of the effects of the Bayh-Dole act of 1980. *Research Policy* 30:99–119.

Nettleton, S., and R. Burrows. 2003. E-scaped medicine? Information, reflexivity and health. *Critical Social Policy* 23 (2): 165–85.

Nicoll, J. A., D. Wilkinson, C. Holmes, P. Steart, H. Markham, and R. O. Weller. 2003. Neuropathology of human Alzheimer disease after immunization with amyloid-beta peptide: A case report. *Nature Medicine* 9 (4): 448–52.

Orgogozo, J. M., S. Gilman, J. F. Dartigues, B. Laurent, M. Puel, L. C. Kirby, P. Jouanny, et al. 2003. Subacute meningoencephalitis in a subset of patients with AD after A{beta}42 immunization. *Neurology* 61 (1): 46–54.

Perry, E. K., B. Gibson, G. Blessed, R. H. Perry, and B. Tomlinson. 1977. Neurotransmitter enzyme abnormalities in senile dementia: Choline acetyltransferase and glutamic acid decarboxylase activities in necropsy brain tissue. *Journal of the Neurological Sciences* 34 (2): 247–65.

Rabeharisoa, V., and M. Callon. 2002. The involvement of patients' associations in research. *International Social Science Journal* 54 (1): 57.

Rabinow, P. 1999. *French DNA: Trouble in purgatory*. Chicago: University of Chicago Press.

Reisberg, B., S. H. Ferris, M. J. de Leon, and T. Crook. 1982. The global deterioration scale for assessment of primary degenerative dementia. *American Journal of Psychiatry* 139 (9): 1136–39.

Scheltens, P., N. Fox, F. Barkhof, and C. de Carli. 2002. Structural magnetic resonance imaging in the practical assessment of dementia: Beyond exclusion. *Lancet Neurology* 1:13–21.

Schenk, D., R. Barbour, W. Dunn, G. Gordon, H. Grajeda, T. Guido, K. Hu, et al. 1999. Immunization with amyloid-beta attenuates Alzheimer-disease-like pathology in the PDAPP mouse. *Nature* 400 (6740): 173–77.

Schenk, D., M. Hagen, and P. Seubert. 2004. Current progress in beta-amyloid immunotherapy. *Current Opinion in Immunology* 16:599–606.

Schmidt, L. A. 1999. *The corporate transformation of American health care: A study in institution building*. Ph.D. diss., Department of Sociology, University of California at Berkeley.

Shapin, S., and S. Schaffer. 1985. *Leviathan and the air-pump: Hobbes, Boyle, and experimental life*. Princeton, N.J.: Princeton University Press.

Sismondo, S. 2004. Pharmaceutical maneuvers. *Social Studies of Science* 34 (2): 149–59.

Stewart, R. 2001. NICE guidelines and the treatment of Alzheimer's disease: Evidence-based medicine may be discriminatory. *British Journal of Psychiatry* 179:367.

Thal, L. J. 1991. Assessment issues in clinical trials of tetrahydroaminoacridine and studies to alter decline in Alzheimer disease. *Alzheimer Disease and Associated Disorders* 5 (suppl. 1): S37–9.

———. 2002. How to define treatment success using cholinesterase inhibitors. *International Journal of Geriatric Psychiatry* 17:388–90.

Whitehouse, P. J. 1997. The international working group on harmonization of dementia drug guidelines: Past, present, and future. *Alzheimer Disease and Associated Disorders* 11 (3): 2–5.

———. 2000. History and the future of Alzheimer disease. In *Concepts of Alzheimer disease: Biological, clinical, and cultural perspectives*, ed. P. J. Whitehouse, K. Maurer, and J. F. Ballenger, 291–305. Baltimore: Johns Hopkins University Press.

Whitehouse, P. J., D. L. Price, R. G. Struble, A. W. Clark, J. T. Coyle, and M. R. Delon. 1982. Alzheimer's disease and senile dementia: Loss of neurons in the basal forebrain. *Science* 215 (4537): 1237–39.

Winblad, B., H. Brodaty, S. Gauthier, J. C. Morris, J. M. Orgogozo, K. Rockwood, L. Schneider, M. Takeda, P. Tariot, and D. Wilkinson. 2001. Pharmacotherapy of Alzheimer's disease: Is there a need to redefine treatment success. *International Journal of Geriatric Psychiatry* 16 (7): 653–66.

Yankner, B. A. 2000. A century of cognitive decline. *Nature* 404:125.

CHAPTER 13

APOE Genotyping, Risk Estimates, and Public Understanding of Susceptibility Genes

MARGARET LOCK, PH.D.
AND ADAM HEDGECOE, PH.D.

More than a decade ago, research carried out in the laboratory of Allan Roses demonstrated that one specific allele of the apolipoprotein E (APOE) gene located on chromosome 19 places individuals at an increased risk for late-onset Alzheimer's disease (AD) (Strittmatter et al. 1993; Roses 1998). This finding has since been verified in more than 100 laboratories. APOE, already implicated in heart disease before its association with AD was established, is a polymorphic protein with three alleles, 2, 3, and 4, that are universally but unequally (clinally) distributed. The APOEε4 variation places individuals at increased risk not only for contracting AD but also for an earlier age of onset of the disease by as much as seven to nine years. Despite consensus on these findings, it is agreed that the allele *determines* nothing with respect to the incidence of AD. All that can be inferred is that the APOEε4 genotype confers a greater degree of *susceptibility* but that it is neither necessary nor sufficient to cause the disease. It is estimated that at least 50 percent of patients diagnosed with AD do not have the APOEε4 genotype and that about 50 percent of individuals with the ε4 allele do not develop AD (Selkoe 2000). The presumption of by far the majority of researchers is that combinations of gene/gene and gene/protein interactions as well as interactions with environmental variables must also be implicated, and a great deal of time and energy is currently being invested into establishing what contribution these other variables make to the disease occurrence and its age of onset (Tilley, Morgan, and Kalsheker 1998; Bertram and Tanzi 2004). The latest effort to make some progress on this front is to carry out genome-wide association studies (GWAS), in which a dense array of genetic markers thought to capture a substantial proportion of common variation in genome sequence is genotyped using extremely large samples of DNA from at least several thousand people. The purpose of GWAS is to map susceptibility effects through detection of associations between genotype frequency in the sample of certain markers and the expression of the disease in question, in this instance, AD. Provisional results are just beginning to be made available and thus far confirm only the findings already well known about the APOE gene.

At present there is universal agreement among involved professional organizations and health policy–making institutions that genetic testing should not be routinely performed in connection with late-onset AD (although it is used at times to confirm a clinical diagnosis). The Alzheimer's societies of the United States, Canada, and the United Kingdom take a similar position. These recommendations are easily justified given that knowledge about the APOE status of a patient has absolutely no effect on clinical care. However, several private companies offer testing; for example, an "Early Alert Alzheimer's Home Screening Test" kit is marketed directly to consumers (Kier and Molinari 2003), and at least one nursing home in North Carolina is on record as not accepting applicants that have not submitted to an APOE test. Potential residents who test positive for APOEε4 are turned down on the grounds that they are likely to become demented and troublesome (Thomas et al. 1998). Furthermore, an NIH-approved randomized controlled trial named REVEAL (risk evaluation and education for Alzheimer's disease) has been carried out. Individuals from families where one or more member has been affected by late-onset AD are subjects of this research. One justification for the REVEAL project is to assess how people respond to being informed that they have a gene that puts them at increased risk for AD.

Of course, blood is routinely drawn for hundreds of research projects in connection with AD, at which time DNA testing is often carried out. With informed consent, research subjects agree to participate, fully aware that they will not gain access to their test results on the grounds that scientific knowledge is not sufficiently advanced for findings to be meaningful for individual cases. However, *should* it be convincingly demonstrated that one or more medication for AD proves to be differentially effective according to APOE genotype, it is likely that the guidelines for testing and disclosure will be changed.

Pressures from the private sector, increased demand on the part of individual patients and families to know about their genotype, and the possibility of a breakthrough in pharmacogenetics all point to the likelihood that routinized testing for APOE may well become reality in the not-too-distant future. In this chapter we draw on three bodies of knowledge that have a bearing on testing for APOE genotypes. First, findings from a portion of the epidemiological and cross-cultural research on APOEε4 and its relationship to AD will be summarized to demonstrate the difficulties involved in making predictions about individual risk on the basis of population-based data. Second, discussion of the current situation with respect to the pharmacogenetics of APOE will be presented. The final portion of the chapter will present findings from semistructured open-ended interviews with 55 people who participated in the REVEAL study. These three windows onto data that has a bearing on APOE testing clearly show, in our opinion, that much more systematic work needs to be done before APOE genotyping is routinely undertaken.

Cross-cultural Research: Dementia, Alzheimer's Disease, and APOE

Cross-cultural research into dementia is fraught with methodological difficulties. For example, local diagnostic criteria and methods of identifying cases frequently differ among epidemiological surveys, making meaningful comparison unreliable (Corrada, Brookmeyer, and Kawas 1995; Prince 2000). Furthermore, formal tests for cognitive ability are culture dependent; in the United States, English speakers and those with higher levels of education score above average on neuropsychological testing, whereas illiterate individuals and those with only a few years of formal education are at a great disadvantage.

Among the best of the epidemiological research examining dementia cross-culturally is that of the 10/66 Dementia Research Group. This is an international consortium of researchers centered on the Institute of Psychiatry in the United Kingdom who argue forcefully that research is urgently needed into dementia and its management in developing countries, where more than two-thirds of the world's elderly presently live—a number that is rapidly increasing (Prince 1997). A statement by this group suggests that studies showing low reporting of AD in some developing countries may well simply reflect a nonrecognition of dementia as anything other than "normal" aging, possibly resulting in early deaths for many people with dementia because their plight is not brought to public attention. Research carried out in India is used to support this claim (Consensus Statement from the 10/66 Dementia Research Group 2000). It has also been noted that widespread social stigma about dementia results in significant underreporting. High rates of comorbidity mask functional decline, and high mortality rates combined with little or no access to medical services for large numbers of people result in artificially low prevalence rates (Ineichen 1998; Henderson 2002). On the other hand, in spite of these shortcomings, many researchers conclude that differences in the incidence of dementia among ethnic groups are well demonstrated.

It has been shown that a constant rate of increase of risk for dementia with age is essentially the same worldwide. For example, the odds ratio between the age of onset and AD is the same in Ibadan, Nigeria, and in Indianapolis, Indiana, although the prevalence is quite different (Hall et al. 1998). Findings of this kind strongly suggest that the biological processes of normal aging are implicated but that genetic and environmental factors shift the absolute level of risk up or down and significantly alter age-specific rates of onset.

One study found that the greater the "genetic degree" of Cherokee ancestry (as documented in tribal records), the greater the protection against developing AD (Rosenberg et al. 1996). This research was carried out with 26 AD patients ages 65 or older and a control group of 26, both selected from the Cherokee community. It was confirmed that the control group had a "higher degree of Cherokee ancestry." This "protective factor" was independent of the APOE allele and was shown to diminish with age. The study, frequently cited, is similar to one involving 192 Cree ages 65 and over in which only one case of dementia was found. Among the obvious difficulties with this type of research is the sample size, the conflation of tribal identity with something variously labeled as race or ethnicity presumed to correlate with specific biological characteristics, and the use of "standardized dementia evaluations" to assess AD that were originally developed for use among middle-class urban populations.

An assumption about a uniformity in APOEε4 function adds to the difficulty, because this polymorphism has been shown to work in unexpected ways in certain populations. For instance, among Pygmies and other groups of people whose subsistence economy was until relatively recently predominantly that of hunting and gathering, possession of an APOEε4 genotype apparently *protects* against AD. This finding holds when controlled for age (Corbo and Scacchi 1999).

Farrer et al. carried out a meta-analysis based on data obtained from 40 research teams on nearly 6,000 patients diagnosed with probable AD (1997). The control group comprised 8,607 individuals without dementia recruited from clinics and communities as well as autopsy-based studies. Subjects came from four ethnic groups (African American, Hispanic, Caucasian, and Asian American [specifically, Japanese American]), and the findings were controlled for age of onset of the disease and sex. It was shown that the APOEε4 allele represents a major risk factor for AD in all four ethnic groups, across all ages between 40 and 90, and in both men and women. African Americans had higher frequencies of APOEε4 than the other groups, but the presence of the allele appears not to pose as great a risk for dementia as it does in Caucasian populations, although increased risk is still significant.

A large proportion of African Americans have a shared genetic ancestry with present-day Nigerians. Low rates of AD have been reported for parts of Nigeria, despite a high frequency of the APOEε4 allele. Researchers acknowledge limitations to the methodologies used, but even so, the data appear sufficiently robust to conclude that risk-reducing factors (lower cholesterol levels and less coronary heart disease (CHD) among Nigerians as compared to African Americans) *and* risk-enhancing factors (in North America) must be implicated, among them other genes and their products, diet, environment, and possibly yet other factors such as exposure to viruses (Farrer 2000; Graff-Radford et al. 2002).

The Indo-U.S. Cross-national Dementia Study found that among a sample of 4,450 people aged 55 and older living in Ballabgarh, Northern India, the prevalence of AD and other dementias was low indeed. The frequency of APOEε4 in this population is significantly lower than in a comparable U.S. sample. Nevertheless, APOEε4 is associated with an increased risk for AD in both populations and the *effects* of the allele appear to be similar. The apparent difference in prevalence of dementia may therefore be due to the lower APOEε4 frequency in India (Ganguli et al. 2000).

These studies, together with others from different areas of the world, make it clear that the specific role of APOEε4 and its molecular products in connection with AD is far from well understood. Similarly, the contribution of epigenetics—of interactions at the cellular level and the influence of macroenvironments—remain obscure, as does that of history and culture. For example, the APOEε4 allele is implicated in placing individuals at increased risk not only for AD but also for serious illness associated with lipid metabolism and heart disease. This particular allele exhibits what is known as "antagonistic pleiotropy" in that it has protective properties early in life that become detrimental in postreproductive life, particularly in unfavorable environments or when the diet is high in sugar and/or fats, as is the case in virtually all modernized societies (Gerber and Crews 1999).

The above findings strongly suggest that in a globalized, mobile world of multicultural societies, creating risk estimates for AD based on APOE genotyping is highly problematic. As noted above, establishing prevalence and incidence rates is a major challenge; the conflation of socially recognized ethnic groups with biological populations poses another intransient problem, and the importance of situating and understanding the functioning of the APOE gene in the nexus of specific cpigenetic contexts brings about a complexity that is possibly insurmountable when attempting to make reliable predictions of risk.

Pharmacogenetics and APOE Genotyping

As the most robust finding linking a gene to late-onset AD, APOEε4 has become the focus of considerable attention on the part of pharmaceutical companies and researchers exploring pharmacogenetics.[1] Interest in this area was stimulated by the findings by a group of scientists led by Judes Poirier of McGill University, who in 1995 published a paper suggesting that APOEε4 was an indicator of response to the drug tacrine (Poirier et al. 1995). At the time, tacrine was the only available treatment for AD; although by no means a cure, it slowed down the onset of the condition in about 50 percent of patients. The Poirier paper suggested that more than 80 percent of non-APOEε4 carriers responded to tacrine, while only 40 percent of ε4 carriers gained any benefit.

Since then, this result has been supported by other work carried out by the same group (Farlow et al. 1996, 1998) and by other researchers (MacGowan et al. 1995; Wilcock et al. 1995; Almkvist et al. 2001; Sjögren et al. 2001). There has been research involving other drugs from the same family (Poirier 1999; Oddoze, Michel, and Lucotte 2000) as well as research into APOE4-dependent response to other kinds of Alzheimer's drugs (Richard et al. 1997; Riekkinen, Koivisto, and Reinikaianen 1998; Álvarez et al. 1999; Cacabelos 2002). From reading review articles and commentaries about pharmacogenetics, one might gain the impression that APOE-based pharmacogenetics is "the best current illustration of the power of pharmacogenomics" (Marshall 1997, p. 1249) and that such testing is used in the clinic to guide prescribing (Emilien et al. 2000; Maitland-van der Zee et al. 2000; McLeod and Evans 2001; Crentsil 2004). Yet this is far from the case. In interviews (conducted by

Hedgecoe)[2] with Alzheimer's researchers and clinicians, it is hard to find any-
one (other than those involved in the original research results) who takes
APOE4-based response to tacrine (and subsequent results) seriously. Responses range from the vague: "My understanding is that there's no consistent effect of APOE status on cholinesterase response," to the definitive: "I
think the Poirier paper is nonsense."

Understanding the reasoning underpinning these responses is important if
pharmacogenetic testing for AD is to become a serious therapeutic option
(similar reasoning is likely to apply to other genes for complex diseases). Obvi-
ously there are technical, scientific factors involved: for example, for many clinicians, the problem with the link between APOEε4 and tacrine is that there
is a perceived lack of replication: "I'm not sure that study's ever been replicated. In fact, I don't think it has. I dimly remember reading someone tried to
and failed." For UK-based clinicians, studies involving tacrine are largely irrel-
evant anyway because the drug was refused a license by the Committee on
Safety of Medicines (CSM) in 1995 (Hall 1995; Hunt 1996). Although, as already mentioned, there are some studies with the second generation AChEIs,
for clinicians the most important research was carried out in the clinical trials for these drugs. Coming in the wake of the original 1995 study, these trials
stratified patient groups according to APOE status and found no association.
As one informant put it: "there was one study with galantamine . . . and they
looked to APOE and said that the response wasn't affected by APOE genotype
at all . . . I mean I can't think offhand of studies with donepezil or rivastigmine
but I'm sure that they must be there too" (see also Wilcock et al. 2000; Winblad et al. 2001).

In addition to these points, significant social and ethical factors also underpin concerns about APOE-based pharmacogenetics. For clinicians, a pharmacogenetic test has to provide useful discrimination between those who should
be treated with a particular drug and those who should not. Yet the kinds of
"numbers" offered up by the original Poirier research on tacrine, with 40 percent of APOEε4 carriers still responding, do not justify denying treatment to
any patients. As one interviewee put it, "I'd have thought that if I got a 40 percent response in my kind of field, that would be good." Many clinicians responded along the following lines: "If you're going to have something, you have
to have it up in the mid to high 90s in terms of your sensitivity of your test if it's
going to be helpful." Thus, on the basis of current knowledge, APOE-based
pharmacogenetics is not specific enough for clinicians to want to deny treatment to a group of patients, many of whom may well respond to specific drugs.

But beyond these points is the hurdle that APOEε4 itself presents to clinical uptake of testing. As noted earlier, the professional consensus around APOE testing is that while it may be suitable for research purposes, it should not take place in a clinical context. The American Academy of Neurology suggests, for example, that "routine use of ApoE genotyping in patients with suspected AD is not recommended at this time" (Knopman et al. 2001, p. 1149). Yet clearly, these concerns about APOE testing in the clinic will carry over into its use as a pharmacogenetic test: "That's the problem with the ε4, it's not just a pharmacogenetic tool, it's also a risk factor for the disease." And given this "overlap" between pharmacogenetics and disease-susceptibility genetics, it is not surprising to find that clinicians are reluctant to adopt APOE-based pharmacogenetic testing because of the additional kinds of information it might reveal. As one researcher put it: "The same sort of reservations that have been applied to disease risk are now being applied to any purely pharmacogenetic application of APOE."

Clinicians' concerns about APOE center on nonspecialists' inability to understand the uncertain nature of the information contained in an APOE result: "When you say vague things about relative risk at an individual case level, and all you can say to somebody is, you're three times more at risk than you would have been if you didn't have one ε4 allele, or you're six or eight times more at risk than if you didn't have two ε4 alleles, but then because I don't know what your risk was individually before, it's three times more. People can't understand that, they say, no, it must be three times the population risk. We say, no, it's not. Even with very bright people, you end up in a position that is not helping them, I don't think." Clinicians believe that it is difficult to explain this complexity not just to "bright" laypeople, but also to other medical professionals: "It's difficult for me to even impart this information to psychiatrists. In fact, just before you came, someone said 'Oh, I've got someone who's got a family history, can we do their ε4?' And I said, 'Well, why?' Literally they've got the blood in their hand, and I said, 'Well why are you doing it?' And I'd just given a talk on this, a week ago. They can't work it out, they can't work out why I'm saying it's of no value."

Thus, a core factor in clinicians' reluctance to employ APOE-based pharmacogenetics is professionals' concerns about how some of their colleagues as well as patients and their families interpret the results of an APOE test. But of course, a professional consensus, like that against clinical APOE testing, is not fixed. A survey in 1999 noted that more than 90 percent of clinicians rejected the use of such testing (Gifford et al. 1999, p. 242), and a more recent study supported the idea that clinicians are reluctant to use predictive APOE testing, with more than 90 percent of those asked in a 2002 study suggesting they were "unlikely" to offer such a test to an asymptomatic individual over 65 with no family history of AD (Chase et al. 2002, p. 300). Yet this research also noted that 47.2 percent of clinicians asked were "likely" to offer an APOE test to a *symptomatic* person over the age of 65 currently being evaluated for memory problems (that is, as a diagnostic adjunct). In addition to these reports of possible future behavior, this paper noted the "nontrivial rate at which physicians used ApoE testing in asymptomatic individuals, possibly in response to patient demand. Almost one sixth of respondents [15.5 percent] had been asked to order this test under circumstances in which testing is not recommended, and of these, nearly one-third [5.3 percent] had indeed done this" (Chase et al. 2002, pp. 301–2).

Whatever the original strength of the norm against clinical APOE genotyping, U.S.-based professionals at least are now more willing to offer such testing, a change that becomes more serious in light of the empirical findings presented in the last part of this chapter. These findings show clearly that, even with careful preparation and dissemination of information about the APOE gene by genetic counselors, for the most part, individuals remain bemused by this type of information and many have no idea of what use it might be to them.

Individual Responses to APOE Testing

Subjects for the REVEAL trial were recruited either through systematic ascertainment from American AD research registries kept at Boston, Case Western Reserve, and Cornell universities or through self-referral at each site (Cupples et al. 2004). The 160 participants who took part in the first round of this randomized controlled trial known as REVEAL I came from families in which late-onset AD had been diagnosed in one or more first-degree relatives, and upon recruitment they were randomized into intervention and control groups. Participants attended an education session about AD in the form of a Power Point presentation, with emphasis on theories about causation, including genetic susceptibility, after which they were asked to return to the research site at a later date for a blood draw. People in the intervention arm were informed a few weeks later about their APOE status.[3] Individuals assigned to be controls were not given this information. Reactions of REVEAL subjects who were informed of their APOE status were systematically monitored by means of three follow-up structured interviews conducted by genetic coun-selors over the course of twelve months. Their reactions were then compared with the reactions of individuals in the control group whose blood had been stored but not tested. A subset of the sample, 55 individuals, volunteered to return after the completion of the basic REVEAL study to participate in a follow-up project involving semistructured, open-ended interviews carried out by anthropologists between 2002 and 2003.

The concept of "blended inheritance" proved to be helpful in discussing the interview findings. "Blended inheritance" refers to a prevalent understanding among the public that involves thinking about inheritance as a "mixing or blending of influences from each parent," rather than as entailing a Men-delian transmission of genes (Richards 1996, p. 222). Ideas about inheritance stem from a long tradition of such reasoning evident as early as classical times (Turney 1995, p.12). Martin Richards suggests that today the notion of blended inheritance not only conflicts with professional genetic explanations about single-gene disorders but also works to reduce acceptance of those same explanations, both in the classroom and the clinic (1996).

The data presented below make it clear that the idea of blended inheritance is drawn on by families, not only in connection with diseases transmitted in a Mendelian mode but also, not surprisingly, in accounting for who is at risk for complex diseases. For example, when a disease such as AD occurs in a family, there is a consistent tendency to identify a family member who in some way resembles the afflicted person as the individual most likely to be at risk for de-veloping the disorder, whether individual genotypes are known or not. Kerr et al. (1998) comment that, in effect, individuals act as their own authority about the interpretation of genomic information.

Participants in the REVEAL study were exposed to a genetic educational session and individual genetic counseling. As part of the counseling sessions, they were provided with "personalized risk assessments" of their AD risk (based on age, family history, gender, and, for those people in the experimen-tal arm of the project, DNA typing). The interview results show that the ma-jority of these research subjects had a complex, intermingled understanding of "heredity," "inheritance," and "genetics" that they continued to hold even after completion of the REVEAL project. By the time the open-ended inter-views were carried out, more than twelve months after being told of their es-timated risk, individuals had transformed the estimates they had been given into accounts that "fit" with their experience of being a relative of someone with AD, personal assessments of their own family history, and the accumulated knowledge about the disease that they had gathered from a variety of sources. In other words, risk estimates provided in the REVEAL study did not displace "lay knowledge" that participants brought with them to the project. Rather, this "scientific" information is nested into existing knowledge, permitting the creation of idiosyncratic personalized risk estimates. This may in part account for the relatively small number of REVEAL participants (25 percent) who were able to recall with accuracy the risk estimates that they were given—particularly noteworthy when 91 percent of the informants stated that "wanting to know" their genotype was a major motivation for participation in the REVEAL study.[4] Furthermore, many were confused about the meaning of their results and made few if any behavioral changes after receiving them.

For example Carolyn, 52, a psychiatric nurse whose mother has AD, when asked specifically about her reaction to her result of an APOEε3/3 genotype responded: "I didn't think one way or the other when I found out my risk factor . . . I guess I don't recall an awful lot." Yet she also justified her participation in REVEAL as reflecting her desire to know about her genotype: "Knowledge is power. I really believe that. I mean, I don't think you can necessarily change your destiny, but certainly to go through life with your eyes only half open doesn't help you at all." But Carolyn remains unsure of what kinds of actions such power might motivate: "I think (REVEAL) provides useful information . . . Just don't ask me how I would use it . . . I honestly don't know."

Perhaps this response by Carolyn is a partial answer to why, a year after testing, 75 percent of the participants had forgotten or mixed up their risk estimates: "Is it the 3/4 that's the least likely to get it? I don't even remember. But it was good news. Whatever it was" (66-year-old female, APOEε3/3).

"I would come in—from one meeting to the next, I would come in and I couldn't remember what my risk was. And to this day, I'm not 100 percent sure. But I know that it's elevated" (54-year-old female, control).

"I don't remember much . . . to be truthful, not much. I'm sure I have (my risk estimate) somewhere, but I don't remember where" (45-year-old female, control).

However, participants have not forgotten everything that they were taught as part of the REVEAL educational program, and they take away more than a collection of numbers from the experience. Individuals appear to be particularly receptive to what they were taught about the fallibility of genetic risk estimates and about the uncertainties in connection with the relationship of genes to the onset of AD. Participants applied this knowledge to their own life

risk. Despite attending sessions with genetic counselors, participants discussed "genes" and "alleles" with much less facility than they did their beliefs about inheritance of personality and physical type or constitution from one's parents. The results of genetic testing did not apparently elevate anxiety in most cases, or at least did so for only a few weeks, in part because genetic or "science-based" explanations do not displace common sense explanations, and in part because those people who already believed they were at 100 percent risk for AD were reassured that this is not the case (something that surely their family practitioner could do effectively).

The above windows onto the complexities associated with genetic testing for the APOE gene strongly suggest, in our opinion, that such testing should not be routinized at this time. Calculations of risk estimates do not allow for education levels, ethnic differences, comorbidity, or for the way in which APOEε4 can function differently at different stages of the life cycle and in different environmental contexts. Systematic collection of broader-based population databases is clearly needed, but even then, conversion of these estimates for use in clinical situations raises numerous problems. In contrast to controlling for cholesterol levels, nothing can be done to change one's genome, and we have little insight, as yet, into what individuals believed to be at an increased risk for AD should do to delay or avoid the onset of the disease. Given the prevalence of AD with increasing age, every one of us should, in effect, be taking whatever precautions are currently recommended.

The qualitative part of the REVEAL study has shown that individuals draw extensively on the concept of "blended inheritance" to make sense of the probabilistic information that they receive about AD risk. In all likelihood, given that the only responsible way to impart risk estimates for late-onset Alzheimer's disease is with considerable caution and acknowledgement of all that is not yet known, people will continue to draw on nonscientific ideas about what "runs in the family." Even if major changes are made in the way genetics are taught in high school and college, such beliefs are likely to persist in the face of uncertainty with respect to the action of susceptibility genes.

Finally, interviews with clinicians show clearly that, given the current state of research in connection with medication for AD, the majority will remain conservative for some time to come about APOE disclosure. However, it is increasingly apparent that their hand is going to be forced by the private sector as more testing for the APOE gene is made available. For example, in March 2008, a Philadelphia-based company called Smart Genetics began to market its "Alzheimer's Mirror" service for $399, which provides APOE genotyping as well as education about risk and post-test genetic counseling, direct to the public. A few months earlier, the "genomic medicine" firms 23andme, Navigenics, and deCODEme launched, with their use of DNA chips to simultaneously screen customers' DNA for thousands of different polymorphisms. One of the variations all three companies screen for is APOEε4. The question remains, however, to what extent will the public want to know whether or not they have the "bad" gene?

ACKNOWLEDGMENTS

Funding for this research was provided by the Social Science and Humanities Research Council of Canada (SSHRC), grant no. 22447900223 and the Wellcome Trust, grant no. GR061491MA.

NOTES

1. Pharmacogenetics (and its more recent formulation, pharmacogenomics) involves the use of genetic testing to either focus the prescription of current drugs on those people most likely to respond well to a product or to develop new drugs targeted at genetically defined subpopulations.

2. These interviews were conducted between April 2001 and June 2003. See Hedgecoe 2006 for detailed description.

3. The findings presented here are based on the portion of the REVEAL study known as REVEAL I. The protocol was changed somewhat in later parts of the REVEAL trial. To carry out the "risk disclosure" portion of the study, all subjects were shown a "risk curve." These curves were developed by first drawing on gender- and age-specific incidence curves of first-degree relatives of persons with AD that had already been calculated from a meta-analysis of studies involving large samples of Caucasian subjects (Green et al. 1997). In addition, the curves were further subdivided by incorporating APOE genotype-specific odds ratio estimates for gender and age, reported in a second meta-analysis of 50 studies worldwide (Farrer et al. 1997). This gave a total of 12 curves based on the six possible combinations of APOE alleles for both males and females. Risk curves for the control group were based on gender, age, and family history alone. Based on their genotyping, the researchers showed the appropriate risk curve to each trial participant and then discussed with them their estimated increased risk for AD as they aged. Creating these risk curves entailed exceedingly complex mathematical formulations (Cupples et al. 2004). No other variables, such as ethnicity or education, were factored in, nor were such variables discussed informally during time with genetic counselors. To date virtually everyone enrolled in the trial had been white, but the second part of the REVEAL project, begun in 2005, includes at one of its sites, African American individuals recruited through Howard University. The risk estimates to be used with these volunteers are currently being estimated (Green et al. 2002).

4. Two major motivations for participating in the REVEAL study were cited by interviewees: the desire to know their own risk, as indicated above, as well as the desire to help further research on AD (74 percent).

REFERENCES

Almkvist, O., V. Jelic, K. Amberla, E. Hellstrom-Lindhal, L. Meuling, and A. Nordberg. 2001. Responder characteristics to a single oral dose of cholinesterase inhibitor: A double-blind placebo-controlled study with tacrine in Alzheimer patients. *Dementia and Geriatric Cognitive Disorders* 12 (1): 22–32.

Álvarez, X. A., R. Mouzo, V. Pichel, P. Perez, M. Laredo, L. Fernandez-Novoa, and L. Corzo, et al. 1999. Double-blind placebo-controlled study with citicoline in APOE genotyped Alzheimer's disease patients. Effects on cognitive performance, brain bioelectrical activity and cerebral perfusion. *Methods and Findings in Experimental and Clinical Pharmacology* 21 (9): 633–44.

Bertram, L., and R. E. Tanzi. 2004. Alzheimer's disease: One disorder, too many genes? *Human Molecular Genetics Advance Access*, February 5 (online). http://hmg.oxfordjournals.org/cgi/content/abstract/13/suppl_1/R135.

Cacabelos, R. 2002. Pharmacogenomics for the treatment of dementia. *Annals of Medicine* 34: 357–79.

Chase, G., G. Geller, S. Havstad, N. Holtzman, and S. Spear Bassett. 2002. Physicians' propensity to offer genetic testing for Alzheimer's disease: Results from a survey. *Genetics in Medicine* 4 (4): 297–303.

Consensus Statement from the 10/66 Dementia Research Group. 2000. Dementia in developing countries. *International Journal of Geriatric Psychiatry* 15:14–20.

Corbo, R. M., and R. Scacchi. 1999. Apolipoprotein E (ApoE) allele distribution in the world: Is ApoEε4 a "thrifty" allele? *Annals of Human Genetics* 63:301–10.

Corrada, M., R. Brookmeyer, and C. Kawas. 1995. Sources of variability in prevalence rates of Alzheimer's disease. *International Journal of Epidemiology* 24:1000–1005.

Crentsil, V. 2004. The pharmacogenomics of Alzheimer's disease. *Ageing Research Reviews* 3:153–69.

Cupples, L. A., L. A. Farrer, A. D. Sadovnick, N. Relkin, P. Whitehouse, and R. C. Green. 2004. Estimating risk curves for first-degree relatives of patients with Alzheimer's disease: The REVEAL study. *Genetics in Medicine* 6:192–96.

Emilien, G., M. Ponchon, C. Caldas, O. Isacson, and J. M. Maloteaux. 2000. Impact of genomics on drug discovery and clinical medicine. *Quarterly Journal of Medicine* 93 (7): 391–423.

Farlow, M., D. K. Lahiri, J. Poirier, J. Davignon, L. Schneider, and S. Hui. 1998. Treatment outcome of tacrine therapy depends on apolipoprotein E genotype and gender of the subject with Alzheimer's disease. *Neurology* 50:669–77.

Farlow, M., D. K. Lahiri, J. Poirier, J. Davignon, and S. Hui. 1996. Apolipoprotein E genotype and gender influence response to tacrine therapy. *Annals of the New York Academy of Science* 802:101–10.

Farrer, L. A. 2000. Familial risk for Alzheimer disease in ethnic minorities: Nondiscriminating genes. *Archives of Neurology* 57:28–29.

Farrer, L. A., L. A. Cupples, J. L. Haines, B. Hyman, W. A. Kukull, R. Mayeux, R. H. Myers, M. A. Pericak-Vance, N. Risch, and C. M. van Duijn. 1997. Effects of age, sex, and ethnicity on the association between apolipoprotein E denotype and Alzheimer's disease: A meta-analysis. *JAMA* 278:1349–56.

Ganguli, M., V. Chandra, M. I. Kamboh, J. M. Johnston, H. H. Dodge, B. K. Thelma, R. C. Juyal, R. Pandav, S. H. Belle, and S. T. DeKosky. 2000. Apolipoprotein E polymorphism and Alzheimer's disease: The Indo-US Cross-National Dementia Study. *Archives of Neurology* 57:824–30.

Gerber, L. M., and D. Crews. 1999. Evolutionary perspectives on chronic degenerative diseases. In *Evolutionary Medicine*, ed. W. R. Trevathan, E. O. Smith, and J. J. McKenna, 443–69. Oxford: Oxford University Press.

Gifford, D. R., R. G. Holloway, M. R. Frankel, C. L. Albright, R. Meyerson, R. Griggs, and B. Vickrey. 1999. Improving adherence to dementia guidelines through education and opinion leaders: A randomized control trial. *Annals of Internal Medicine* 131 (4): 237–46.

Graff-Radford, N., R. C. Green, R. C. P. Go, M. L. Hutton, T. Edeki, D. Bachman, and J. L. Adamson, et al. 2002. Association between apolipoprotein E genotype and Alzheimer disease in African American subjects. *Archives of Neurology* 59:594–600.

Green, R. C., V. C. Clarke, N. J. Thompson, J. L. Woodard, and R. Letz. 1997. Early detection of Alzheimer disease: Methods, markers, and misgivings. *Alzheimer Disease and Associated Disorders* 11:S1–5.

Green, R. C., L. A. Cupples, R. Go, K. S. Benke, T. Edeki, P. A. Griffith, and M. Williams, et al. 2002. Risk of dementia among white and African relatives of patients with Alzheimer's disease. *JAMA* 287:329–36.

Hall, C. 1995. Makers appeal for Alzheimer's drug licence. *Independent*, March 22, 4.

Hall, K., O. Gureje, S. Gao, A. Ogunniyi, S. L. Hui, O. Baiyewu, F. W. Unverzagt, S. Oluwole, and H. C. Hendrie. 1998. Risk factors and Alzheimer's disease: A comparative study of two communities. *Australian and New Zealand Journal of Psychiatry* 32:698–706.

Hedgecoe, A. 2006. Pharmacogenetics as alien science: Alzheimer's, core sets, and expectations. *Social Studies of Science* 36 (5): 723–52.

Henderson, J. N. 2002. The experience and interpretation of dementia: Cross-cultural perspectives. *Journal of Cross-Cultural Gerontology* 17:195–96.

Hunt, L 1996. Unravelling the tangles of dementia. *Independent on Sunday,* Sunday Review, April 28, 42.

Ineichen, B. 1998. The geography of dementia: An approach through epidemiology. *Health and Place* 4 (4): 383–94.

Kerr, A., S. Cunningham-Burley, and A. Amos. 1998. The new human genetics and health: Mobilizing lay expertise. *Public Understanding of Science* 7:41–60.

Kier, F. J., and V. Molinari. 2003. "Do-it-yourself" dementia testing: Issues regarding an Alzheimer's home screening test. *Gerontologist* 43:295–301.

Knopman, D. S., S. T. DeKosky, J. L. Cummings, H. Chui, J. Corey-Bloom, N. Relkin, G. W. Small, B. Miller, and J. C. Stevens. 2001. Practitioner parameter: Diagnosis of dementia (an evidence based review). Report of the Quality Standards Subcommittee of the American Academy of Neurology. *Neurology* 56:1143–53.

MacGowan, S., M. Scott, M. Agg, and G. Wilcock. 1995. Influence of apolipoprotein E genotype on response to tacrine in male and female patients with Alzheimer's disease. Abstract presented at the International Psychogeriatrics Association conference, Apolipoprotien E et Maladie d'Alzheimer, May 29, Paris.

Maitland-van der zee, A. H., A. de Boer, and H. Leufkens. 2000. The interface between pharmacoepidemiology and pharmacogenetics. *European Journal of Pharmacology* 410:121–30.

Marshall, A. 1997. Getting the right drug into the right patient. *Nature Biotechnology* 15:1249–52.

McLeod, H., and W. Evans. 2001. Pharmacogenomics: Unlocking the human genome for better drug therapy. *Annual Review of Pharmacology and Toxicology* 41:101–21.

Oddoze, C., B.-F. Michel, and G. Lucotte. 2000. Apolipoprotein E epsilon 4 allele predicts a better response to donepezil therapy in Alzheimer's disease. *Alzheimer's Report* 3 (4): 213–16.

Poirier, J. 1999. Apolipoprotein E4, cholinergic integrity and the pharmacogenetics of Alzheimer's disease. *Journal of Psychiatry and Neuroscience* 24 (2): 147–53.

Poirier, J., M.-C. Delisle, I. Aubert, M. Farlow, D. Lahir, S. Hui, P. Bertrand, J. Nalbantoglu, B. Gilfix, and S. Gauthier. 1995. Apolipoprotein E allele as a predictor of cholinergic deficits and treatment outcome in Alzheimer disease. *Proceedings of the National Academy of Sciences* 92: 12260–64.

Prince, M. 1997. The need for research on dementia in developing countries. *Tropical Medicine and International Health* 2 (10): 993–1000.

———. 2000. Methodological issues for population-based research into dementia in developing countries: A position paper from the 10/66 Dementia Research Group. *International Journal of Geriatric Psychiatry* 15:21–30.

Richard, F., N. Helbecque, E. Neuman, D. Guez, R. Levy, and P. Amouyel. 1997. ApoE genotyping and response to drug treatment in Alzheimer's disease. *Lancet* 349:539.

Richards, M. 1996. Lay and professional knowledge of genetics and inheritance. *Public Understanding of Science* 5:217–30.

Riekkinen, P. J., K. Koivisto, K. J. Reinikainen, T. Hänninen, M. Hallikainen, P. Kilkku, E. L. Helkala, and E. Heinonen. 1998. Can apo-4 subtype predict response to selegiline treatment in Alzheimer's disease? In *Proceedings of the 5th International Geneva/Springfield Symposium on Advances in Alzheimer's Therapy*, ed. E. Giacobini, A. Nordberg. J.-P. Michel, B. Winblad, and R. Becker, 91. Springfield: Southern Illinois University.

Rosenberg, R. N., R. W. Richter, R. C. Risser, K. Taubman, I. Prado-Farmer, E. Ebalo, J. Posey, et al. 1996. Genetic factors for the development of Alzheimer disease in the Cherokee Indian. *Archives of Neurology* 53:997–1000.

Roses, A. D. 1998. A new paradigm for clinical evaluations of dementia: Alzheimer disease and apolipoprotein E genotypes. In *Genetic testing for Alzheimer disease: Ethical and clinical issues*, ed. S. G. Post and P. J. Whitehouse. Baltimore: Johns Hopkins University Press.

Selkoe, D. J. 2000. The pathophysiology of Alzheimer's disease. In *Early diagnosis of Alzheimer's disease*, ed. L. F. M. Scinto and K. R. Daffner. Totowa, N.J.: Humana Press.

Sjögren, M., C. Hesse, H. Basun, G. Köl, H. Thostrup, L. Kilander, J. Marcusson, et al. 2001. Tacrine and rate of progression in Alzheimer's disease: Relation to ApoE allele genotype. *Journal of Neural Transmission* 108:451–58.

Strittmatter, W. V., et al. 1993. Apolipoprotein E: High-avidity binding to beta-amyloid and increased frequency of type 4 allele in late-onset familial Alzheimer disease. *Proceedings of the National Academy of Sciences* 90:1977–81.

Thomas, A. M., G. Cohen, R. M. Cook-Deegan, J. O'Sullivan, S. G. Post, A. D. Roses, K. F. Schaffner, and R. M. Green. 1998. Alzheimer testing at silver years. *Cambridge Quarterly of Healthcare Ethics* 7:294–307.

Tilley, L., K. Morgan, and N. Kalsheker. 1998. Genetic risk factors in Alzheimer's disease. *Journal of Clinical Pathology: Molecular Pathology* 51:293–304.

Turney, J. 1995. The public understanding of genetics: Where next? *European Journal of Genetics in Society* 1:5–20.

Wilcock, G., S. Lilienfeld, and E. Gaens, on behalf of the Galantamine International-1 Study Group. 2000. Efficacy and safety of galantamine in patients with mild to moderate Alzheimer's disease: Multicentre randomised controlled trial. *British Medical Journal* 321:1–7.

Wilcock, G., S. MacGowan, M. Scott, and D. Dawbarn. 1995. Apolipoprotein E genotype and response to tacrine in Alzheimer's disease. Poster presented at the International Psychogeriatrics Association conference, Apolipoprotein E et Maladie d'Alzheimer, May 29, Paris.

Winblad, B., K. Engedal, H. Soininen, F. Verhey, G. Waldemar, A. Wimo, A. L. Wetterholm, R. Zhang, A. Haglund, and P. Subbiah. 2001. A 1-year, randomized, placebo-controlled study of donepezil in patients with mild to moderate AD. *Neurology* 57:489–95.

CHAPTER 14

Developing Drugs for Dementia

Hope, Hype, and Hypocrisy

PETER V. RABINS, M.D., M.P.H.

For as long as there have been written medical texts, old age has been associated with cognitive decline. As translated by Loza and Milad (1990), a papyrus from the ninth century BCE states: "My sovereign master, old age is here. Senility has descended upon me . . . My mouth is mute, it can no longer speak . . . My spirit is forgetful and I can no longer remember yesterday . . . What causes senility in men is bad in every way." Extant medical writings from the ancient Greek and Roman worlds further document this association. Thus, for millennia, aging was seen as a causal agent of later-life cognitive decline. Not until the 1890s, when Alois Alzheimer described the neuropathology of vascular dementia (made possible by the technological advance afforded by Nissl's discovery of the staining of neuronal processes by aniline dyes), or perhaps a decade later when he identified plaques and tangles in the brain of a woman who died of "premature senility" (Berrios and Freeman 1991), did disease, rather than being considered an expected consequence of the aging process, seem a possible explanation for late-life cognitive changes. However, throughout the first half of the twentieth century, neuropathological studies did not always confirm the association between dementia and neuropathology, and the matter remained controversial (see, for example, Rothschild 1941).

While noted neuropathologists such as Raymond Adams taught that senile dementia was characterized by the neurofibrillary tangles and plaques described by Alzheimer (Paul McHugh, personal communication, 2000) in the 1950s, it was not until the pioneering work of Roth, Corsellis, and Tomlinson in the 1960s that the matter was settled in the minds of most scholars. Their finding that most individuals with senile dementia had plaques and tangles throughout their brains at autopsy and that the number of these abnormal structures was much greater in cognitively impaired individuals than in age-matched cognitively normal individuals convinced most scientists that dementia was due to brain disease, not usual aging (Corsellis 1962; Roth et al. 1967; Tomlinson et al. 1968).

It is important to note that this change from "senility" as an expected consequence of aging to "dementia" as a disease that becomes increasingly common in later life was as much a sociological as a biomedical change—perhaps even a sociological revolution. It came at a time in human history when living to old age became the norm rather than the exception and when the economic and political power of elderly people became increasingly prominent and had begun to change the concept of aging itself.

By the early 1980s, this reconceptualization of "senility" as dementia—a syndrome characterized by declines in multiple cognitive capacities and normal alertness/attention—and the subdivision of dementia into specific diseases based on associations with various pathologic abnormalities in the brain such as Alzheimer's disease, Creutzfeldt-Jacob disease, vascular dementia, and Pick disease, became accepted within the medical community and, increasingly, the population at large. Gradually, decline in memory and the progressive impairment of other cognitive capacities such as language, judgment, and the performance of everyday activities such as dressing and bathing became identified as the symptoms of disease rather than an expected accompaniment of aging.

This reconceptualization has had many benefits. Redefining senility as dementia has led to a widespread appreciation of the suffering caused by cognitive decline and of the need for the kinds of services and resources that society makes available to the "sick." It has been paralleled by a reconceptualization of commonly associated neuropsychiatric symptoms such as wandering, aggression, agitation, hallucinations, suspiciousness, and delusions as being the result of a dementing brain disease, not simply a common "second childhood" or final stage of life.

The reconceptualization of late-life cognitive decline as dementia also brought notice to the impact of the caregiving process on the caregiver, most commonly a family member (Rabins, Mace, and Lucas 1982). While dementia is not the only chronic illness for which individuals are provided care, much of the research on caregiving has focused on those providing care to an individual with dementia. This has led to a body of research documenting the adverse emotional and physical sequelae associated with caregiving as well as the fulfillment that can result. It is unlikely that this would have occurred without a focus on dementia as a disease. These findings have undoubtedly increased the services available to both caregivers and patients, fostered the development of support organizations that provide emotional, social, and financial support to caregivers, and encouraged the development of alternate care resources that address the needs of both caregivers and persons with the disease.

As in all situations, this relabeling has had negative effects as well. They include the "depersonalization" of the patient (referring to an individual as a "dement" or a "diabetic," for example), the stigma that accompanies being identified as different ("sick," a negative consequence of moving from "normal aging" to "pathological aging"), and the loss of privilege that can come from being included in a group (for example, the cancellation of drivers' licenses even for individuals who retain the skills to drive).

One of the benefits of the reconceptualization of senility is the emergence of a worldwide biomedical research effort aimed at discovering treatments and strategies for eradication. This effort has been fostered by an appreciation of the public health implications of these diseases. For example, the number of individuals with significant cognitive disorder will double in the United States and many countries in the next 25 years because of the increasing life expectancy of the population. Data such as these have also resulted in the a recognition by pharmaceutical companies that dementia and Alzheimer's disease are prevalent problems and that a large amount of money could be made were an effective treatment or prevention developed.

The Current Status of Dementia Research

By the mid-1970s, seven or eight years after the Roth group demonstrated that senile dementia was most commonly due to Alzheimer's disease, several groups reported that individuals who died with Alzheimer's disease had deficiencies in the brain neurotransmitter acetylcholine (actually, an enzyme that degrades the neurotransmitter and serves as a "marker" for the neurotransmitter). This suggested, based on an analogy with Parkinson's disease, that boosting the levels of this chemical might improve the symptoms. Initial efforts at doing so met with failure, but by the mid-1990s, four compounds, tacrine, donepezil, galantamine, and rivastigmine, were shown to modestly improve cognitive function in individuals with dementia. While arguments about the strength of this improvement ("effect size") and the long-term benefits of these modest improvements continue, there is little doubt that cognitive performance improves modestly in approximately one-third of individuals clinically diagnosed with Alzheimer's disease who take these medications and that such benefits might also occur in individuals with vascular dementia and dementia with Lewy bodies.

The availability of these modest treatments has raised a number of questions. For regulators, what outcome measures should be used to determine if a drug is approved when cures or treatments that result in dramatic improvement are not available? In the case of the dementias, cognitive improvement has been chosen as the outcome because cognitive decline is the primary characteristic that defines dementia, but, if the cognitive improvements do not result in improved function in everyday activities or in the quality of life of the ill person, is that adequate? Furthermore, once the metric of benefit is agreed upon, how long should such treatments be continued for individuals who do not initially show a measurable benefit?

From the point of view of the patient, family, and society, how does one balance the cost of the drug with the modest benefits that accrue? Also, should benefit to the family or caregiver be considered a basis for approval or for long-term use if clear benefit to the patient cannot be demonstrated? This issue is particularly relevant to the dementias because much of patients' care is provided by family members and professional caregivers and much of the financial burden is borne by families and society.

For health professionals, how does one balance therapeutic optimism with the reality that treatments are only modestly effective? How important is "doing something" to the caring process, and can the prescription of a modestly effective treatment ever be justified because it addressed the desire of many patients and their families to "do everything they could"? Also, how does one temper the influence of marketing that is directed toward clinicians and consumers in the face of modest benefit in a society that values free speech?

For pharmaceutical companies, who have a fiduciary responsibility to maximize profit as well as obligations to function ethically and follow the laws governing the industry, a major goal is to increase the use of their product. While marketing is constrained by the language of the approval notice, the goal of advertising is to sell product, not provide balance or nuance. What responsibility do they have, then, to limit expectations?

The challenge of placing therapeutic benefit in the context of modest gains is not unique to dementia. Indeed, it is true for the treatment of many common disorders including hypertension, type II diabetes, depression, and many forms of cancer. Thus, the challenge presented in prescribing and marketing modestly beneficial therapies for chronic diseases is a broad issue that deserves a wide general debate. The currently available therapies for dementia provide but one example and should not be singled out as an unusual case. At present, many therapies for chronic disease require treatment of a large number of individuals to achieve a small benefit (a small effect size).

At the same time, therapeutic nihilism inappropriately demoralizes patients and caregivers and dissuades individuals from using effective nonpharmacological therapies. I believe clinicians best serve patients by discussing all treatments in the context of their potential benefits and side effects, by informing potential users of the range of therapies available, by individualizing the treatments offered based on the needs of the ill person and their caregivers, and by encouraging patients and caregivers to use their values in making these challenging decisions.

Hype, Hope, and Raised Expectations

As someone who has been involved in both clinical care and clinical research since the late 1970s, I have observed several recurring themes that are problematic and should be guarded against. First, scientists have repeatedly predicted since the 1970s that "cures" or "major breakthroughs" would occur within five years. This has been wrong thus far and is unconscionable. I hope the prediction will be correct some day, but making such pronouncements in public is self-serving and offers nothing but false hope to those experiencing the disease (Rabins 1987).

The lack of dramatically effective pharmacologic or surgical therapies has led some clinicians to be needlessly and inappropriately nihilistic about what can be done. Providing a balanced view of the efficacy and drawbacks of all available treatments, nonpharmacologic and pharmacologic, helps patients appreciate the likely prognosis while providing them the means to act in accordance with their goals. Therapeutic nihilism undervalues the benefits of education, caregiver support, environmental management, and activity-based treatments. Clearly, though, exaggerating the modest benefits of pharmacologic and nonpharmacologic therapies can harm patients and their caregivers.

The development of treatments for the neuropsychiatric (also called behavioral and psychological) symptoms commonly associated with dementia has trailed behind the development of methods for testing efficacy. In general, randomized trials in which the entry criteria are both a specific level of cognitive impairment and a specific level of the targeted neuropsychiatric symptom are almost nonexistent and are sorely needed. Without them, claims of efficacy cannot be judged. Ideally such treatments would not adversely impair cognition or function, and these should be measured in all trials.

Another disturbing trend is the tendency to exaggerate the prevalence of the dementias, the burden imposed on caregivers, the failure of families to provide care, and the failure of institutional facilities to provide good care. While there is no doubt that the dementias are a devastating group of illnesses, and there is truth to each of these claims, exaggerating the negatives harms those who have the illness and those providing care. It diminishes the sacrifices and joys that can result from caregiving, takes away the hope and affirmation that can accompany caring, and dismisses the efforts of family and professional caregivers to better the life of the person with dementia. Balanced reporting of data is crucial to planning, resource allocation, and establishing research priorities.

Reflections on the Treatment of Chronic Illness

I have argued that the treatment of dementia is but one example of the challenges inherent in treating chronic illness. For most of human history, medical professionals had little to offer but a prognosis, support, and occasional symptom relief. We now know that many of the nostrums used to treat patients with chronic diseases over the millennia were ineffective and sometimes even harmful. We live in an era in which dramatic breakthroughs in medical treatment have become commonplace and seem to have changed the valence and expectations of patients and practitioners alike. And yet most individuals identified as patients suffer from common conditions for which dramatic treatments are unavailable. Guarding against undocumented or exaggerated claims has always been the provenance of the clinician and remains so today. Giving hope and providing accurate evaluations of available treatments is as much a part of the caring professions as it has always been.

The reconceptualization of senility as dementia has led to social, psychological, and biological benefits accruing to those who have the disease and those caring for them. Nonetheless, the dangers of the disease model and the objectification of the individual must be continuously guarded against.

The extensive focus on understanding the neurobiology of dementia, particularly of Alzheimer's disease, has led to an explosion of knowledge about normal brain function and the function of the brain in dementia. However, few treatments have emerged from these advances in knowledge, and repeated predictions of impending breakthroughs have been unfulfilled. Research should continue apace, but soothsaying should be left to psychics, portfolio managers, and company executives devising research agendas.

The core and defining deficits of dementia are in the cognitive realm, so the *sine qua non* of response to treatment should be an improvement in cognition. However, given the high prevalence of neuropsychiatric symptoms, the decline in activities-of-daily-living function that parallels the cognitive decline, the fact that care is usually provided by others and that this care can adversely affect a carer's psychological and physical well-being, and impairment of quality of life caused by dementia, questions remain of what outcomes should be used to determine benefit of treatments for dementia once it has developed.

Balanced presentations of what is and isn't known, of what can and cannot be done, and what is likely but not definitely going to happen remain cornerstones of the treatment of dementia and many other chronic diseases.

REFERENCES

Berrios, G. E., and H. L. Freeman, eds. 1991. *Alzheimer and the dementias.* London: Royal Society of Medicine.

Blessed, G., B. Tomlinson, and M. Roth. 1968. The association between quantitative measures of dementia and senile changes in cerebral grey matter of elderly subjects. *British Journal of Psychiatry* 114:797–811.

Corsellis, J. A. N. 1962. *Mental illness and the ageing brain: The distribution of pathological change in a mental hospital population.* London: Oxford University Press.

Corsellis, J. A. N., C. J. Bruton, and D. Freeman-Bowen. 1973. The aftermath of boxing. *Psychological Medicine* 3:270–303.

Loza, N., and G. Milad. 1990. Notes from ancient Egypt. *International Journal of Geriatric Psychiatry* 5:403–5.

Rabins, P. V. 1987. Science and medicine in the spotlight: Alzheimer's disease as an example. *Perspectives in Biology and Medicine* 31:161–70.

Rabins, P. V., N. L. Mace, and M. J. Lucas. 1982. The impact of dementia on the family. *JAMA* 248:333–35.

Roth, M., B. E. Tomlinson, G. Blessed. 1967. The relationship between quantitative measures of dementia and of degenerative changes in the cerebral grey matter of elderly subjects. *Proceedings of the Royal Society of Medicine* 60 (3): 254–60.

Rothschild, D. 1941. The clinical differentiation of senile and arteriosclerotic psychosis. *American Journal of Psychiatry* 98:324–33.

Tomlinson, B. E., G. Blessed, M. Roth. 1968. Observations on the brains of non-demented old people. *Journal of the Neurological Sciences* 7 (2): 331–56.

Index

Dementia (*cont.*)
194–95; public awareness of, 211, 220;
reconceptualization of senility as, 186,
214, 251–52, 256; staging of, 219;
stigma of, 234, 252
Depersonalization of patients, 252
Deprenyl, 34, 203
Depression, 29–30, 78, 118–19; efficacy of
treatment for, 76, 77; among family care-
givers, 106, 114
Dexamphetamine, 26
Diagnosis of AD, 44–45; fear of, 119, 177;
NINCDS-ADRDA criteria for, 126, 215,
218–19; tests for, 126, 128–29, 215, 219
*Diagnostic and Statistical Manual of Mental
Disorders* (DSM), 9, 11, 12, 13, 33, 79,
126
Diet and nutrition, 20, 121, 195
Dihydroergotamine (Hydergine), 26, 27, 29,
196, 198
Disease concept of dementia, 177–80,
199–201, 251
Disease-modifying drugs, 210, 221–25
Donepezil (Aricept), 18, 31–32, 59, 81, 86,
91n. 4, 92n. 21, 104, 105, 106, 119,
153, 154, 205, 253; advertising of, 206;
assessing symptomatic benefit of, 139–40;
clinical trials of, 138–41; discontinuation
of, 107–8; disease stabilization with,
142–43; effectiveness vs. benefit of, 141;
ethics of withholding, 140–41; ignoring
nonpromotional studies of, 144; research
literature and promotion of, 134–35,
137–45; "spinning" negative trial of,
134, 137, 141–42
L-Dopa, 31, 202, 203, 213
Dopamine, 29, 202
Drug development, 135, 136, 147–64,
214–15, 250–56; consumer influence
on, 185; drugs defining disease, 152–55;
expectations about future of, 171–72;
FDA guidelines for drug evaluation, 204,
215–17; multiple routes of, 155–56;
ontological disease concept and, 148–52,
164nn. 1–2, 165nn. 3–6; profiling drugs
and diseases, 148, 156–59, 165nn. 7–8;
science and ethics of, 161–64; social context of, 184, 189; truth and hope in, 184,

210–26; as two-way process, 148, 154,
160–64
Drug Efficacy Study Implementation, 26
Drug therapy. *See* Pharmacotherapy for AD

Eating/feeding, 121, 122
Educational programs, 195
Efficacy of psychotropics for dementia: ADLs
as measure of, 81–82, 85–87, 92n. 14,
101, 104, 108–10, 216, 217–18; for
behavioral and psychological symptoms,
76–77, 89, 104, 109, 216; clinical trials
as measure of, 125, 216; evaluation of
disease-modifying therapies, 221–23;
evidence for, 3, 26–27, 32, 104, 184,
197–99, 202–5, 253; QOL as measure of,
81, 86, 89, 90n. 2, 92n. 14, 109, 169–75,
218; reformulation of evaluative framework for, 216–18
Electroconvulsive therapy, 195
Environmental factors, 179, 180, 234
Estrogen, 153
Ethical concerns, 140–41, 161–64, 177,
184, 237
Ethnicity, APOE, and AD risk, 234–35
Exelon (rivastigmine), 18, 31, 59, 85, 88,
91n. 4, 104, 105, 110, 253
Extrapyramidal symptoms (EPS), 91n. 8

Familial AD, 43, 47–49, 240
Family/caregivers: burden on, 112, 186,
252; burnout of, 112; depression in, 106,
114; perspective of, 100–101, 116–24;
pharmacotherapy and needs of, 99, 101,
111; research on, 252
FDA drug evaluation guidelines, 204, 215–17
Fear, 119, 177
Federal funding: for AD research, 120,
124n. 1, 201; for nursing home place-
ment, 194
Fluoxetine (Prozac), 33
Food, Drug, and Cosmetics Act, 3, 26
Freud, Sigmund, 192

Gabapentin (Neurontin), 119
Galantamine (Reminyl), 18, 31, 59, 86–87,
91n. 4, 93n. 23, 104, 105, 237, 253
Gene therapy, 174